# Glucose, Insulin, Potassium and the Heart:

## Selected Aspects of Cardiac Energy Metabolism

### Richard J. Kones, M.D.

*Assistant Professor of Clinical Medicine (Cardiology), New York Medical College, New York, N.Y.*

*Director of Electrocardiology and Cardiologist, Northern Westchester Hospital Center—Cornell Medical College Affiliate, Mt. Kisco, N.Y.*

**FUTURA
PUBLISHING COMPANY
1975**

*TO SANDI, KIM, AND ROBIN*

*WHOSE GENEROUS LOVE WAS SO APPARENT AND NECES-
SARY DURING THE WRITING OF THIS BOOK*

# ACKNOWLEDGMENTS

I wish to thank Dr. John H. Phillips, Chief of Cardiology and Professor of Medicine at Tulane University School of Medicine for his continued support, guidance and encouragement over the years. My gratitude is also extended to Drs. Morton Ziskind and Hans Weill, also of Tulane University, for their sponsorship, sincere kindness, and advice.

My appreciation goes to Barbara Gaynor for her talented secretarial help, Sylvia Birbrower, R.N. for her assistance, Pat Isom for her library aid, and Sandra Riccio for supportive secretarial work. Finally, the generous help and continuing good judgment of the staff of Futura Publishing Company is gratefully acknowledged.

# FOREWORD

Since books, beyond synthesizing the experience acquired in the past, aspire to mold the future, the analysis of a specialized technical book from this point of view may shed light both on the scope of problems that a book encompasses and the creative imagination and courage of the author in trying to solve them and to indicate the road that should be followed in the future. In this book, Dr. Kones succeeds in presenting the most important events of myocardial metabolism and he relates them successfully not only to other fields of cardiovascular science, such as cardiac electrophysiology and mechanics, but most importantly, all of these events are linked masterfully to clinical observation. In this way, on the one hand, the clinical observations are presented and may be understood by the metabolic reactions and, on the other hand, the importance of the metabolic changes are emphasized by indicating their clinical consequences. This is an enormous task at this time, since the sphere of knowledge is expanding continuously, both the technologic aspects, where new instruments and new methods are constantly devised and the scientific aspects, where phenomena that previously could be only superficially analyzed, today can be examined on the molecular and ultrastructural levels. The latter open new avenues to the understanding of many fundamental events that determine both the physiologic regulation of cellular events and their alterations under pathologic conditions. The correct interpretation of these changes when a pathologic process occurs and the ensuing treatment can be accomplished only with a thorough understanding of all the biological events.

The lucid, comprehensive analysis of the effects of glucose on myocardial ischemia starting from subcellular levels and then advancing to the cellular level, the isolated heart, the intact animal, and ending in clinical observation on patients with ischemic heart disease offers the so often searched for but so rarely reached bridge between the basic sciences and their clinical application. The richness in detail and the well-researched subjects turn this into a book that not only transmits the view of the author but that permits the reader to judge the controversial points for himself. Most certainly, therefore, this book should have an important and salutary effect on cardiology, since the progress in this field in the next decade will depend on physicians who are knowledgeable both in clinical medicine and in basic science. This book lays the foundations for this approach.

Peter R. Maroko, M.D.
*Associate Professor of Medicine (Cardiology)*
*Harvard Medical School*

# PREFACE

Energy metabolism and the effects of glucose, insulin, and potassium (GIK) on the heart have received much attention over the years and it is still unknown, despite the impressive literature, what these actions are and whether they may be used clinically to advantage. As is true in many areas of cardiology today, a thoughtful consideration of the actions of these substances—alone or in combination—on the myocardium soon leads to very basic questions about cellular properties and function. This trend is reflected in the progressively greater proportion of cardiology literature space devoted to cellular events. It behooves the clinician to once again direct his attention to cellular physiology and pharmacology for an in-depth understanding of various problems in cardiology of current interest.

This book does not defend GIK treatment for heart disease. It does attempt to bridge the gap between the physical biochemist's and cardiologist's knowledge of the actions of GIK on the heart. In general, these fall into two categories—electrophysiologic and intermediary metabolic changes. The function of the heart as a pump is affected by changes in both categories, and therefore excitation-contraction coupling is briefly discussed. Myocardial energy metabolism is basic to all considerations, and is a common theme throughout this volume. For those readers interested in the fundamentals of physical chemistry applicable to intermediary metabolism, such as the meaning of free energy, high-energy bond, etc., an appendix is provided.

# TABLE OF CONTENTS

## CHAPTER III—POTASSIUM AND CALCIUM

# CHAPTER 1

# GLUCOSE

Available now. LINEAR MOTOR. Rugged and dependable: design optimized by worldwide field testing over an extended period. All models offer the economy of "fuel-cell" type energy conversion and will run on a wide range of commonly available fuels. Low stand-by power but can be switched within msecs to as much as 1 KW mech/Kg (peak, dry). Modular construction, and wide range of available sub-units, permit tailor-made solutions to otherwise intractable mechanical problems.

Choice of two control systems:

(1) *Externally triggered mode.* Versatile, general-purpose units. Digitally controlled by picojoule pulses. Despite low input energy level, very high signal-to-noise ratio. Energy amplification: $10^6$ approx. Mechanical characteristics: (1 cm modules) max. speed: optical between 0.1 and 100 mm/ sec. Stress generated; 2 to $5 \times 10^{-5}$ newtons m$^{-2}$.

(2) *Autonomous mode with integral oscillators.* Especially suitable for pumping applications. Modules available with frequency and mechanical impedance appropriate for

    (a) solids and slurries (0.01-1.0 Hz).
    (b) Liquids (0.5-5 Hz): lifetime $2.6 \times 10^9$ operations (typ.), $3.6 \times 10^9$ (max.)-independent of frequency.
    (c) Gases (50-1,000 Hz).

Many optional extras, *e.g.,* built-in servo (length and velocity) where fine control is required. Direct piping of oxygen. Thermal generation, etc.

> —*Notice of a lecture on muscle to the Institution of Electrical Engineers in London, Feb. 11, 1969, Prof. D. R. Wilkie*

## I. INTRODUCTION

The function of the heart as a pump critically depends upon the oxidation of substrate, from which energy is derived for the performance of work. In this chapter selected aspects of intermediary metabolism will be reviewed. The dependence of cardiac metabolism upon glucose during ischemia—the so-called "glucose hypothesis"—will also be discussed. Finally, other topics of importance in the understanding of the

1

metabolism of the heart and the potential influence of glucose, insulin and potassium will be considered.

As an introduction, an analysis of events that occur after the entire organism ingests an evening meal serves to illustrate the extent of coordination between metabolic events in order to insure sufficient substrate for cellular function (Fig. 1). Glucose absorption first raises plasma glucose levels, with an attendant stimulation of the beta cells of the pancreas. D-glucose, rather than L-glucose, is the more important insulin secretagogue, with the α anomer of D-glucose more potent than the β anomer in this respect.[187] There is a ten-fold rise in plasma insulin

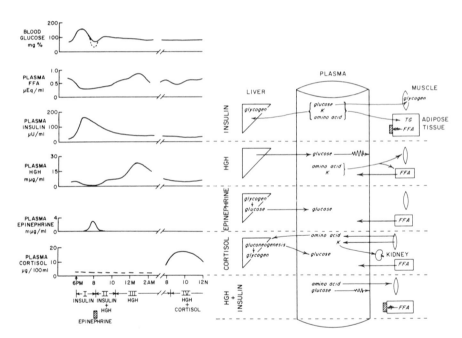

**Figure 1**   An example of extrinsic hormonal rhythm. The response to a meal containing carbohydrate at 6 p.m. Changes in blood glucose and plasma free fatty acid (FFA) concentrations are shown. Average plasma levels of insulin, growth hormone (HGH), epinephrine, and cortisol over the next 18 hours are given. This enables division into various phases, dominated by one or several of these hormones. Phase I (insulin); phase II (insulin and HGH); phase III (HGH); phase IV (cortisol); emergency phase (epinephrine). The actions of these hormones on liver, muscle, and adipose tissue are diagrammed. Reproduced with permission from Rabinowitz, D., *Principles and Practice of Medicine*, edited by Harvey, A.M., Cluff, L.E., et al., Appleton-Century-Crofts, New York, 17th edition, 1968.

levels, and growth hormone (HGH) secretion is inhibited. After plasma glucose concentration peaks and begins to fall, insulin secretion decreases and HGH levels begin to rise. By the fourth postprandial hour, HGH concentration is high and the insulin level has fallen to its preprandial value.

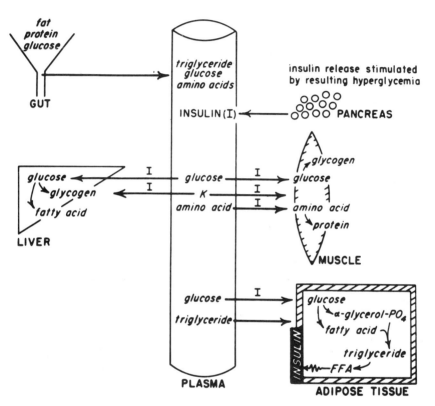

**Figure 2** Some metabolic events in the postprandial period. Absorption of glucose has resulted in hyperglycemia which in turn is associated with enhanced insulin release from the pancreas. The postprandial package of insulin (I) (plasma insulin levels reaching a peak of 100 $\mu$U per ml or greater) promotes glucose translocation from plasma, net potassium uptake by several organs, and inhibition of FFA release from adipose tissue. The incorporation of amino acids into protein is accelerated. Uptake of triglyceride by adipose tissue is increased postprandially. This is a complex process, in which insulin's participation may not be prominent. Reproduced with permission, from Rabinowitz, D., *Principles and Practice of Medicine*, Harvey, A. M., Cluff, L. E., et al., Appleton-Century-Crofts, New York, 17th edition, 1968.

Since each hormone is secreted for a given period, several metabolic phases may be discerned following a glucose meal. During phase I, arterial insulin is high, HGH is low and therefore an insulin effect predominates. Glucose uptake by insulin sensitive tissues—cardiac and skeletal muscle, adipose, and liver—increases at the appropriate time when glucose is being absorbed from the intestine. Glycogen is deposited in muscle, the liver, and to a lesser extent in adipose tissue. Potassium and amino acids move into muscle and fat cells. Triglycerides are synthesized in adipose tissue and free fatty acid release from adipose is inhibited. Simultaneously, the absorbed triglyceride is deposited in adipose tissue, which appears to be related to glucose and perhaps insulin availability [1] (Fig. 2).

During phase II, two to four hours after the meal, both HGH and insulin are present in appreciable amounts. HGH alone would mediate mobilization of free fatty acid from adipose tissue into the circulation and would enhance free fatty acid uptake by muscle. However, HGH also inhibits glucose translocation from the plasma space (Fig. 3). The net effect is a defense of the plasma glucose level and presentation

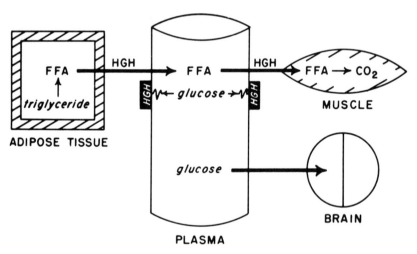

**Figure 3** Summary of effects of HGH on muscle and on adipose tissue. HGH enhances hepatic glucose output and blocks glucose translocation into muscle and adipose tissue. HGH enhances mobilization of FFA and uptake of FFA by skeletal muscle. The overall effect is the preservation of blood glucose and presentation to the tissues of easily oxidizable fatty acids in the face of carbohydrate lack. Reproduced with permission from Rabinowitz, D.: *Principles and Practice of Medicine*, edited by Harvey, A. M., Cluff, L. E. et al., Appleton-Century-Crofts, New York, 17th edition, 1968.

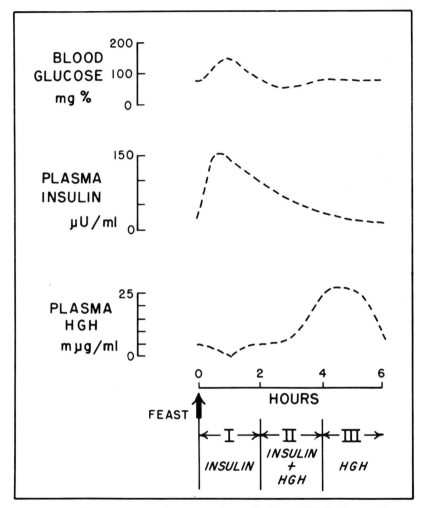

**Figure 4** Fluctuations in plasma insulin and plasma HGH after a glucose meal. In the first hour or two after a glucose meal, insulin circulates at high concentration, and HGH levels are zero (phase I); two hours or so after the meal, both HGH and insulin circulate together in moderately high concentration (phase II); after the fourth hour, plasma HGH is high, insulin has returned to low basal values (phase III). Reproduced with permission from Rabinowitz and Zierler: *Nature* (London), **199**:913, 1963.

of oxidizable fatty acids to the muscle mass at a time when glucose availability is waning. The gradual preservation of plasma glucose probably modulates the anticipated overshoot in insulin's action on blood glucose. Insulin action on blocking free fatty acid release "overcomes" that of HGH's tendency to effect free fatty acid mobilization (Fig. 1). Potassium and amino acid translocation into muscle continues in phase II, and therefore this phase of both insulin and HGH presence is thought to favor protein anabolism.

After the fourth hour postprandially, HGH levels persist as insulin secretion falls (Fig. 4). By this time, gastrointestinal absorption of substrate is completed and HGH reduces glucose uptake by muscle and adipose tissue. Plasma glucose is further supported by hepatic release of glucose. Potassium translocation across muscle is minimal. The synthesis of polypeptides is also relatively modest, most likely due to the lack of insulin. Under the influence of HGH, free fatty acid release from adipose tissue provides substrate for muscle. If the organism fasts for a prolonged period, HGH levels return to their basal values.

Phase IV is characterized by high plasma cortisol values during the early morning hours. Potassium and amino acids are lost from skeletal

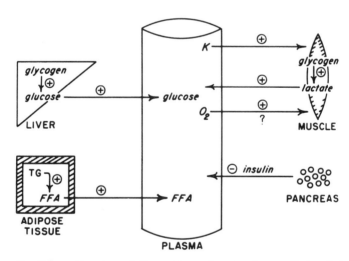

**Figure 5**  Schematic view of the actions of epinephrine. Epinephrine enhances (+) glucose release from the liver, FFA release from adipose tissue, and lactate output from skeletal muscle. Epinephrine inhibits (−) insulin release from the pancreas. Epinephrine induces net movement of potassium into muscle. Reproduced with permission from Rabinowitz, D., *Principles and Practice of Medicine*, edited by Harvey, A. M., Cluff, L. E., et al., Appleton-Century-Crofts, New York, 17th edition, 1968.

muscle; the potassium is cleared by the kidney, while amino acids are transaminated in the liver. A net increase in liver glycogen occurs. Thus, phase IV is catabolic for nitrogen and potassium, but hepatic glucose output and inhibition of peripheral glucose uptake defend the blood glucose level. The intrinsic diurnal rhythm of plasma cortisol ensures that cells remain in net potassium and nitrogen balance over a long period of time.[2]

If blood glucose falls excessively, epinephrine secretion increases abruptly to restore the glucose level, thus providing an emergency means for the organism to provide substrate during stress (Fig. 5).

Despite the drawback of oversimplification, the foregoing discussion provides a useful overview of metabolism. For instance, the ill effects of insulin lack may be understood more clearly with these principles in mind (Fig. 6).[3] Specifically, the panmetabolic nature of insulin deprivation in the organism affects carbohydrate metabolism (Fig. 7A), fat metabolism (Fig. 7B) and protein metabolism (Fig. 7C).

Each of the events described will be discussed in greater detail in this chapter, the specific metabolic pathways will be outlined and finally cardiac glucose metabolism will be considered.

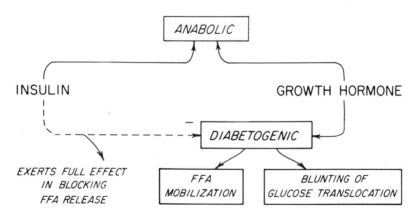

**Figure 6** Suggested model whereby HGH can act as an anabolic and diabetogenic agent. It is proposed that this may be determined by the simultaneous availability of insulin. Thus, when insulin levels are low, HGH acts chiefly as a fat-mobilizing hormone and serves to retard glucose translocation from plasma; in the presence of insulin, the fat-mobilizing effects of HGH are inhibited, insulin and HGH together, serving as anabolic agents. Reproduced from Rabinowitz, Merimee, and Burgess, *Diabetes*, **15**:905, 1966.

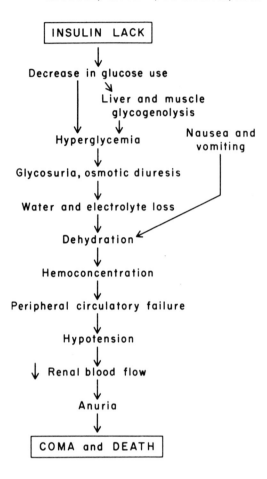

**Figure 7A**   The effect of insulin lack on carbohydrate metabolism. Reproduced with permission.[30]

## II. GENERAL SCHEME OF INTERMEDIARY METABOLISM

Energy for a number of purposes is produced by nonautotrophs from the metabolism of foodstuffs via several "pathways" involving enzymatically catalyzed sequences of reactions. Each pathway accomplishes a specific goal, *e.g.*, the tricarboxylic acid cycle, $\beta$-oxidation of fatty acids, the Embden-Meyerhoff pathway. These sequences are summarized in Figure 8. *Anaerobic glycolysis* refers to the conversion of glucose and carbohydrate to lactate via pyruvate. Although no oxygen is consumed, glycolysis is an oxidative reaction in that an internal oxidation-reduction occurs with the carboxyl group of lactate

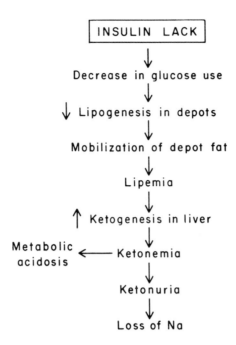

**Figure 7B**    The effect of insulin lack on fat metabolism.

being the product of oxidation and its methyl group the product of reduction. *Aerobic glycolysis* involves the conversion of carbohydrate to carbon dioxide and water via pyruvate, for which oxygen is utilized. Glucose, the key carbohydrate, is formed from and in turn used to form the polymer glycogen which may function as a substrate reserve, or may serve a structural role, for example, as hyaluronidase.

Acetate is a common intermediate of both carbohydrate and lipid metabolism, and the tricarboxylic acid cycle—leading acetate to its final product $CO_2$ and $H_2O$—is a common pathway in the metabolism of carbohydrates, lipids and amino acids. Acetyl CoA is formed from pyruvate decarboxylation in the liquid phase of the mitochondria. Acetyl CoA is also derived from long chain fatty acids which enter the mitochondrion esterified to carnitine. Once inside the mitochondrion FFA are reesterified with coenzyme A and then oxidized at the $\beta$ position to yield acetyl-CoA moieties. Finally, certain amino acids may contribute to the acetate pool after deamination and partial degradation.

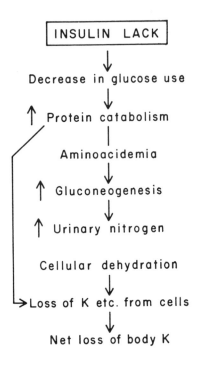

**Figure 7C**    The effect of insulin lack on protein metabolism.

The reactions in intermediary metabolism of especial interest in this discussion are further diagrammed in Figure 9, in which a cell is depicted with the compartments cytosol (cell fluid), mitochondrion liquid phase and mitochondrion solid phase. The intracellular sites where reaction sequences occur are of importance and are outlined in Table I. The tricarboxylic acid cycle enzymes are found in the aqueous phase of the mitochondria which generate nicotinamide adenine dinucleotide ($NAD^+$, formerly termed $DPN^+$), and flavin adenine dinucleotide (FAD) from the oxidation of acetate. These carriers enter the (solid) mitochondrial cristae, where high energy phosphate bonds are formed (see appendix), and hydrogen and oxygen combine to form water. Under normal conditions, for each oxygen molecule consumed, three high energy phosphate bonds are generated.

Tissues differentiated for particular functions have differing activities of metabolic pathways which are integrated with the feeding phases illustrated in Figures 1-5. In the postprandial state, glucose metabolism leads to fat deposition in adipose tissue and glycogen

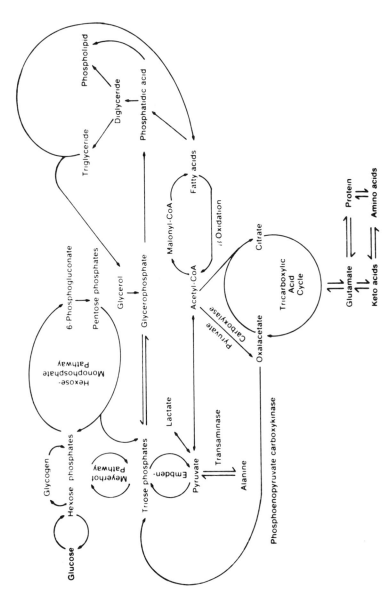

**Figure 8** An overall view of the metabolism of carbohydrates, lipids and amino acids. Note that acetate is a common intermediate of carbohydrate and lipid metabolism and that the tricarboxylic acid cycle is the common pathway for oxidation of carbohydrates, lipids, and amino acids.

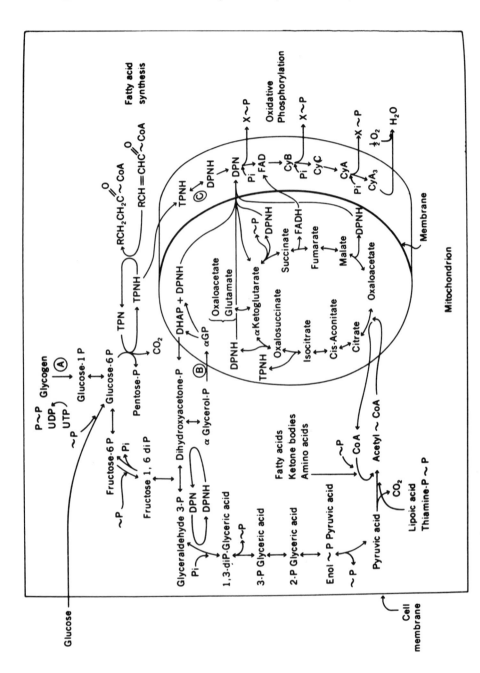

Figure 9    General scheme of intermediary metabolism.

**Table I**  Subcellular distribution of enzymes

| Metabolic Sequence | Principal Subcellular Distribution |
| --- | --- |
| Glycolysis | Cytosol<br>May be glycogen bound |
| Gluconeogenesis | Mitochondria<br>Cytosol<br>Microsomes |
| Pentose pathway | Cytosol |
| Tricarboxylic acid cycle<br>(isocitrate dehydrogenase TPN<br>requiring) | Mitochondria<br>Cytosol |
| $\beta$-Oxidation | Mitochondria |
| Fatty acid synthesis | Cytosol |
| Cholesterol synthesis | Microsomes |

storage in the liver (Figs. 10 and 11). During fasting these processes are appropriately altered (Figs. 10B and 11B). Nervous tissue may utilize only glucose as its substrate which must be continually supplied, since little storage capability exists (Fig. 12B). Muscle tissue is much more versatile in that several substrates may be utilized, *i.e.*, muscle is omniverous (Fig. 12A). In addition to the ability to metabolize fatty acids, glucose, ketone bodies and some amino acids to furnish energy, muscle serves as a storage site for amino acids. Insulin, apart from its celebrated action on glucose utilization, also stimulates the incorporation of amino acids into muscle protein by a different mechanism. In the absence of insulin, this process is slowed or reversed, and may be opposed by ACTH. The details of these processes will be discussed in Chapter II.

## III. GLUCOSE METABOLISM

Glucose is an important substrate in both heart muscle and cells of other tissues, but the myocardium may utilize a variety of substances as sources of energy.[1-9] Free fatty acids are the other fuels of major importance but the heart may utilize lactate, pyruvate, ketone bodies (acetoacetate, $\beta$-hydroxyacetate, from the incomplete combustion of fatty acids in the liver), and amino acids to provide ATP. The relative proportions of these substrates actually utilized at a given time is a function of the availability of the substrates, *i.e.*, their relative plasma concentrations; the inotropic state of the heart; hormonal influences;

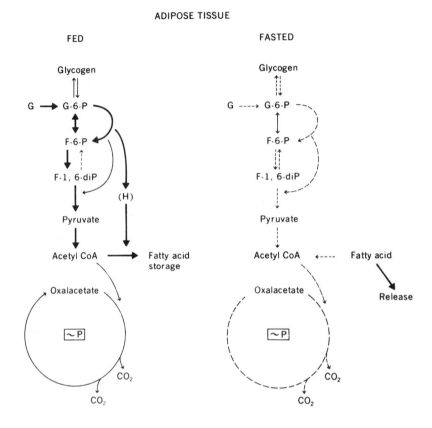

**Figure 10**   Comparison of flow of substrate across metabolic pathways in adipose tissue in the fed and fasted state. In the former, glucose (G) is metabolized to acetyl CoA, which is then resynthesized to fat and stored. During fasting, glucose metabolism is limited, and fatty acids are released for fuel for the remainder of the body. Reproduced with permission.[18]

and the rate of oxidative respiration, in turn dependent upon the rate of perfusion. When the oxygen supply is not limited, all of the substances mentioned may be oxidized in the tricarboxylic acid cycle, and NADH is produced by this means or by $\beta$-oxidation of free fatty acids (Fig. 13).[10] However, in well oxygenated myocardium, fatty acids rather than carbohydrate are the preferred substrate, and under certain circumstances can account for 100 percent of total oxidative phosphorylation.[11-15] Under more physiologic conditions, fatty acid metabolism accounts for 60 to 70 percent of oxidative phosphorylation.[16, 17]

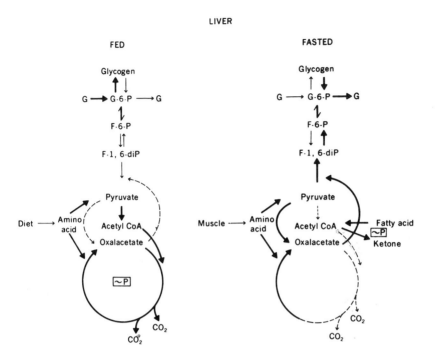

**Figure 11** The liver in the fed animal stores glucose as glycogen and derives its own energy from amino acid metabolism. During fasting its energy ($\sim$P) is derived from the conversion of fatty acids to ketone and amino acids are diverted into glucose synthesis. Reproduced with permission.[18]

In hearts perfused with glucose as the only substrate, glucose oxidation accounts for approximately 40 percent of the oxygen consumption at low workloads, but up to 80 percent of the oxygen consumption at high workloads.[19] Again, however, under normal conditions in which the heart may "select" among available substrates, fatty acids are preferentially oxidized at all levels of energy utilization, even though the uptake of both glucose and fatty acids are both accelerated. A number of fatty acid substrates suppress glucose utilization by inhibition of several steps in the glycolytic pathway. Since this action disappears under anaerobic conditions, oxidation of the fatty acid seems to be the necessary process.

Of particular importance are the changes that occur in myocardium deprived of adequate energy supply. Experimentally, this may occur in one of two ways: (i) reducing the oxygen tension in the perfusate of

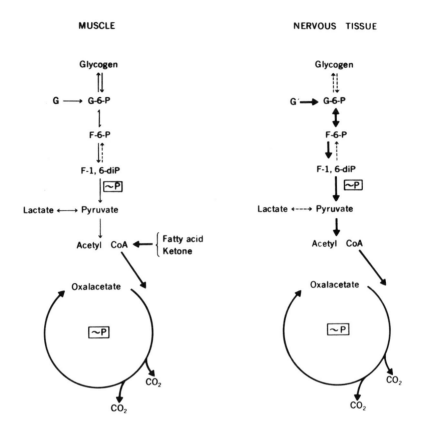

**Figure 12**   Muscle tissue utilizes predominantly fatty acid or ketone as a source of fuel, but it is also able to derive limited amounts of energy ($\sim$P) from the conversion of glucose to lactate (anaerobic glycolysis). Nervous tissue is able to utilize only glucose as its metabolic fuel, and requires a constant supply of oxygen for total combustion of the glucose to $CO_2$ in order to derive energy for adequate function. Reproduced with permission.[18]

the heart, thereby producing *hypoxia*, and (ii) lowering the rate of perfusion, to produce *ischemia*. The precise biochemical changes accompanying these two conditions will be considered in a later secton.

## A. Glucose transport

### 1. *The "carrier hypothesis:" introduction*

Studies on the transport of glucose across the heart cell membrane are in accord with the notion that this process may be facilitated by

## CORONARY CIRCULATION

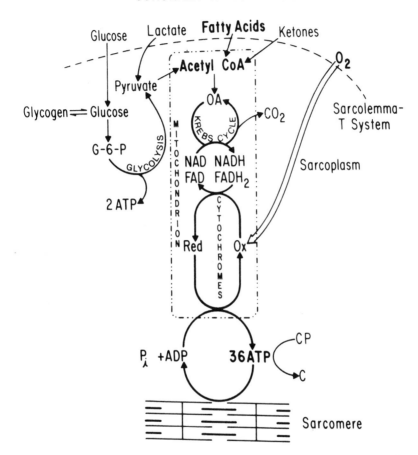

**Figure 13**  Diagram of metabolic pathways of energy (adenosine triphosphate) production within the cardiac cell. Complete oxidation of a substrate such as glucose yields a total of 36 moles of adenosine triphosphate per mole of glucose, whereas glycolysis alone provides only 2 moles of adenosine triphosphate. ADP=adenosine diphosphate; ATP=adenosine triphosphate; C=creatine; CP=creatine phosphate; CoA=coenzyme A; FAD and FADH =flavin adenine dinucleotide and its reduced form, respectively; OA=oxaloacetic acid; OX=oxidation; $P_i$=inorganic phosphate; Red=reduction. Reproduced with permission.[10]

means of a "carrier," an hypothesized mobile protein moiety in the membrane. The "carrier" is presumed to combine with glucose on the extracellular side, and the glucose-carrier complex is supposed to pass through the membrane to dissociate on the intracellular side to liberate free glucose. This process is reversible, does not require energy and only equilibrates the glucose concentrations on either side of the membrane, i.e., glucose is not transported "against" an electrochemical gradient.[20] Facilitated diffusion of glucose is also saturable, stereospecific, and demonstrates the phenomena of countertransport and competitive inhibition.

The concept of a "carrier" was introduced by Danielli [21] in order to explain the apparent high permeability of substances with low solubilities in the membrane. The large deviation in these systems from Fick's law and the property of saturation suggested a specific interaction of permeant with a selective "carrier" with a limited total number of binding sites. Glucose molecules are thought to reversibly adsorb to a membrane surface, under the influence of a residual field of force at the surface site.[22]

If the mass or quantity of molecules adsorbed at a given time is $Q$ and the maximum which can be adsorbed by the surface is $Q_{max}$, and the concentration of substrate is denoted $[S]$, then at equilibrium

$$\frac{Q}{Q_{max}} = \frac{[S]}{[S] + K_s} \qquad \text{where}$$

$Q/Q_{max}$ is the proportion of surface occupied, $K_s$ is a constant representing the relationship between association and dissociation (and hence it determines the proportion of surface occupied at different values of $[S]$). This equation describes a rectangular hyperbola which is plotted in Figure 14. At low concentrations of $[S]$ relatively few sites are occupied, and a rise in $[S]$ raises the number of sites occupied almost proportionally. When a great number of sites are occupied, there are fewer sites available for a net increase in association and an increase in $[S]$ produces little change in the proportion of surface saturated.

A "carrier" transporting glucose across the heart cell membrane may be regarded kinetically as a number of mobile adsorption sites.[23, 24] Assuming the number of carrier sites on each side of the membrane to be equal, and on each side the sites are in adsorption equilibrium, and that equal numbers of sites move in each direction in unit time, and that substrate molecules adsorb on sites in an equimolar fashion, and that binding does not change the rate of movement of sites, we may write:

$$v = \frac{v_{\max}\,[S]}{[S] + K_m}$$

where $v_{\max}$ is the maximal rate of transport and $K_m$ is a constant. Transport described by this equation is said to follow Michaelis-Menton kinetics because of the relation to the equation describing enzyme reaction rates (see appendix) (Fig. 15).

Studying a more generalized model, Blumenthal and Katchasky [25] have kinetically described transport in a two compartment system shown in Figure 16.

## 2. A theoretical model

The membrane system is composed of two compartments separated by a membrane permeable to the carrier, C, the permeant, S, and to the permeant-carrier complex, denoted CS. Equilibrium

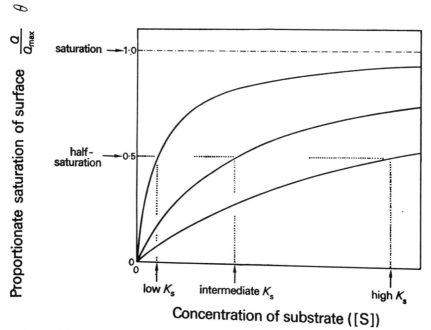

**Figure 14** Progressive saturation of adsorption surface with increase in concentration of substrate. $K_s$, the equilibrium constant, has a value equal to the concentration at which the surface is half-saturated. When the value of $K_s$ is lower, a greater proportion of available sites is occupied at all concentrations of substrate than when it is higher. By adjustment of the scale of the abscissa all curves can be made to appear the same, since proportionate relationships are the same for all curves.

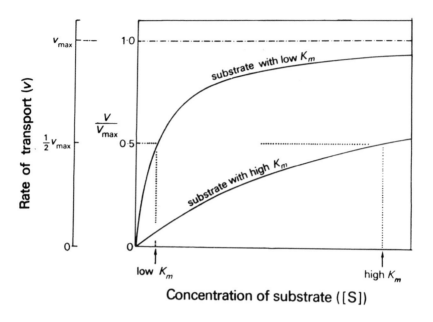

**Figure 15** Relationship between rate of transport and Michaelis constant ($K_m$). Transport may be expressed as a rate or as a proportion of $v_{max}$ (*i.e.*, $v/v_{max}$, which is equivalent to $\theta$, or the proportionate saturation of sites). The Michaelis constant has a value equal to the concentration of substrate at which half the maximal rate of transport is developed, and hence at which the carrier system may be assumed to be half-saturated. A substrate with a higher value of $K_m$ occupies less sites and hence is transported less rapidly at a particular concentration than one with a lower value of $K_m$.

is assumed between permeant in compartment (1) and the external reservoir concentration, $S_1$, and similarly for compartment (2). The outer membranes, $\alpha$ and $\beta$ are considered impermeable to the carrier and the permeant-carrier complex. Assuming simple rate laws the reaction rates $J^1_{Ch}$ and $J^2_{Ch}$ may be expressed

$$J^1_{Ch} = K_1 C_1 S_1 - K_{-1} CS_1$$

and

$$J^2_{Ch} = K_1 C_2 S_2 - K_{-1} CS_2.$$

Where $K_1$ and $K_{-1}$ are the rate constants for the reactions

$$C_i + S_i \underset{K_{-1}}{\overset{K_1}{\rightleftharpoons}} CS_i \qquad i = 1 \text{ or } 2$$

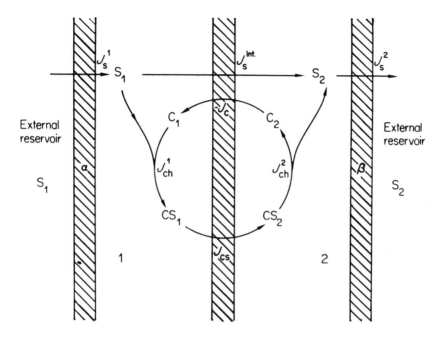

**Figure 16** "Circulation of carrier" in a composite membrane-facilitated transport system. From Katchalsky and Spangler, 1968.

If the flows of C and CS are assumed to be simply proportional to their concentration differences across the membrane we have

$$J_C = P(C_1 - C_2)$$

$$J_{CS} = P(CS_1 - CS_2).$$

The flow of free permeants, $J_S^{int}$ is given by

$$J_S^{int} = P(S_1 - S_2), \qquad \text{where}$$

the permeability coefficient P is assumed to be the equal for C and CS. In the steady state

$$-J_{Ch}^1 - J_C = 0$$

$$J_C - J_{Ch}^2 = 0$$

$$J_{Ch}^1 - J_{CS} = 0$$

$$J_{CS} - J_{Ch}^2 = 0$$

and for the circulation process,

$$J_{S_1} - J_S^{int} - J_{Ch}^1 = 0$$

and

$$-J_{S_2} + J_S^{int} - J_{Ch}^2 = 0.$$

Applying the stationary state conditions to concentrations and flows:

$$J_C = J_{Ch}^2 = -J_{CS} = J_{Ch}^1$$

$$J_{S_1} = J_S^{int} + J_{CS} = J_{S_2} = J_S^{ext}.$$

This system involves five diffusional flows and two reaction flows. In a macroscopic examination one would simply observe an external driving force $\Delta\mu_S^{ext}$ and one flow $J_S^{ext}$, so that the dissipation function would be

$$\Phi = J_S^{ext} \Delta\mu_S^{ext}$$

while the more detailed mechanism would contain all elements of the model:

$$\Phi = J_{S_1}\Delta\mu_{S_1} + J_S^{int}\Delta\mu_S + J_{S_2}\Delta\mu_{S_2} + J_C\Delta\mu_C + J_{CS}\Delta\mu_{CS} + J_{Ch}^1 A_1 + J_{Ch}^2 A_2$$

and from the previous relation

$$\Phi = J_S^{ext}(\Delta\mu_{S_1} + \Delta\mu_S + \Delta\mu_{S_2}) + J_{CS}(\Delta\mu_{CS} - \Delta\mu_C - \Delta\mu_S + A_1 - A_2).$$

Expanding the changes of chemical potentials one obtains the expression

$$\Phi = J_S^{ext} \Delta\mu_S^{ext}$$

The corresponding phenomenological equation may be written

$$J_S^{ext} = L\Delta\mu_S^{ext}$$

and expansion of L in terms of the model shows that

$$L = (L_p + L_f)$$

where $L_p$ is the term for passive transport independent of carrier mechanism and proportional to the permeability of S, $P_S$. $L_f$ is the contribution due to circulation increasing the overall permeability of the membrane to S. The phenomenon of saturation may also be described by this model.

## 3. Regulation of glucose transport

In heart muscle the regulation of glucose transport is governed by the presence of insulin, growth hormone, catecholamines, hypoxia, and level of cardiac work, all of which tend to accelerate glucose transport.[17] Kinetic data support the contention that the "carrier-mediated" stage of glucose permeation is stimulated, rather than a diffusion component.

When insulin is not present, transport is the rate limiting step for glucose utilization in myocardium.[26, 27] This major action of insulin in regulation of glucose uptake is similar to that suggested in other tissues (Fig. 17).[28] When insulin is lacking, the formation of glucose-6-phosphate, catalyzed by hexokinase, is limited by the availability of free intracellular glucose. However, in the presence of insulin, the rate limiting step of glucose uptake shifts from glucose transport to glucose phosphorylation.[31] Further discussion of the role of insulin in substrate transport appears in Chapter 2.

The actual mechanisms of alteration in glucose transport remain unknown. Part of the inhibition in glucose utilization associated with fatty acid oxidation is accomplished by diminished glucose transport,[32, 33] which is accentuated in the presence of insulin.[34] It is hypothesized that alterations in glucose transport are mediated by

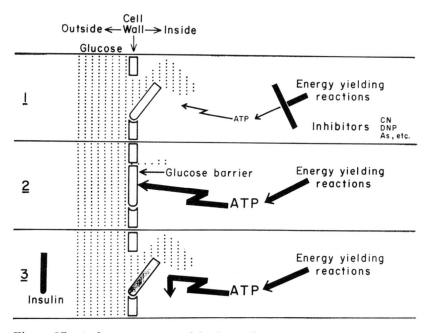

**Figure 17** A diagrammatic model of Randle and Smith's theory of the mechanism of insulin's action on glucose transport. Reproduced with permission.[30]

various substances, yet to be indentified. Thus, there may be specific inhibitors or accelerators of glucose transport to account for the effects of hypoxia,[35] increased muscular work [36] and fatty acid oxidation.[17, 37] One such mediator, NADH, has been identified as an activator of transport under anaerobic conditions in noncardiac tissue.[38]

The role of calcium and guanyl cyclase in sugar transport is also uncertain. There is evidence to suggest that a specific membrane-bound $Ca^{++}$ pool mediates the effect of various factors regulating sugar transport in muscle.[138, 191] Calcium ion is involved in the cyclic GMP system and in fact calcium is also a stimulant of guanyl cyclase in the heart.[139] These relations are not mentioned to imply a connection, but simply serve to show there is much yet to be learned about sugar transport.

## B. Glycolysis

Glycolysis, or the dissolution of sugar to three carbon fragments, may be written:

$$C_6H_{12}O_6 + 2\,P_i + 2ADP \rightleftharpoons 2CH_3\overset{\displaystyle OH}{\underset{\displaystyle |}{CH}} - \overset{\displaystyle OH}{\underset{\displaystyle |}{C}} = O + 2ATP + 2H_2O$$

and occurs in the following sequence:

$$
\begin{array}{cccccc}
1 & 2 & 3 & 4 & 5 & 6 \\
\end{array}
$$
C—C—C—C—C—C
Glucose
$\downarrow$

$$
\begin{array}{ccccccc}
1 & 2 & 3 & & 4 & 5 & 6 \\
\end{array}
$$
C—C—C   +   C—C—C
Trioses
$\downarrow$

1 $CH_3$         6 $CH_3$
   |                |
2 CH—OH   +   5 CH—OH
   |                |
3 COOH         4 COOH

If the overall equation is broken into two parts: glucose→lactate, which is exergonic, and the formation of ATP, which is endergonic, we have

$$\text{Glucose} \rightarrow 2 \text{ Lactate} \qquad \Delta G_1^{0\prime} = -47.0 \text{ kcal}$$

$$2 P_i + 2ADP \rightarrow 2ATP + 2H_2O \qquad \Delta G_2^{0\prime} = 7.3 \times 2 = +14.6 \text{ kcal}$$

For the entire reaction (see appendix):

$$\Delta G_s^{0\prime} = \Delta G_1^{0\prime} + \Delta G_2^{0\prime} = -32.4 \text{ kcal},$$

or approximately 31% of the free-energy decrease during breakdown of glucose to lactate is conserved as $\sim$P in ATP. At the actual steady state concentrations of reactants and products, using $\Delta G'$ instead of $\Delta G^{0\prime}$, the actual energy recovery is closer to 53%.

Glycolysis may be regarded as comprising two major stages (Fig. 18).[39] In the first, several hexoses may enter the pathway, are phosphorylated using ATP, and form glyceraldehyde-3-phosphate. In a second stage, the oxidation-reduction steps and reformation of ATP occur. It is evident that the reactions may be analyzed from three points of view: pathway of carbon, pathway of phosphate and pathway of electrons.

The general reactions in glycolysis are as follows (Fig. 19):

*Reaction 1*—Glucose is converted to glucose-6-phosphate (G-6-P) under the influence of hexokinase and adenosine triphosphate (ATP). This is an irreversible reaction because a high-energy phosphate group in ATP is used to form a low-energy ester phosphate bond in G-6-P.

*Reaction 2*—G-6-P is converted back to glucose in the liver by glucose-6-phosphatase, not by reversal of reaction 1. Muscle does not have this phosphatase.

*Reaction 3*—G-6-P is converted to glucose-1-phosphate (G-1-P) by phosphoglucomutase.

*Reaction 4*—This summarizes a series of reactions resulting in the formation of glycogen, as follows:

$$\text{G-1-P} + \text{UTP} \xrightarrow{\text{Pyrophosphorylase}} \text{UDPG} + \text{pyrophosphate}$$

$$\text{UDPG} \xrightarrow[\text{Branching enzyme}]{\text{Glycogen synthetase}} \text{Glycogen} + \text{UDP}$$

$$\text{UDP} + \text{ATP} \xrightarrow{\text{Phosphokinase}} \text{UTP} + \text{ADP}$$

UTP = uridine triphosphate
UDP = uridine diphosphate
UDPG = uridine diphosphate-glucose

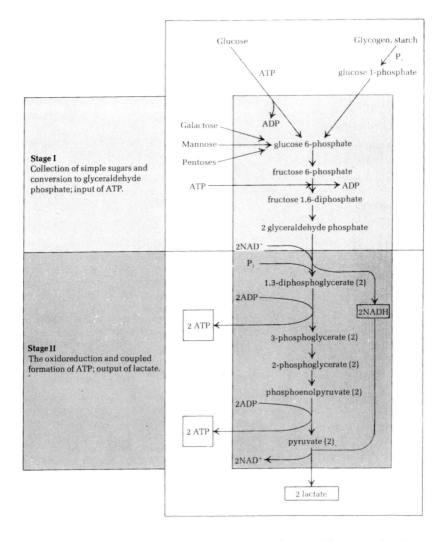

**Figure 18**   The two stages of glycolysis. Reproduced with permission.[39]

Glycogen synthetase:  forms 1,4-linkages between glucose moieties, making straight chains.
Branching enzyme:  forms 1,6-linkages between glucose moieties, making branches between straight chains.

*Reaction 5*—Glycogen is broken down to G-1-P in the presence of a debranching enzyme (breaks 1,6-linkages) and phosphorylase (breaks 1,4-linkages). Reaction 3 converts G-1-P to G-6-P. If required for blood sugar, G-6-P can be converted back to glucose by reaction 2.

*Reaction 6*—G-6-P is converted to fructose-6-phosphate (F-6-P) in a reversible reaction catalyzed by phosphohexose isomerase.

*Reaction 7*—F-6-P is phosphorylated to fructose-1,6-diphosphate (F-1,6-P$_2$) in an irreversible kinase reaction in the presence of phosphofructokinase.

*Reaction 8*—Reaction 7 can be biologically reversed by way of a phosphatase reaction.

*Reaction 9*—F-1,6-P$_2$ is split into two triose phosphate molecules, glyceraldehyde-3-phosphate (glyceralde-3-P) and dihydroxyacetone phosphate [(OH)$_2$-acetone-P], in a reversible reaction catalyzed by fructose diphosphate aldolase.

*Reaction 10*—The triose phosphates, glyceralde-3-P and (OH)$_2$-acetone-P, are in equilibrium with each other in the presence of an isomerase. Thus, both halves of the original glucose molecule are available for subsequent reactions.

*Reaction 11*—The conversion of glyceralde-3-P to 1,3-diphosphoglycerate (1,3-P$_2$-glycerate) is catalyzed by glyceralde-3-P-dehydrogenase in a reversible reaction. The carboxyl phosphate bond is a high-energy bond, the energy coming from the oxidation of the aldehyde to a carboxyl group.

*Reaction 12*—In the conversion of 1,3-P$_2$-glycerate to 3-phosphoglycerate (3-P-glycerate) under the influence of phosphoglycerate kinase, the energy of the carboxyl phosphate bond is captured in the concomitant conversion of ADP to ATP.

*Reaction 13*—3-P-glycerate forms 2-P-glycerate in the presence of phosphoglyceromutase in a reversible reaction.

*Reaction 14*—The dehydration of 2-P-glycerate to phosphoenolpyruvate (P-E-pyr) with the production of a high-energy phosphate bond is catalyzed by enolase.

*Reaction 15*—The high energy in P-E-pyr is captured in the formation of ATP from ADP in an irreversible reaction in the presence of pyruvate kinase, resulting in the formation of pyruvate.

*Reaction 16*—Under anaerobic conditions, pyruvate is converted to lactate in the presence of lactate dehydrogenase in a reaction which reverses itself under aerobic conditions. This concludes the glycolysis reactions.

*Reaction 17*—In the liver, reaction 15 can be reversed (bypassed) with a set of two reactions with the expenditure of energy.

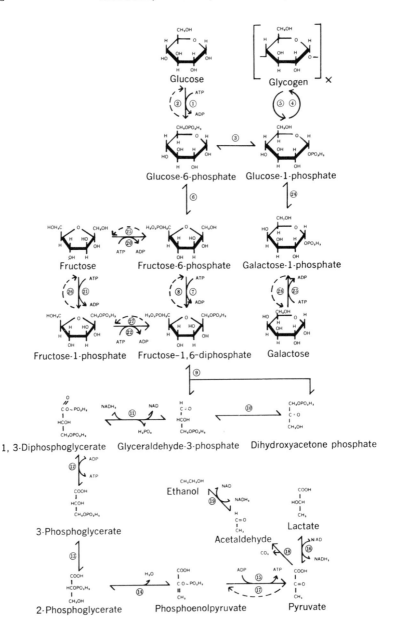

**Figure 19** Anaerobic metabolism of glucose (glycolysis) and related hexoses (∼ = high energy bond). The solid line arrows indicate the reactions in the direction of glycogenesis and the anaerobic metabolism of glucose to the pyruvate or lactate stage (glycolysis). A singleheaded arrow (→) indicates a

$$\text{Pyruvate} \xrightarrow{\text{Pyruvate carboxylase}} \text{Oxaloacetate}$$

$$\text{Oxaloacetate} \xrightarrow[\text{carboxykinase}]{\text{Phosphoenolpyruvate}}$$

*Reaction 18*—In the presence of a kinase, fructose (F) can be converted to F-6-P, which is directly on the glycolytic pathway.

*Reaction 19*—In another kinase reaction, F can be converted to F-1-P.

*Reaction 20*—F-1-P, in the presence of a phosphofructokinase, is converted to F-1,6-P$_2$, also directly on the glycolytic pathway.

*Reaction 21*—Galactose (Gal) is converted to Gal-1-P in a kinase reaction.

*Reaction 22*—Gal-1-P can be converted to G-1-P in a reaction involving uridine diphosphate glucose and a transferase. G-1-P can then be converted to G-6-P by reaction 3.

*Reactions 23 to 26*—All the phosphorylations in reactions 18 to 21 can be biologically reversed with appropriate phosphatase reactions.

From studies done in the erythrocyte, an energy profile of glycolysis may be constructed (Fig. 20). First the actual steady state concentrations of all intermediates of glycolysis are determined. Then the free energy change ($\Delta G'$ rather than $\Delta G^{o'}$) of each step may be calculated with the equation (see appendix):

$$\Delta G' = \Delta G^{o'} + RT \ln \frac{[C][D]}{[A][B]}.$$

The free energy profile is then constructed which shows that eight of the reactions of glycolysis are very close to equilibrium (Fig 20). Three reactions in particular involve large decreases in free energy and hence are far from equilibrium—the hexokinase, phosphofructokinase, and

---

reaction which is irreversible as written. A double-headed arrow ($\leftrightarrow$) indicates a reversible reaction. A broken arrow ($--\rightarrow$) indicates a reaction which has the effect of reversing an irreversible reaction by a reaction which is different from the forward reaction. Thus there is complete biologic reversibility, but it occurs at the price of a loss of energy, *i.e.*, since the reactions in the direction of glucose to pyruvate generate energy, the reactions in reverse must require an input of energy. The individual reactions are listed in the text by numbers corresponding to those in this figure. From Toporek: *Basic Chemistry of Life*, 1968. Courtesy of Appleton-Century-Crofts, Inc.

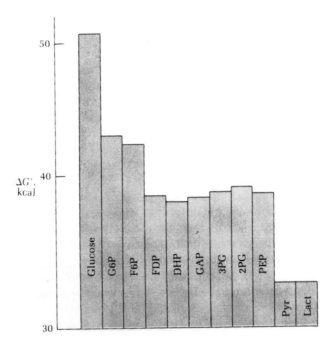

**Figure 20**   Energy profile of glycolysis in human erythrocyte. All the reactions are at or near equilibrium except those catalyzed by hexokinase, phosphofructokinase, and pyruvate phosphokinase, at which large decreases in ΔG′ occur. Reproduced with permission.[39]

pyruvate kinase catalyzed reactions. From these data the calculated free energy of hydrolysis of ATP is −13.3 kcal at intracellular conditions and the efficiency of energy recovery is about 53%, a figure much greater than that calculated from standard free energy data.

## C. The tricarboxylic acid cycle

The process of cellular respiration (Fig 9) in which glucose is oxidized completely to carbon dioxide and water yields a great deal more energy than glycolysis:

$$\text{glucose} \rightarrow 2 \text{ lactate} \qquad \Delta G^{0\prime} = -47 \text{ kcal}$$
$$\text{glucose} + 6 \text{ O}_2 \rightarrow 6 \text{ CO}_2 + 6 \text{ H}_2\text{O} \qquad \Delta G = -686 \text{ kcal}$$

When pyruvate is the electron receptor in glycolysis, less energy is liberated and carbon remains in the same oxidation state in lactate as it was in the glucose molecule. However, when oxygen is the electron acceptor in respiration, nearly fifteen times as much energy is released.

The reactions of the tricarboxylic acid cycle are outlined in Figure 21:

*Reaction 1*—Acetyl-CoA is taken into the tricarboxylic acid cycle in an irreversible reaction by way of a condensation with oxaloacetate

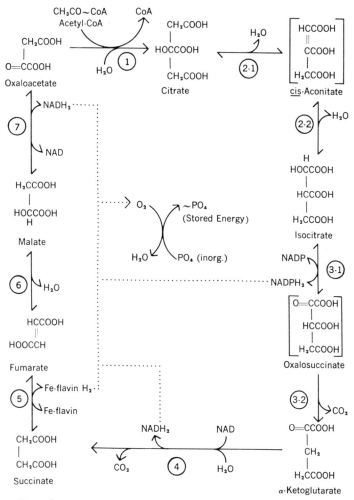

**Figure 21** The tricarboxylic acid cycle (also known as the citric acid cycle or the Krebs cycle). ($\sim$ = high energy bond). From Toporek: *Basic Chemistry of Life*, 1968. Courtesy of Appleton-Century-Crofts, Inc.

to form citrate as CoA is regenerated. Oxaloacetate is a member of the cycle which is regenerated with each turn of the cycle.

*Reactions 2-1 and 2-2*—These reactions involve an equilibrium between citrate, cis-aconitate, and isocitrate. The net result, under the influence of aconitase, is the production of isocitrate, an isomer of citrate, by moving the $=OH$ group from the central carbon atom to an end carbon atom.

*Reactions 3-1 and 3-2*—In this two-stage reaction, apparently catalyzed by a single enzyme, isocitrate dehydrogenase, the net reaction is an oxidative decarboxylation of isocitrate to α-ketoglutarate, the oxalosuccinate apparently not being free during the reactions and mediated by *threo*-D-(2R:3S) isocitrate. The decarboxylation makes the net reaction irreversible.

*Reaction 4*—α-Ketoglutarate is oxidatively decarboxylated to succinate in an irreversible reaction involving NAD, vitamin $B_1$, and CoA.

*Reaction 5*—In a reversible reaction catalyzed by succinic dehydrogenase and iron-flavin prosthetic groups acting as hydrogen acceptors (instead of NAD), succinate is oxidized to fumarate.

*Reaction 6*—The reversible hydration of fumarate to malate is catalyzed by fumarase.

*Reaction 7*—Malate is dehydrogenated in a reversible reaction involving malate dehydrogenase and NAD, and oxaloacetate is regenerated as a result, in preparation for the next turn of the cycle.

The dotted lines in Figure 21 indicate the production and capture of energy as high-energy phosphate bonds as the hydrogen atoms are fully oxidized to $H_2O$ by way of the oxidative chain.

## IV. GLYCOLYSIS IN THE HEART

### A. General remarks

Because of the constraints imposed by the lack of all enzymes, not every reaction outlined in Figure 19 takes place in the heart. However, the general scheme of major events is similar (Fig. 22).[40] This pathway is self-regulating in that rates of substrate utilization are controlled by several allosteric feedback mechanisms, of particular importance in the myocardium. As in other mammalian tissues, these reactions occur in the cytoplasm. Under "normal" conditions (adequate coronary blood flow and arterial oxygen content), glucose is rapidly transported into the myocyte, and is irreversibly phosphorylated to glucose-6-phosphate (G-6-P). The enzyme hexokinase catalyzes this reaction, which uses

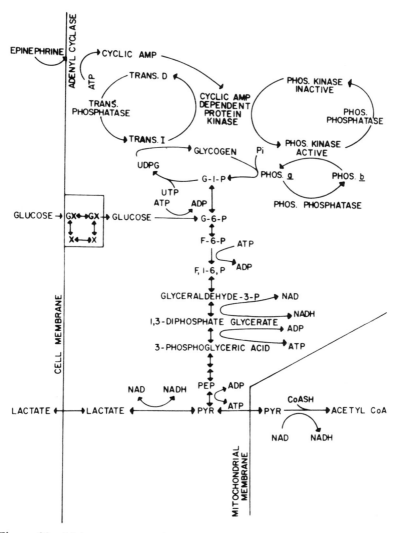

**Figure 22** Major steps in pathways of glucose and glycogen metabolism in heart muscle. Reproduced with permission.[40]

one molecule of ATP during the process, $\Delta G^{0'} = -4.0$ kcal. There is a good correlation between the rate of glucose phosphorylation and the intracellular concentration of G-6-P.[31, 40] G-6-P accumulation inhibits hexokinase [41] and thus G-6-P regulates its own production if the end product is not consumed. G-6-P buildup also inhibits phosphorylase, thereby protecting glycogen stores as well. As mentioned, in the absence of insulin, glucose transport is the rate-limiting step for glucose utilization in the heart.[26, 27] In the presence of insulin, the rate-limiting step shifts to the hexokinase reaction.[31]

Conversion to the isomer, fructose-6-phosphate (F-6-P) is catalyzed by phosphoglucoisomerase with a $\Delta G^{0'}$ of $+0.4$ kcal. The next step, the second of the two "primary" reactions of glycolysis, invests an additional molecule of ATP to phosphorylate F-6-P to fructose-1,6-diphosphate, with a $\Delta G^{0'} = -3.4$ kcal. The enzyme involved at this step, phosphofructokinase (PFK), is an allosteric or regulatory enzyme whose activity controls the overall rate of glycolysis in a number of circumstances.[42, 43] The rate of this reaction is affected by a variety of smaller molecules and hence PFK is called a multivalent allosteric enzyme. The negative $\Delta G^{0'}$ shows that PFK, as most regulatory enzymes of its type, catalyzes a nearly irreversible reaction. The activity of PFK is inhibited by ATP[44] or citrate,[45-47] and is accelerated by inorganic phosphate, $(P_i)$, AMP, ADP, adenyl cyclate, and fructose diphosphate.[48-51] Fatty acid oxidation is accompanied by low levels of AMP and $P_i$, high levels of citrate and ATP, and glycolysis is inhibited.[45-47, 52] Augmented cardiac work also accelerates PFK activity.[52, 53] Finally, when oxidative metabolism is limited, PFK is activated by low tissue ATP levels and high levels of $P_i$ and AMP.[31, 54-56]

Cleavage of F-1,6-diP, catalyzed by aldolase, and yielding glyceraldehyde-3-phosphate and dihydroxyacetone phosphate, has a $\Delta G^{0'}$ of $+5.73$ kcal. Since the intracellular concentration of F-1,6-diP is generally low in comparison with the standard conditions at which $\Delta G^{0'}$ is calculated (see appendix), a large fraction of reactant is cleaved before equilibrium is reached. The equilibrium position is strongly affected by the concentration of F-1,6-diP.

Only one of the triose phosphates—glyceraldehyde-3-phosphate (G-3-P)—can proceed in glycolysis. Dihydroxyacetone phosphate is reversibly converted to G-3-P by the enzyme triose phosphate isomerase, with a $\Delta G^{0'} = +1.83$ kcal. In the heart, the product of the mass action ratios of the aldolase and triose phosphate isomerase reactions is near the equilibrium value.[57]

An important step in the second "stage" of glycolysis is the oxidation of glyceraldehyde-3-phosphate to 1,3-diphosphoglycerate, the only oxidative reaction in the pathway. This reaction is catalyzed by glyceraldehyde-3-phosphate dehydrogenase and has a $\Delta G^{0'} = +1.5$ kcal. $NAD^+$ is required as an oxidizing agent and unless NADH is continuously oxidized to $NAD^+$, lack of $NAD^+$ will inhibit this step. When oxygen and blood flow are adequate, mitochondrial oxidative phosphorylation provides such regeneration; a number of "shuttles" transport electrons from cytoplasmic to intramitochondrial sites. Glyceraldehyde-3-P dehydrogenase activity is rate-controlling in hearts perfused under anoxic or ischemic conditions after PFK is activated, since fructose-1,6-diP and triose-P accumulate at this level.

The energy from the oxidation step is transferred to ADP to form ATP as 1,3-diP-glycerate forms 3-phosphoglycerate ($\Delta G^{0\prime} = -4.5$ kcal). Enolase catalyzes the dehydration of 3-phosphoglycerate ($\Delta G^{0\prime} = +0.44$ kcal) and pyruvate kinase then catalyzes the transfer of a phosphate group to ADP ($\Delta G^{0\prime} = -7.5$ kcal).

The resulting pyruvate may be reduced to lactate at the expense of electrons originally donated by glyceraldehyde 3-phosphate and carried by NADH. $NAD^+$ is regenerated in this reaction, catalyzed by lactate dehydrogenase, with a $\Delta G^{0\prime} = -6.0$ kcal. In heart muscle, pyruvate may also be converted to acetyl CoA or alanine. Whether pyruvate is reduced to lactate or converted to acetyl-CoA depends upon the activity of the enzymes involved and the levels of NADH and acetyl CoA. Pyruvate dehydrogenase, which catalyzes the reaction

$$\text{pyruvate} + \text{CoASH} + \text{NAD}^+ \rightarrow \text{acetyl CoA} + CO_2 + \text{NADH} + H^+,$$

is subject to allosteric inhibition by the products: NADH, CoA [58] and ATP.[59] Oxidation of fatty acids results in inhibition of this enzyme from increased levels of NADH and acetyl CoA.[60] In "anaerobic hearts," inhibition of pyruvate dehydrogenase by high NADH levels may divert pyruvate to lactate, thereby increasing oxidation of NADH and allowing glycolytic production of ATP to proceed. In addition, regulation of pyruvate dehydrogenase activity is controlled by a phosphorylation-dephosphorylation system involving pyruvate dehydrogenase kinase and phosphatase. Phosphorylation decreases activity while dephosphorylation restores it.

## B. Control of glycolysis

Glycolysis and mitochondrial oxidative phosphorylation are closely integrated. With a rise in oxidative phosphorylation, ATP and creatine phosphate (CP) are plentiful and PFK activity diminishes. Citrate production by the oxidation of fatty acids also inhibits PFK. This action partially accounts for the lowered aerobic glycolysis rate of 350 $\mu$mole/glucose/hour as opposed to the anaerobic glycolysis rate of 900 $\mu$mole/glucose/hour, and helps explain the preference of the well-oxygenated heart for fatty acids for energy production.

**Table II**    Rate-controlling reactions and regulatory factors during glycolysis in the heart

| RATE-CONTROLLING STEP | REGULATORY FACTOR ($\uparrow$=ACTIVATION; $\downarrow$=INHIBITION) |
|---|---|
| GLUCOSE TRANSPORT | $\uparrow$INSULIN, $\uparrow$ANOXIA, $\uparrow$AUGMENTED CARDIAC WORK $\downarrow$FFA |
| HEXOKINASE | $\uparrow$ATP, $\uparrow$ADP, $\uparrow$P$_i$ $\downarrow$G-6-P |
| PFK | $\uparrow$F-6-P, $\uparrow$P$_i$, $\uparrow$AMP, $\uparrow$ADP, $\uparrow$F-1,6-diP $\downarrow$ACIDOSIS, $\downarrow$CP, $\downarrow$ATP, $\downarrow$CITRATE |
| GLYCERALDEHYDE-P-DEHYDROGENASE | $\downarrow$NADH, $\downarrow$1,3di-P-GLYCERATE |
| PYRUVATE DEHYDROGENASE | $\downarrow$PHOSPHORYLATION $\downarrow$ACETYL CoA, $\downarrow$NADH |

The inhibitors and accelerators of the major rate-controlling enzymes appear in Table II. In the well-oxygenated heart, which reaction is rate-controlling depends upon the work level and presence of insulin (Table III). The effect of increased cardiac work affects different rate-controlling steps, also a function of substrate (Table IV).

## C. Aerobic metabolism

The importance of aerobic metabolism in the myocardium is reflected by the number of mitochondria in the heart; over 35% of the myocardial volume is occupied by mitochondria.[61] In addition to hormonal influences the rate of glycolysis is tuned to the rate of mitochondrial oxidation.[62] Chance and co-workers [63] have shown that electron transport is dependent upon the presence of a phosphate acceptor, namely ADP. Oxidation of substrate is inhibited in the absence of ADP at three separate loci, probably those for coupled high

**Table III**    Control of glycolysis in well-oxygenated hearts

| CONDITION OF HEART | RATE-CONTROLLING STEP | REGULATORY FACTOR |
|---|---|---|
| LOW PEAK SYSTOLIC PRESSURE | GLUCOSE TRANSPORT PFK | INSULIN LEVEL FFA SUPPLY CITRATE |
| INSULIN AVAILABLE | HEXOKINASE PFK | G-6-P CITRATE |

**Table IV**   Effect of increased cardiac work level on glycolysis

| SUBSTRATE | REACTIONS AFFECTED | REGULATORY FACTORS |
|---|---|---|
| GLUCOSE | ↑GLUCOSE TRANSPORT ↑HEXOKINASE ↑PFK | UNKNOWN G-6-P UNKNOWN |
| GLUCOSE AND FFA | ↓GLUCOSE TRANSPORT ↓HEXOKINASE ↓PFK | FFA OXIDATION G-6-P CITRATE, CP |

energy phosphate bond synthesis. The presence of ADP, from the hydrolysis of ATP used for muscle contraction or other energy-requiring process, releases the inhibition of electron transport, and ATP synthesis resumes. Thus the rate of ATP production is governed by its disappearance. A prolonged increase in cell energy requirements may be met by an enlarged mitochondrial mass and growth of other intracellular constituents.[61]

As mentioned, in the normal heart, free fatty acid oxidation exerts a negative feedback on glucose metabolism, chiefly by increasing levels of intracellular citrate and reducing the activity of phosphofructokin-ase. Recent evidence suggests that free fatty acid accumulation within the cell may directly inhibit membrane hexose transport as well.[65-67]

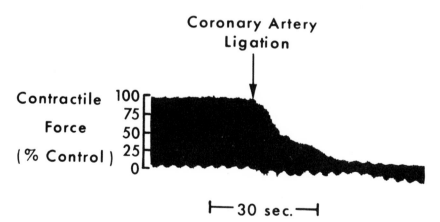

**Coronary Artery Ligation**

Contractile Force (% Control)

├─ 30 sec. ─┤

**Figure 23**   Left ventricular contractile force measured by an isometric strain gauge arch sutured into the myocardium of a dog. Note the rapid decline in force after ligation of the left anterior descending coronary artery. Reproduced with permission.[10]

## D. Anaerobic metabolism

In the hypoxic (low oxygen tension, blood flow maintained) or ischemic (low blood flow, oxygen tension normal) heart, the electron transport chain is inhibited and ATP replenishment is likewise reduced. There is an immediate fall in tension (Figs. 23 and 24) as reduced flavin and nicotine coenzymes and reduced cytochrome substances accumulate and the redox potential falls.[6, 8, 9, 68-73] Levels of creatine phosphate fall and parallel the fall in tissue ATP (Fig 25). Oxygen consumption is of course greatly restricted (Fig 26). Free fatty acids are converted to lipids rather than be oxidized. Glucose utilization and glycogenolysis increase and the rate of glycolysis may rise 15- to 20-fold. Accelerated glucose transport, activation of hexokinase, a decrease in the apparent phosphorylation $k_m$ (see appendix) and a reduction in the inhibition of hexokinase by glucose-6-P by an increase in $P_i$ level all participate in this process. The resulting pyruvate generated cannot be oxidized (Figs. 27A and B). Together with high concentrations of reduced nicotinamide adenine dinucleotide (NADH), lactate is produced by the hypoxic heart and cell potassium is lost (Fig. 28).[74, 75] In the intact heart, oxygen extraction may increase, but most often cannot fully compensate for reduced coronary blood flow and/or arterial hypoxemia. Lactate production may be used clinically to assess the degree of myocardial hypoxia, and is a function of myocardial glucose extraction [75, 77, 78] (Fig. 29).

Glycogen is normally not used as a substrate by the intact working heart. In contrast with liver and skeletal muscle, fasting accelerates myocardial glycogen synthesis mediated by FFA mobilization, citrate inhibition of PFK, and elevated glucose-6-P levels. Glycogenolysis is accelerated after an acute increase in cardiac work even in the face of adequate glucose supply, which is dependent upon $P_i$ levels. Parenthetically, the chronically exercised heart is protected against ischemia by relatively augmented glycogen stores. Hence, glycogen utilization in the "aerobic heart" is determined by the availability of other substrates and by the level of heart work demanded. During ischemia glycogenolysis follows oxidation of endogenous triglyceride and may account for up to 20 per cent of total oxygen consumption.[52] In the anoxic working heart, glycogen stores are soon exhausted.[79] Glycogenolysis is regulated by the enzymes glycogen phosphorylase, usually present in its inactive "b" form because of low concentrations of cofactors AMP and $P_i$, and by inhibition induced by ATP, glucose-6-P, and possible ADP.[80] When phosphorylated to the "a" form by a kinase system, the aforementioned inhibitory factors no longer affect the

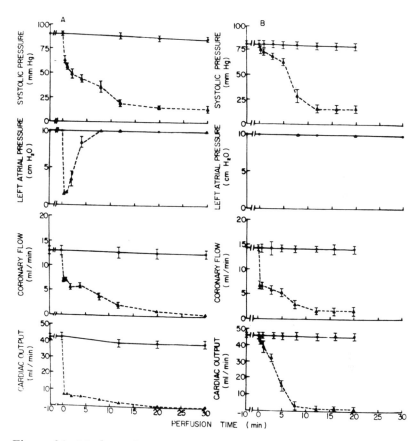

**Figure 24** Mechanical performance of control (solid lines) and ischemic rat hearts (dashed lines). Each heart received a 10-min washout perfusion as a Langendorff preparation. At −10 min in the figure, hearts were switched to a recirculation perfusion as a working heart with a left atrial filling pressure of 10 cm $H_2O$. This control period of perfusion as a working heart was continued for an additional 10 min. At zero time in the figure ischemia was induced by the low cardiac output, high aortic resistance procedure (A) or by one-way aortic valve procedure (B). Perfusion as an ischemic heart was continued for 30 min. Volume of perfusate recirculated was 100 ml in each case. Perfusate was Krebs-Henseleit buffer containing 11 mM glucose and gassed with 95% $O_2$:5% $CO_2$. Each point represents mean ±SE for 8-10 hearts. Reproduced with permission.[68]

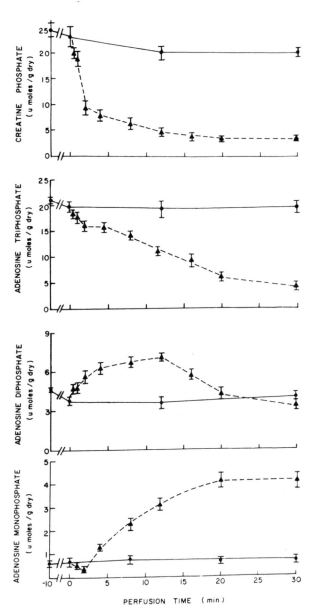

**Figure 25** Tissue levels of creatine phosphate, ATP, ADP, and AMP in control (solid lines) and ischemic hearts (dashed lines). Hearts were perfused as described in Figure 24. Each value represents mean ±SEM for 10 to 12 hearts. Reproduced with permission.[68]

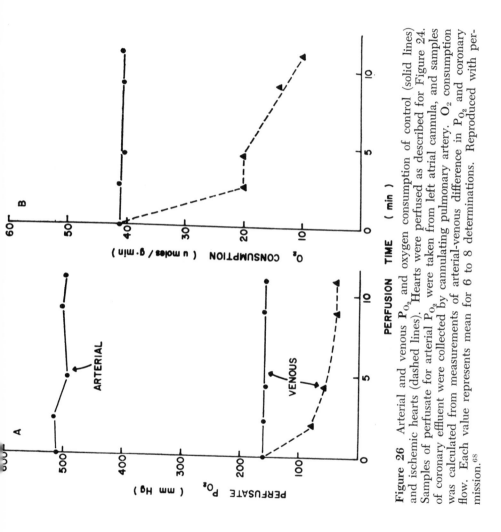

**Figure 26** Arterial and venous $P_{O_2}$ and oxygen consumption of control (solid lines) and ischemic hearts (dashed lines). Hearts were perfused as described for Figure 24. Samples of perfusate for arterial $P_{O_2}$ were taken from left atrial cannula, and samples of coronary effluent were collected by cannulating pulmonary artery. $O_2$ consumption was calculated from measurements of arterial-venous difference in $P_{O_2}$ and coronary flow. Each value represents mean for 6 to 8 determinations. Reproduced with permission.[68]

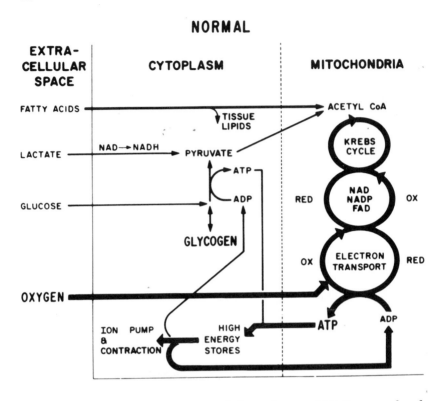

**Figure 27** Relative activities of metabolic pathways of (A) the normal and (B) hypoxic heart contrasted. Reproduced with permission from Scheuer.[76]

enzyme (Figs. 30 and 31). Within seconds after the onset of anoxia or ischemia, phosphorylase *b* kinase is activated and rapid transformation of glycogen phosphorylase from the *b* to the *a* form occurs, possibly related to the modest rise in pH coincident with creatine phosphate disappearance.[81] In addition, during hypoxia the activity of phosphorylase *b* is increased by falling ATP and glucose-6-P levels as well as by increased levels of AMP and $P_i$. Further information about the enzymes involved in glycogen synthesis and breakdown may be found in several recent reviews.[82-85]

Conversion of cardiac metabolism from aerobic to anaerobic pathways during hypoxia is accompanied by a great loss of efficiency. Whereas approximately 36 moles of ATP are formed from the complete oxidation of 1 mole of glucose, only 2 moles of ATP are formed from its glycolysis. Such a drastic reduction in ATP available does not meet the energy demands of contracting mammalian myocardium.[86, 87] The

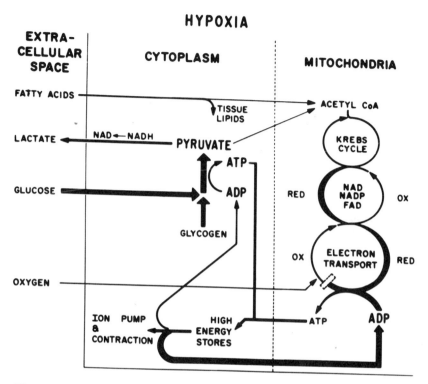

**HYPOXIA**

**Figure 27(B)**—continued

improvement in myocardial performance following various cardio-plegic procedures directly depends upon the concentrations of ATP and CP prior to recovery.[188] Glycogen is 30 percent more efficient than glucose as a substrate and has a net glycolytic yield of 3 moles of ATP per mole of glucose equivalent metabolized.

The maximum glycolytic flux (glucose + glycogen) of working per-fused hearts when insulin is available is 3.5 μmoles glucose/min/gm (wet), which is much less than the peak capacity (42-60 μmoles) of PFK.[79] If these later rates were achieved, glycolytic flux could provide enough energy to sustain the beating heart, as it does in the turtle heart. The exact mechanisms of limitation in glycolytic flux in the mammalian heart have yet to be detailed.

## E. Myocardial ischemia versus hypoxia

The importance of distinguishing between myocardial ischemia and hypoxia has recently been stressed by several workers.[88-90] Oxygen available to the isolated heart may be altered by reducing the oxygen

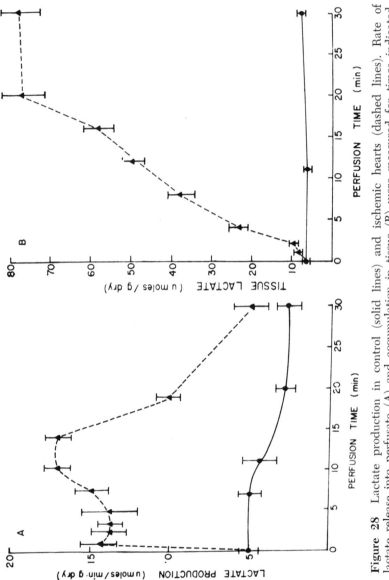

**Figure 28** Lactate production in control (solid lines) and ischemic hearts (dashed lines). Rate of lactate release into perfusate (A) and accumulation in tissue (B) were measured for times indicated. Perfusion conditions were same as for Figure 24, except that perfusate was not allowed to recirculate. Each value represents mean ±SE for 12 hearts. Reproduced with permission.[68]

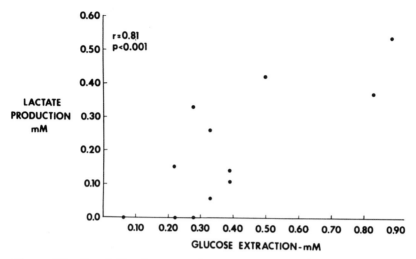

**Figure 29** Correlation between glucose extraction and lactate production during myocardial ischemia. Reproduced from Gorlin [75] with permission.

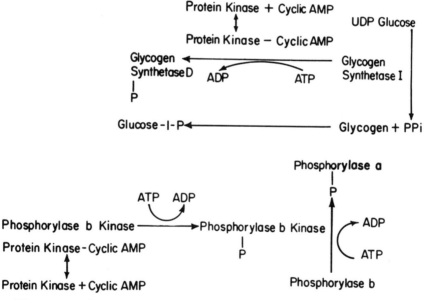

**Figure 30** The reactions involved in the hormonal activation of phosphorylase in cardiac muscle, resulting in glycogenolysis. Cyclic AMP affects a protein kinase, which activates phosphorylase-*b*-kinase. In turn, phosphorylase *b* is converted to phosphorylase *a*, leading to glycogen cleavage.

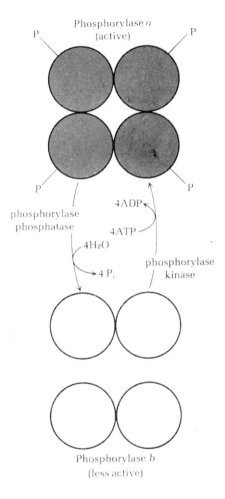

**Figure 31**   Conversion of phosphorylase *a* to phosphorylase *b* by phosphorylase phosphatase and reactivation of phosphorylase *b* by phosphorylase kinase. Reproduced with permission.[39]

tension of the perfusate to produce anoxia, or by restricting the flow of perfusate containing normal or high oxygen tensions. In other preparations, ischemia may be produced by coronary artery ligation. Rovetto and associates[91] reported that in both instances—ischemia and hypoxia—the rate of glycolysis was increased, but the rate was doubly fast in the anoxic preparation. During ischemia lactate produced was ten times that observed during anoxia, and the onset of mechanical failure correlated with lactate accumulation. These investigators postulated that the acidosis inhibited PFK activity and accounted for their observations, although Bing and associates [92] found that acidotic hearts following hypoxia recovered nearly all their contractility.

Differences in carbohydrate metabolism between ischemic and hypoxic myocardium were also noted by Kubler and Spieckermann.[93] In both instances, glycolytic metabolism was insufficient to maintain high energy phosphate stores, lactate was produced, glycolysis increased over 20-fold, and many glycolytic reactions progressed at less than 10 per cent maximum rate because of allosteric kinetic limitations. In *ischemic* tissue, PFK became rate-limiting, and hexokinase was inhibited by glucose-6-phosphate. Later, phosphoglucomutase, which requires ATP as a cofactor, became rate-limiting. When ATP concentrations fell further, glycolytic flux stopped, since insufficient ATP was present to phosphorylate fructose-6-phosphate.

In the *anoxic* perfused heart, glycolysis was activated, beginning at the PFK level, the glucose-6-phosphate concentration decreased (contrast with ischemia where it increased), and hexokinase was stimulated. Total glycolytic flux in the anoxic tissue met 90 per cent of the energy demands, but only 70 per cent of the needs of the ischemic heart. The fall in high energy phosphate stores is therefore tempered by glycolytic ATP production, which may be significant in the anoxic or ischemic heart.[94] Thus energy for the steady-state performance of stroke work may be derived in part from anaerobic metabolism.[95] Thus, in hypoxic or anoxic hearts, fatty acid oxidation is suppressed and glycolysis is accelerated as much as 10- to 20-fold. Ischemia results in only a transient increase in the glycolytic rate lasting for 3-4 minutes, followed by inhibition. Fatty acid oxidation is also limited in ischemic preparations which results in long-chain-CoA and triglyceride buildup. The reactions affected during anoxia and ischemia and the regulatory factors involved are contrasted in Table V.

The mechanisms of activation of cardiac glycogen phosphorylase under ischemic and anoxic conditions also differ.[29] Normally, the percentage of phosphorylase activated (y) bears a monotone relationship to the energy turnover or metabolism in millicalories/gm (M):

$$y = \theta M$$

which shows that muscle is capable of pacing energy production in such a way that it approaches energy needs. In the well-oxygenated heart ATP concentration is high, $P_i$ concentration is low, and glycogen is not a major substrate for energy production.

**Table V** Comparison of rate-controlling steps during anoxia and ischemia in the heart

| CONDITION | STEP AFFECTED (↑=ACTIVATION, ↓=INHIBITION) | REGULATORY FACTOR |
|---|---|---|
| ANOXIA ⎛↓pO₂ ⎞ ⎜FLOW ⎟ ⎝ADEQUATE⎠ | GLUCOSE TRANSPORT↑ | UNKNOWN |
| | HEXOKINASE↑ | ↓G-6-P |
| | PFK↑ | ⎧↑ADP, ↑AMP, ↑Pᵢ ⎨↓ATP, ↓CP, ↑F-1,6-diP |
| | GLYCERALDEHYDE-3-P-DEHYDROGENASE↓ | ↑NADH |
| ISCHEMIA ⎛↓FLOW ⎞ ⎝pO₂ ADEQUATE⎠ | GLUCOSE TRANSPORT↑ | UNKNOWN |
| | HEXOKINASE↓ | ↑G-6-P |
| | PFK↑ | ⎧↑ADP, ↑AMP, ↑Pᵢ ⎨↓ATP, ↓CP, ↑F-1,6-diP |
| | GLYCERALDEHYDE-3-P-DEHYDROGENASE↓↓ | NADH↑↑ |

In an open-chest rat preparation, ischemia (produced by reduction in coronary blood flow) and anoxia (produced by $N_2$ breathing) both resulted in increased cyclic AMP levels and phosphorylase activity. Phosphorylase kinase activity increased during ischemia but not during anoxia. Beta-receptor blockade with practolol prevented a rise in cyclic AMP levels and phosphorylase activity only during ischemia. Treatment with epinephrine enhanced cyclic AMP levels as much as did anoxia, associated with augmented contractility (dP/dt) during $N_2$ breathing. These data are consistent with the view that in the intact working heart ischemia causes phosphorylase $a$ formation through a cyclic AMP-dependent transformation of phosphorylase kinase. During anoxia, however, phosphorylase $a$ formation depends only upon the regulation of phosphorylase kinase activity without conversion of the enzyme to its activated form. The absolute requirement for $Ca^{++}$ may be another mechanism of regulation of phosphorylase kinase. An increase in cyclic AMP levels during anoxia would not be accompanied by a positive inotropic response even though epinephrine could produce enhanced contractility. According to Mayer [186] cyclic AMP is not involved in glycogenolysis during anoxia, but does mediate glycogenolysis in association with catecholamine action during cardiac ischemia.

## F. Coronary blood flow, substrate preference and the "adenosine hypothesis"

Three recent interesting reports bear on the relationship between coronary blood flow and intermediary metabolism in the heart. Rovetto, Neely and Whitmer [140] studied glycolytic flux in the ischemic isolated rat heart. During the first two minutes of ischemia, glycolysis and glycogenolysis were stimulated but were limited by PFK activity. After sixteen minutes of ischemia when coronary blood flow was 20 per cent of control, glycolysis was depressed, and glyceraldehyde-3-P dehydrogenase activity was the rate-limiting step. Tissue lactate and $\alpha$-glycerophosphate rose sharply 12-fold; intracellular pH and coronary effluent pH decreased. In anoxic hearts perfused with control values of coronary blood flow, glycolysis was stimulated and $\alpha$-glycerophosphate achieved the same concentration as did ischemic hearts which received 20 per cent control flow with tissue lactate rising 2-fold. Reduction of coronary blood flow by 85 per cent in anoxic hearts resulted in inhibition of glycolysis.

Spitzer and co-workers,[141] varied the afterload in isolated dog left ventricle. After four hours of 50 mm Hg afterload (control, 100 mm Hg afterload), coronary sinus blood flow decreased from 45 to 33 ml/min, and oxygen consumption decreased from 194 to 138 $\mu$moles/min. Prolonged severe hypotension in this model also caused a relative preference of FFA oxidation by the heart with associated decreases in glucose and lactate uptake.

Moravec and associates [142] studied the fluorescent emission of the isolated rat heart perfused with the Langendorff technique. The perfusion (containing $\beta$-hydroxybutyrate 5 mM as substrate in fasted rats) minimized glycolytic flux, and the cytoplasmic NAD pool was unchanged, as reflected by perfusate and tissue lactate/pyruvate ratios. It was concluded that the observed decrease in fluorescent emission at 481 *nm* resulting from increased perfusion pressure was due to an oxidation of the mitochondrial NAD pool to NAD$^+$, which was also a function of substrate used by the heart.

In response to a negative oxygen balance and/or to ischemia, adenosine is released by the stressed myocardium *in vivo*.[144, 145] This substance is produced from the hydrolysis of 5'-AMP by 5'-nucleotidase, and is a powerful vasodilator, thought to regulate coronary vascular resistance.[146] The "adenosine hypothesis" suggests that the pool of adenosine released by ischemic muscle cells is directly responsible for increased blood flow.[147, 148] In contrast with skeletal muscle, where adenosine is only produced in the vicinity of the blood vessels, adenosine is produced throughout heart tissue, since 5'-nucleotidase is present ubiquitously.[149] The significance of this finding is unclear, but may reflect the survival value of a responsive method regulating coronary blood flow. The interaction between adenosine and hypoxia is also unsettled but it appears as if adenosine is in fact the principal vascular regulator, with hypoxia acting as a sensitizing condition.[177] During recovery from hypoxia, *de novo* synthesis of adenine nucleotides is enhanced,[189] an effect which is similar to that observed after beta-adrenergic stimulation.[190]

## G. Metabolic changes during myocardial ischemia versus infarction

Even if ATP levels are maintained from glycolysis, contractility may decrease. Scheuer [96] has suggested that either ATP is selectively depleted from a small compartment closely related to contraction,[97] or there may be a defect in energy utilization in the hypoxic heart.

Support for the concept of compartmentalization of ATP pools is derived from the work of Gudbjarnason,[98] who examined the relationship between ATP and creatine phosphate (CP) concentrations in acutely ischemic and noninfarcted areas of infarcted myocardium. ATP and CP concentrations fell in infarcted as well as noninfarcted heart muscle, consistent with an increase in energy utilization per unit of surviving muscle, which were out of proportion to the synthesis of high-energy phosphates. CP stores were reduced to a critical level of 7 $\mu$mole/g before ATP concentration fell (Fig. 32).

In acutely ischemic myocardium, the relationship between ATP and CP is very different from that seen in the noninfarcted muscle. A rapid reduction in the CP level occurs in ischemic muscle before a significant drop in ATP concentration is noted (Fig. 33). Ischemic muscle stops contracting at an ATP level of 4.5-4.9 $\mu$mole/g, when only 20 per cent of the ATP is utilized, whereas nonischemic myocardium continues contracting at ATP levels as low as 1.6-2.0 $\mu$mole/g. These data suggest it is not solely the lack of ATP in the ischemic heart that is responsible for its reduced contractility. In ischemic myocardium, the rate of CP breakdown correlates closely with lactate accumulation, but the rate of decrease in ATP stores diminishes with an increase in the rate of lactate production (Fig. 34). This rapid development of intracellular acidosis therefore appears important in the reduction of contractility. Further, the disconcordance of ATP and CP concentra-

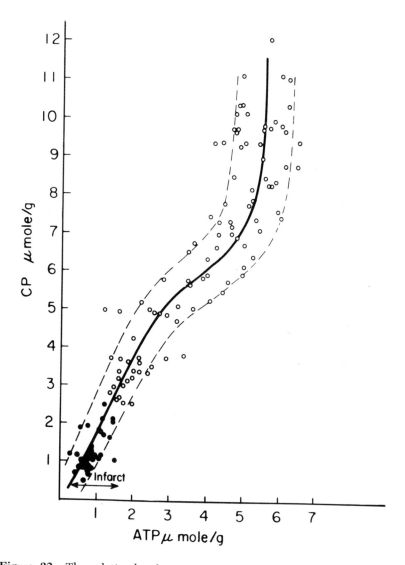

**Figure 32** The relationship between the tissue content of creatine phosphate (CP) and ATP in noninfarcted heart muscle (open circles) and infarcted heart muscle (filled circles) during the post-infarction period. Reproduced with permission from Gudbjarnason.[98]

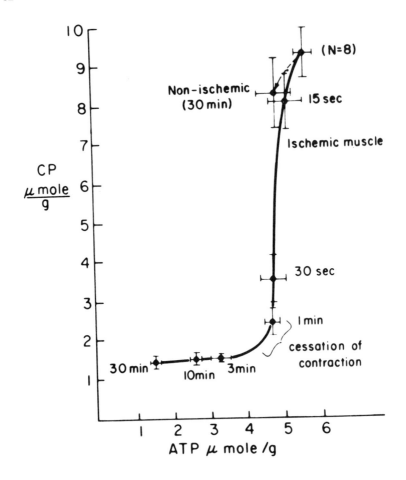

**Figure 33** The relationship between the tissue content of creatine phosphate (CP) and ATP in ischemic heart muscle, following acute coronary artery occlusion. The vertical and horizontal lines represent ± standard error of the mean of CP and ATP determinations.

tions in ischemic heart muscle suggests that a deficient transfer of high energy phosphate bonds from the site of synthesis in mitochondria to the place of utilization—the contractile filaments—may contribute to reduced contractility (Fig. 35).[95, 99]

It should be recognized that irrespective of the mechanism of impairment of contractility mentioned above, the ultimate depletion of high energy phosphate stores in the ischemic or hypoxic heart results

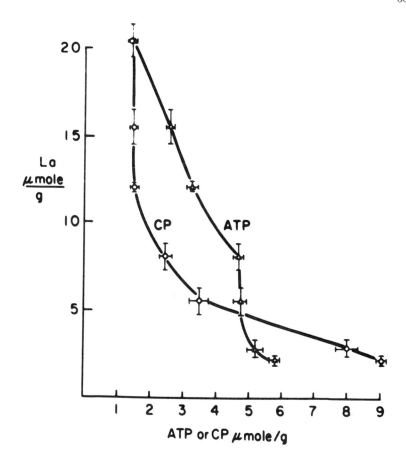

**Figure 34** The relationship between the increase in lactate (la) content of ischemic heart muscle and the decrease in CP and ATP content following acute coronary occlusion. The points correspond to the points in Figure 33.

in mechanical and electrical dysfunction. Restoration of adequate oxygenation replenishes creatine phosphate and ATP to normal levels within 20-30 seconds (Fig. 36).[100]

Changes other than those already discussed occur in the hypoxic heart. The mitochondria may oxidize NADH coupled with fumarate reduction, and may reduce oxaloacetate coupled to alpha-keto-glutarate oxidation, permitting ATP production. Tricarboxylic acid cycle intermediates may maintain ATP stores and glycogen when administered to the hypoxic heart.[101] In "chronic" ischemia (24 hr.), a defect in the activity of carnitine palmityltransferase is also present.[102]

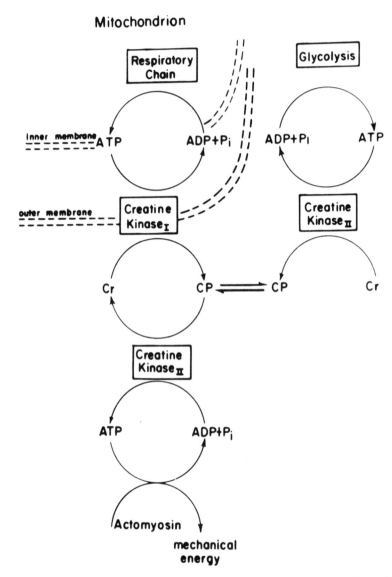

**Figure 35** Compartmentation of ATP and CP in heart muscle and possible paths of high-energy phosphate transfer from the site of synthesis in mito-chondria to the site of utilization by contractile proteins.

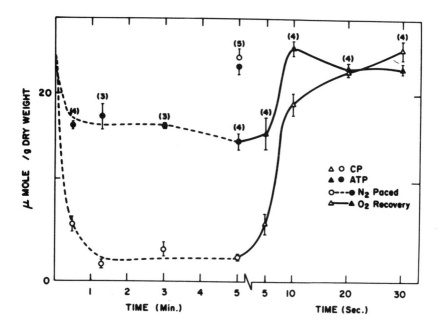

**Figure 36** Changes in myocardial ATP and creatine phosphate with anoxia (N₂, paced) and recovery. Numbers in parentheses indicate the number of hearts (mean ± SE). Rapid restoration of high-energy phosphate stores should be noted. Reproduced with permission from Scheuer.[100]

For a discussion of lipid metabolism during ischemia the reader is referred to two recent reviews.[88, 90]

## H. Intracellular acidosis

Myocardial metabolic acidosis resulting from ischemia and/or hypoxia is well known.[92, 99, 140, 178, 179] A depression in myocardial contractility regularly accompanies hypoxia,[10, 180] which may be reproduced experimentally by a reduction in pH when oxygenation is adequate. A rise in intramyocardial $pCO_2$ in itself may contribute to depressed left ventricular function.[181, 182] Poor myocardial performance is immediately observed even when normal concentrations of high energy phosphates are present. Katz[99, 183, 184] has repeatedly emphasized that anaerobic glycolysis leads to intracellular acidosis, which may impair contractility by increasing the affinity of sacroplasmic reticulum for $Ca^{++}$ (Table VI). Another proposed mechanism for the harmful mechanical effect of acidosis is the displacement of $Ca^{++}$ from its binding site on troponin, which is a necessary event for contraction.

Table VI  The immediate reduction in myocardial contractility from reduced coronary blood flow is most likely due to intracellular acidosis, since
high energy phosphates are normal for a finite period of time when ventricular function is depressed. In turn, an excess of hydronium ion may
compete with calcium for binding sites on troponin and increase the affinity
of the sarcoplasmic reticulum for calcium ion. Diminished activator calcium
ion reduces actomyosin sliding and hence contractility is impaired.

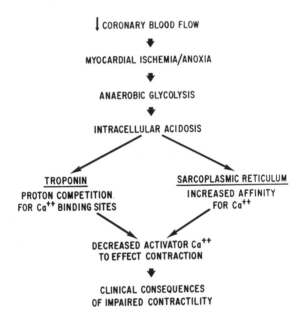

Further intracellular disruption occurs in response to progressive
acidosis. The pH optima of many enzymes is within the normal physiological range, and these enzymes are relatively inhibited at low pH's.
For example, at pH = 6.6, the malate-aspartate shuttle is depressed,
and hydrogen ion transport between cytoplasmal and mitochondrial
pyridine nucleotides is interrupted. PFK is also inhibited by acidosis.
The pH optima of lysosomal proteolytic and hydrolytic enzymes are in
the low pH range and therefore the activity (and release) of such enzymes may be aided at low pH values and lead to cell autolysis (Table
VII).

Although the degree of intracellular acidosis in response to ischemia
may not necessarily be matched by coronary venous effluent pH fluctuations,[185] the buffering capacity of myocardial tissue is relatively poor.
Coronary venous pH does fall, and the response of the myocardium to
inotropic agents may be attenuated. Cardiac electrical function

deteriorates as pacemaker activity is altered and unwanted arrhythmias appear. Coronary flow falls as acidosis progresses, blood coagulability increases and vascular responsiveness to vasoactive agents falters. Acceleration of anaerobic glycolysis by any means would be accompanied by all these ill effects as the severity of acidosis increases.

## V. FATE OF METABOLIC ENERGY IN MYOCARDIUM

The subject of energy metabolism—transport and utilization—in cardiac muscle deserves consideration at this point in the discussion. Thus far energy production has been emphasized in this chapter, and selected aspects of energy storage are covered in the appendix. The next logical question arises: how is the energy stored in ATP and CP used by muscle, *i.e.*, what is its fate? (Fig. 37). The energy from oxidative phosphorylation and/or glycolysis is stored as ATP which is transported through the inner membrane of the mitochrondria. Energy is then delivered to active centers of actinomyosin filaments, the "contractile apparatus," where the chemical energy is transduced into mechanical work.

### A. A phenomenological equation

As a result of Hill's pioneering and now classic experiments,[150-152] Gibbs and associates[153] and Mommaerts[154] offered an expression describing the energy transferred during a single muscle twitch

$$U = A + f(I, t) + \alpha(-\Delta L) + P(-\Delta L),$$

where U is the total energy exchanged, A is the heat of activation,[155] $f(I, t)$ is a term reflecting heat production as a function of duration (t) and intensity (I) of a contraction, $\alpha(-\Delta L)$ is the shortening heat, and $(-P\Delta L)$ is the external work performed during the contraction.

This equation was first developed from heat measurements but subsequently it was shown to have a firm chemical basis as well.[156, 157] The first three expressions of heat [A, $f(I, t)$, $\alpha(-\Delta L)$] are not truly separate, but are mathematical components which reflect different aspects of actinomyosin crossbridge sliding. Hence the terms in the phenomenological equation need not necessarily correspond to the heats of discrete biochemical events. Nonetheless, it is useful to review each term and its possible significance.

A, the activation or tension-independent heat, was investigated by Gibbs and co-workers.[158-160] Lack of correlation between inotropic changes and production of tension-independent heat supported the view that the latter resulted from a process during activation. Gibbs

**Table VII**   Postulated events leading to myocyte death. Lines connecting processes do not necessarily imply an exact temporal sequence, nor a cause and effect relation. The extent of acidosis is proportional to the severity of ischemia and duration of anaerobic metabolism.

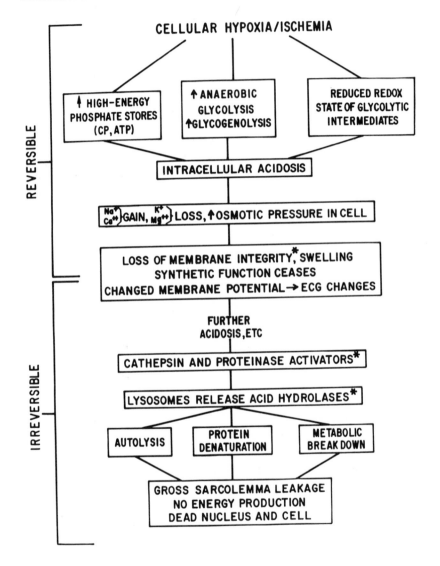

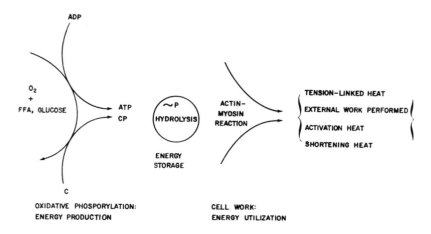

**Figure 37**  The three stages of energy metabolism in the heart are depicted here as energy production, energy storage, and energy utilization.

and associates proposed that the tension-independent heat of cardiac muscle could not be entirely accounted for by the enthalpy of ATP hydrolysis. The magnitude of tension-independent heat correlated with both increasing calcium and sodium concentrations in the perfusate individually and the effects were additive. Therefore, the cardiac tension-independent heat production was thought to be determined in large part by the combined enthalpy of the sodium and calcium pumps.

Such a theory may be examined in the following manner. During the action potential ion movement of $n$ species cross the sarcolemma with the liberation of free energy $\sum_{i=1}^{n} \Delta G_i$ (see appendix). Changes in entropy, $\sum_{i=1}^{n} T\Delta S_i$ occur, such that the enthalpy $\sum_{i=1}^{n} \Delta H_i$ associated with the action potential is nearly zero. During excitation the electrical work performed by ion currents is then matched by the heat absorbed. However, the extrusion of sodium and calcium from the cell against an electrochemical gradient during repolarization requires energy. For sodium alone, this energy would be:

$$ RT \ln \frac{[Na^+]_o}{[Na^+]_i} + F \mathcal{E}_m $$

were R is the gas constant, $[Na^+]_o$ and $[Na]_i$ refer to concentrations of sodium outside and inside the membrane, F is the Faraday, and $\mathcal{E}_m$ is the membrane potential. Using this equation and data relating the energy required to transport calcium from the contractile protein to the sarcoplasmic reticulum, calculations indicate that tension-independent heat production is quantitatively accounted for by calcium and sodium pump activity, the former being of greater importance. The electrochemical $Na^+$-pumping work performed per beat is about 0.2 mcal $g^{-1}$. Since the sarcoreticular calcium pump operates with an efficiency of about 50 percent, and a maximal cardiac contraction is associated with sarcotubular transport of $5 \times 10^{-8}$ mole $Ca^{++}/gm$ muscle, one may calculate a calcium pump enthalpy of about 0.25 mcal $g^{-1}$.[159]

The measurement of A may be obtained by eliminating the contractile response. The value of A is of the magnitude of 1.0 mcal $g^{-1}/$ cycle.[156, 157]

The next term in the phenomenological equation, f(I,t), is a tension-linked heat expression indicating that the generation and maintenance of tension has an associated energy expenditure. f(I,t) may be best isolated by conducting experiments under isometric conditions, although there is some overlap with the third and fourth terms.* Pure isolation of this term in cardiac muscle has not yet been accomplished.

The shortening heat, $\alpha(-\Delta L)$, describes the wasted heat accompanying the contraction, and is proportional to the extent of muscle shortening. Hill's challenge [162] for the biochemical explanation of shortening heat was answered in part by Davies and co-workers.[163] These investigators found no extra ATP breakdown responsible for the heat of shortening. They hypothesized that ATP hydrolysis during shortening [164] was coupled to another reaction with a substantial decrease in entropy. Since the reactions occurred simultaneously, the overall free energy change would have to be negative. The energy change, $d$U, would be given by

$$dU = -TdS - dG - dW$$

where T is the absolute temperature, $d$S the entropy, and $d$G the negative free energy of the coupled reactions. In this instance, total energy

---

* A mechanism for creation of tension-dependent heat during contraction in their model of torsional (rather than linear) filament motion was proposed by Dreizen and Gershman.[161] These workers visualized a torsional movement of thick filaments within a rigid thin filament lattice. ATP hydrolysis caused a conformational and/or quaternary structural change leading to interaction between cross-bridge and thin filament sites. The torsional movement would be associated with the formation of weak enthalpic bonds within the thick filament complex, and thus active contraction would be an exothermic process with the loss of entropy. Finally, the relaxation, or "unwinding" reaction, would be driven by configuration interactions between negatively-charged thick and thin filaments.

change ($d$U) is the same as enthalpy change ($d$H) because pressure, volume, and temperature remain nearly constant in these reactions. Kushmerick and Davies [165] later proposed that an entropy decrease occurred with the first slide of a cross-bridge, thus releasing heat. On recycling, the heat resulting from the entropy change would be resorbed. The overall heat of contraction at any moment would then be a function of the instantaneous positions of each fiber between the two states.

There is little doubt now that the shortening heat "derives from a dissipation of the free energy of the driving reaction plus the entropy term." [166] For a more detailed discussion of this component of the phenomenologic equation in heart muscle, the reader is referred to a recent review by Gibbs. [167]

In 1923, Fenn [168] showed that the amphibian contracting skeletal muscle performs external work, but also that additional heat above that associated with an isometric contraction was produced. Therefore an active muscle has a certain energy "overhead," most easily measured as the isometric heat, in addition to which chemical energy is mobilized exactly equal to the work. In terms of the phenomenologic equation, the sum of the terms A, $f(I,t)$ and $\alpha(-\Delta L)$ is almost constant, and the latter two vary inversely. This relationship also appears to hold for cardiac muscle.[153, 158, 159, 167, 169-172] Under isotonic conditions, additional load-dependent energy utilization above that associated with tension development alone was demonstrated.[153] These results were confirmed more recently by Coleman and associates.[173]

## B. Myocardial efficiency and a model

The work performed by a muscle, $P(-\Delta L)=W$, is the external manifestation of chemicomechanical transduction. For completeness, some remarks should be made regarding muscle efficiency. The definition of efficiency is given by

$$\text{efficiency} = \frac{\text{work performed}}{\text{maximum work possible}} = \frac{-W}{W_{max}} = \frac{e\Delta G}{\Delta G},$$

where $e$ is the coupling efficiency that describes the fraction of free energy manifest as work, $0 \leq e \leq 1$. Since $\Delta$H (see appendix) can be easily measured, the mechanical definition of efficiency is commonly used:

$$\text{efficiency} = \frac{W}{-\Delta H} = \frac{e\Delta G}{-\Delta H}.$$

When part of the free energy $(e\Delta G)$ is transformed into work we have

$$\text{heat produced} = -[T\Delta S + (1-e)\Delta G].$$

At 20°C the maximum efficiency is 10-15 percent, and at 30°C mechanical efficiency is 15-25 percent. This has been attributed to an increased stimulus rate, a decrease in A, and a slight decrease in the slope of the heat versus tension curve.

Chapman and Gibbs [174, 175] recently offered an energetic model of muscle contraction based upon their data. Energy expenditure is visualized as comprising two distinct processes. The first is the calcium pumping of the sarcoplasmic reticulum, with a constant energy requirement. The second is the chemical-mechanical transduction process consisting of a variable number of quantal contractile events, each with a fixed enthalpy exactly matched by the molecular enthalpy of ATP hydrolysis *in vivo*. It is postulated that actinomyosin ATPase activity is velocity-dependent, permitting more contractile events when shortening occurs. Total enthalpy would appear either as heat or work, with total enthalpy varying according to the number of contractile quanta taking place. This model of contraction is equally applicable to different muscles and considers the activation heat, muscle work and residual heat as the three energy terms of primary interest in muscle contraction.

## C. Energy transport in mitochondria

The energy stored in ATP must be delivered to active actinomyosin in order for contraction to occur. In skeletal muscle, ATP is thought to diffuse within the fiber, and the same process was thought to occur in myocardium.[7] However, recent data [96-98] are better explained by hypothesizing two nonexchangeable ATP pools which are located around the mitochondria and the myofibrils respectively. Creatine phosphate could be the molecule responsible for shuttling the energy between the two pools. Saks and associates [176] reported that the kinetics of the mitochondrial isoenzyme creatine phosphokinase permits efficient synthesis of creatine phosphate during oxidative phosphorylation. When creatine is plentiful, all of the ATP synthesized in the mitochondria can be used for creatine phosphate synthesis, and therefore the efficiency of energy supply may depend upon creatine phosphate synthesis rather than on ADP concentration. This sequence of energy transfer is illustrated in Figure 38. Theoretically, since creatine phosphate is smaller than ATP, is would be better suited for diffusion, especially in view of the high adenylate kinase activity in cytoplasm. According to Figure 38, control of the oxidative phosphorylation process would occur via ADP which is shown in the intermembrane space in low concentrations. The behavior of energy transport during ischemia and hypoxia between these postulated ATP pools remains to be fully investigated.

## VI. CLINICAL IMPLICATIONS: THE "GLUCOSE HYPOTHESIS"

A considerable body of experimental data and discussion has revolved about whether glucose is "good," and/or FFA are "bad" for the ischemic myocardium.[103-126] For the organism as a whole, there are changes accompanying myocardial ischemia: depressed insulin response,[127] and augmented catecholamine-,[128-130] corticosteroid-,[130] growth-hormone-,[131-135] and glucagon-levels occur and are responsible for a variety of metabolic alterations (Fig. 39). All these endocrine changes are responsible for relative glucose intolerance and increased FFA levels.

The "glucose hypothesis," recently discussed by Opie[136] postulates that glucose is "good" for the heart, based upon the prediction that glucose availability will enhance the rate of anaerobic glycolysis, will reverse ion losses, will alter impaired membrane electrophysiology, will affect extracellular volume, will decrease plasma free fatty acid concentrations, and will alter plasma osmolarity, all for the better.

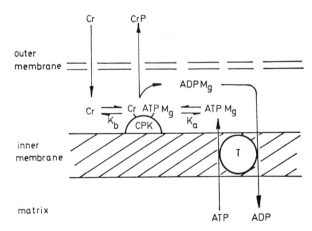

**Figure 38** Scheme relating mitochondrial CPK to oxidative phosphorylation in a myocardial mitochondrion. Contrast with Figure 35. Reproduced with permission.[176]

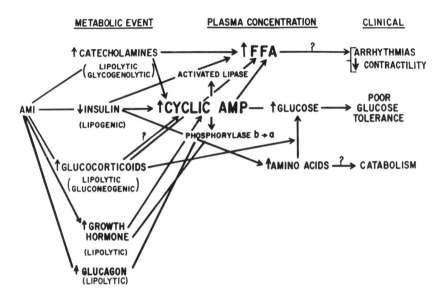

**Figure 39** Systemic metabolic markers of acute myocardial infarction (AMI) mediated by variation in intracellular levels of cyclic AMP (adenosine 3′, 5′-monophosphate).

While it has been postulated that FFA may be "toxic" to the ischemic heart in that arrhythmias are more likely to occur and contractility is depressed, it is not possible to state with authority that FFA are "bad." However, it is true that the well-oxygenated myocardium shifts from FFA as the preferred substrate to glucose during ischemia or anoxia and depends upon the glycolytic pathway for energy production. Extrapolation to the clinical situation is at best tenuous.[137] Even so, pharmacologic agents which reduce plasma levels of FFA have been considered for clinical use in patients with acute myocardial infarction in order to prevent the expected detrimental actions of FFA levels, especially the raised incidence of serious ventricular arrhythmias.[143]

Several of the predicted beneficial actions mentioned above may be enhanced by the simultaneous administration of potassium and/or insulin. In the next three chapters the evidence that these in fact do or do not occur will be presented.

### References

1. Rabinowitz, D., Zierler, K. L.: A metabolic regulating device based on the actions of human growth hormone and of insulin, singly and together, on the human forearm. *Nature* **199**:913-915, 1963.

2. Zierler, K. L., Rabinowitz, D.: Roles of insulin and growth hormone, based on studies of forearm metabolism in man. *Medicine* **42**:385-402, 1963.
3. Catt, K. J.: *An ABC of Endocrinology*, Little, Brown and Co., Boston, 1971, pp. 106-118.
4. Bing, R. J.: The metabolism of the heart, in *Harvey Lecture Series*, Academic Press, New York, **50**:27-70, 1956.
5. McGinty, D. A.: Studies on the coronary circulation. I. Absorption of lactic acid by the heart muscle. *Amer J Physiol* **98**:244-254, 1931.
6. McGinty, D. A.: Cardiac metabolism. *Physiol Rev* **45**:171-213, 1965.
7. Evans, J. R.: Importance of fatty acid in myocardial metabolism. *Circ Res* **14** (Suppl 2): 96-106, 1964.
8. Opie, L. H.: Metabolism of the heart in health and disease. I. *Amer Heart J* **76**:685-698, 1968.
9. Opie, L. H.: Metabolism of the heart in health and disease. II. *Amer Heart J* **77**:100-122, 1969.
10. Amsterdam, E. A.: Function of the hypoxic myocardium. Experimental and clinical aspects. *Amer J Cardiol* **32**:461-471, 1973.
11. Williamson, J. R., Krebs, H. A.: Acetoacetate as fuel of respiration in the perfused rat heart. *Biochem J* **80**:540-547, 1961.
12. Shipp, J. C., Opie, L. H., Challoner, D.: Fatty acid and glucose metabolism in the perfused heart. *Nature* **189**:1018-1019, 1961.
13. Newsholme, E. A., Randle, P., J., Manchester, K. L.: Inhibition of the phosphofructokinase reaction in perfused rat heart by respiration of ketone bodies, fatty acids and pyruvate. *Nature* **193**:270-272, 1962.
14. Most, A. S., Brachfeld, N., Gorlin, R., et al.: Free fatty acid metabolism of the human heart at rest. *J Clin Invest* **48**:1177-1188, 1969.
15. Miller, H. I., Yum, K. Y., Durham, B. C.: Myocardial free fatty acid in unanesthetized dogs at rest and during exercise. *Amer J Physiol* **220**:589-596, 1971.
16. Crass, M. F., III, McCaskill, E. S., Shipp, J. C.: Effect of pressure development on glucose and palmitate metabolism in perfused heart. *Amer J Physiol* **216**:1569-1576, 1969.
17. Neely, J. R., Bowman, R. H., Morgan, H. E.: Effects of ventricular pressure development and palmitate on glucose transport. *Amer J Physiol* **216**:804-811, 1969.
18. Cahill, J. R., Jr.: Intermediary metabolism of protein, fat, and carbohydrate, in *Harrison's Principles and Practice of Internal Medicine* edited by Wintrobe, Wm., Thom, G. W., Adams, R. D., et al., McGraw-Hill Book Co., New York, 7th edition, 1973, pp. 396-408.
19. Neely, J. R., Liebermeister, H., Morgan, H. E.: Effect of pressure development on membrane transport of glucose in isolated rat heart. *Amer J Physiol* **212**:815-822, 1967.
20. Morgan, H. E., Whitfield, C. F.: Regulation of sugar transport in eukaryotic cells. *Curr Topics Membranes Transp:* in press.
21. Danielli, J. F.: Morphological and molecular aspects of active transport. *Symp Soc Exptl Biol* **8**:502-516, 1954.
22. Dixon, M.: The determination of enzyme inhibitor constants. *Biochem J* **55**:170-171, 1953.
23. Wilbrandt, W.: The relation between rate and affinity in carrier transports. *J Cell Comp Physiol* **47**:137-145, 1956.
24. Wilbrandt, W., Rosenberg, T.: The concept of carrier transport and its corollaries in pharmacology. *Pharm Rev* **13**:109-183, 1961.
25. Blumental, R. A., Katchalsky, A.: The effect of the carrier association dissociation rate on membrane permeation. *Biochem Biophys Acta* **173**:357-369, 1969.

26. Park, C. R., Reinwein, D., Henderson, M., et al.: The action of insulin on the transport of glucose through the cell membrane. *Amer J Med* **26**:674-684, 1959.
27. Morgan, H. E., Cadenas, E., Regen, D. M., et al.: Regulation of glucose uptake in muscle. II. Rate-limiting steps and effects of insulin and anoxia in heart muscle from diabetic rats. *J Biol Chem* **236**:262-268, 1961.
28. Randle, P. J., Smith, G. H.: Regulation of glucose uptake by muscle. I. The effects of insulin, anaerobiosis and cell poisons on the uptake of glucose and release of potassium by isolated rat diaphragm. *Biochem J* **70**:490-500, 1958.
29. Dobson, J. G., Mayer, S. E.: Mechanisms of activation of cardiac phosphorylase in ischemia and anoxia. *Circ Res* **33**:412-420, 1973.
30. Tepperman, J.: *Metabolic and Endocrine Physiology*, Year Book Medical Publishers, Chicago, 2nd edition, 1968, p. 169.
31. Post, R. L., Park, C. R.: Regulation of glucose uptake in muscle. III. The interaction of membrane transport and phosphorylation in the control of glucose uptake. *J Biol Chem* **236**:269-272, 1961.
32. Bowman, R. H.: The effect of long-chain fatty acids on glucose utilization in the isolated perfused rat heart. *Biochem J* **84**:14, 1962.
33. Hall, L. M.: Preferential oxidation of acetoacetate by the perfused heart. *Biochem Biophys Res Commun* **6**:177-179, 1961.
34. Randle, P. J., Newsholme, E., Garland, P. B.: Regulation of glucose uptake by muscle. VIII. The effects of fatty acids, ketone bodies and pyruvate and of alloxan-diabetes and starvation, on the uptake and metabolic fate of glucose in rat heart and diaphragm muscles. *Biochem J* **93**:652-665, 1964.
35. Randle, P. J., Smith, G. H.: Regulation of glucose uptake by muscle. II. The effects of insulin, anaerobiosis and cell poisons on the penetration of isolated rat diaphragm by sugars. *Biochem* **70**:501-508, 1958.
36. Morgan, H. E., Neely, J. R., Wood, R. E., et al.: Factors affecting glucose transport in heart muscle and erythrocytes. *Fed Proc* **24**:1040-1045, 1965.
37. Newsholme, E. A., Randle, P. J.: Regulation of glucose uptake by muscle. VI. Effects of anoxia, insulin, adrenaline and prolonged starving on concentrations of hexosephosphates in isolated rat diaphragm and perfused isolated rat heart. *Biochem J* **80**:655-662, 1961.
38. Whitfield, C. F., Morgan, H. E.: Effect of anoxia on sugar transport in avian erythrocytes. *Biochem Biophys Acta* **307**:181-196, 1973.
39. Lehninger, A. L.: *Biochemistry: The Molecular Basis of Cell Structure and Function*, Worth Publishers, Inc., Baltimore, 1970, p. 316.
40. England, P. J., Randle, P. J.: Effectors of rat-heart hexokinases and the control of rates of glucose phosphorylation in the perfused rat heart. *Biochem J* **105**:907-920, 1967.
41. Crane, R. K., Sols, A.: Animal tissue hexokinases, in Colowick, S., and Kaplan, N. O.: *Methods in Enzymology*, Vol. I, Academic Press, New York, 1955, p. 277.
42. Morgan, H. L., Henderson, M. J., Regen, D. M., et al.: Regulation of glucose uptake in muscle. I. The effect of insulin and anoxia on glucose transport and phosphorylation in the isolated, perfused heart of normal rats. *J Biol Chem* **236**:253-261, 1961.
43. Ramaiah, A., Hathaway, J. A., Atkinson, D. E.: Adenylate as a metabolic regulator. Effect on yeast phosphofructokinase kinetics. *J Biol Chem* **239**:3619-3622, 1964.
44. Ahlfors, C. E., Mansour, T. E.: Studies on heart phosphofructokinase desensitization of the enzyme to adenosine triphosphate inhibition. *J Biol Chem* **244**:1247-1251, 1969.
45. Parmeggiani, A., Bowman, R. H.: Regulation of phosphofructokinase activ-

ity by citrate in normal and diabetic muscle. *Biochem Biophys Res Commun* **12**:268-273, 1963.

46. Garland, P. B., Randle, P. J., Newsholme, E. A.: Citrate as an intermediary in the inhibition of PFK in rat heart muscle by FA ketone bodies, pyruvate, diabetes and starvation. *Nature* **200**:169-170, 1963.
47. Passonneau, J. V., Lowry, O. H.: P-fructokinase and the control of the citric acid cycle. *Biochem Biophys Res Commun* **13**:372-379, 1963.
48. Passonneau, J. V., Lowry, O. H.: Phosphofructokinase and the Pasteur effect. *Biochem Biophys Res Commun* **7**:10-15, 1962.
49. Mansour, T. E.: Studies on heart phosphofructokinase: Purification inhibition and activation. *J Biol Chem* **238**:2285-2292, 1963.
50. Newsholme, E. A., Randle, P. J.: Regulation of glucose uptake by muscle. VII. Effects of fatty acids, ketone bodies and pyruvate, and of alloxan-diabetes, hypophysectomy and adrenalectomy, on the concentrations of hexose phosphates, nucleotides and inorganic phosphate in perfused rat heart. *Biochem J* **93**:641-651, 1964.
51. Regen, D. M., Davis, W. W., Morgan, H. E., et al.: The regulation of hexokinase and phosphofructokinase activity in heart muscle. *J Biol Chem* **239**:43-49, 1964.
52. Neely, J. R., Whitfield, D. F., Morgan, H. E.: Regulation of glycogenolysis in hearts: Effects of pressure development, glucose and FFA. *Amer J Physiol* **219**:1083-1088, 1970.
53. Neely, J. R., Denton, R. M., England, P. J., et al.: The effects of increased heart work on the tricarboxylate cycle and its interactions with glycolysis in perfused rat heart. *Biochem J:* in press.
54. Danforth, W. J.: Activation of glycolytic pathways in muscle, in *Control of Energy Metabolism* edited by Chance, B., Estabrook, R., and Williamson, J. R., Academic Press, New York, 1965, p. 287.
55. Morgan, H. E., Randle, P. J., Regen, D. M.: Regulation of glucose uptake by muscle. III. The effects of insulin, anoxia, salicylate and 2:4-dinitrophenol on membrane transport and intracellular phosphorylation of glucose in the isolated rat heart. *Biochem J* **73**:573-579, 1959.
56. Williamson, J. R.: Glycolytic control mechanisms. II. Kinetics of intermediate changes during the aerobic-anoxic transition in perfused rat heart. *J Biol Chem* **241**:5026-5036, 1966.
57. Williamson, J. R.: Glycolytic control mechanisms. I. Inhibition of glycolysis by acetate and pyruvate in the isolated perfused rat heart. *J Biol Chem* **240**:2308-2321, 1965.
58. Garland, P. B., Newsholme, E. A., Randle, P. J.: Regulation of glucose uptake by muscle. IX. Effects of fatty acids and ketone bodies and of alloxan-diabetes and starvation on pyruvate metabolism and on lactate/pyruvate and 1-glycerol 3-phosphate/dihydroxyacetone phosphate concentration ratios in rat heart and rat diaphragm muscles. *Biochem J* **93**:665-678, 1964.
59. Linn, T. C., Pettit, F. H., Reed, L. J.: α-Keto acid dehydrogenase complexes. X. Regulation of the activity of the pyruvate dehydrogenase complex from beef kidney mitochondria by phosphorylation and dephosphorylation. *Proc Nat Acad Sci USA* **62**:234-241, 1969.
60. Garland, P. B., Randle, P. J.: Regulation of glucose uptake by muscle. X. Effects of alloxan-diabetes, starvation, hypophysectomy and adrenalectomy, and of fatty acid, ketone bodies and pyruvate, on the glycerol output and concentrations of free fatty acids, long chain fatty acyl-coenzyme A, glycerol phosphate and citrate-cycle intermediates in rat heart and diaphragm muscles. *Biochem J* **93**:678-687, 1970.
61. Page, E., Polimeni, P. I., Zak, R., et al.: Myofibrillar mass in rat and rabbit

muscle. Correlation of microchemical with steriological measurements in normal and hypertrophied heart. *Circ Res* **30**:430-439, 1972.

62. Kones, R. J.: The catecholamines: reappraisal of their use for acute myocardial infarction. *Crit Care Med* **1**:203-220, 1973.

63. Chance, B., Williams, G. R.: The respiratory chain and oxidative phosphorylation, in *Advances in Enzymology*, edited by Nord, F. F., Interscience Publishers, New York, **17**:65-134, 1956.

64. Rabinowitz, M.: Control of metabolism and synthesis of macromolecules in normal and ischemic heart. *J Mol Cell Cardiol* **2**:277-292, 1971.

65. Neely, J. R., Bowman, R. H., Morgan, H. E.: Effects of ventricular pressure development and palmitate on glucose transport. *Amer J Physiol* **216**:804-811, 1969.

66. Gross, M. F., III, McCaskill, E. S., Ship, J. C.: Glucose-free fatty acid interactions in the working heart. *J Appl Physiol* **29**:87-91, 1970.

67. Carlson, L. A., Lassers, B. W., Wahlquist, M. L., et al.: The relationship in man between plasma free fatty acids and myocardial metabolism of carbohydrate substances. *Cardiology* **57**:51-54, 1972.

68. Neely, J. R., Rovetto, M. J., Witmer, J. T., et al.: Effects of ischemia on function and metabolism of the isolated working rat heart. *Amer J Physiol* **225**:651-658, 1973.

69. Jennings, R. B.: Myocardial ischemia-observations, definitions and speculations. *J Mol Cell Cardiol* **1**:345-349, 1970.

70. Kubler, W., Spieckermann, P. G.: Regulation of glycolysis in the ischemic and anoxic myocardium. *J Molec Cell Cardiol* **1**:351-377, 1970.

71. Williamson, J. R.: Metabolic control in the perfused rat heart, in *Control of Energy Metabolism*, edited by Chance, B., Estabrook, R. W., Williamson, J. R., Academic Press, New York, 1965, p. 333.

72. Scheuer, J., Brachfeld, N.: Myocardial uptake and fractional distribution of palmitate-1-14 by the ischemic dog heart. *Metabolism* **15**:945-954, 1966.

73. Rabinowitz, M.: Control of metabolism and synthesis of macromolecules in normal and ischemic heart. *J Molec Cell Cardiol* **2**:277-292, 1971.

74. Case, R. B., Nasser, M. G., Crampton, R. S.: Biochemical aspects of early myocardial ischemia. *Amer J Cardiol* **24**:766-774, 1969.

75. Gorlin, R.: Assessment of hypoxia in the intact heart. *Cardiology* **57**:24-34, 1972.

76. Scheuer, J.: Myocardial metabolism in cardiac hypoxia. *Amer J Cardiol* **19**:385-392, 1967.

77. Gudbjarnason, S.: The use of glycolytic metabolism in the assessment of hypoxia in human hearts. *Cardiology* **57**:35-46, 1972.

78. Mueller, H., Ayres, S. M., Giannelli, S., Jr., et al.: Cardiac performance and metabolism in shock due to acute myocardial infarction in man: response to catecholamines and mechanical cardiac assist. *Trans NY Acad Sci* **34**:309-333, 1972.

79. Opie, L. H.: Substrate utilization and glycolysis in the heart. *Cardiology* **56**:2-21, 1971.

80. Wollenberger, A., Krause, E. G.: Metabolic control characteristics of the acutely ischemic myocardium. *Amer J Cardiol* **22**:349-359, 1968.

81. Danforth, W. H.: Activation of glycolytic pathways in muscle, in *Control of Energy Metabolism*, edited by Chance, B., Estabrook, R. W., Williamson, J. R., Academic Press, New York, 1965, p. 287.

82. Graves, D. J., Wang, J. H.: Glucan phosphorylases-chemical and physical basis of catalysis and regulation. *Enzymes* **7**:435-482, 1972.

83. Fischer, E. H., Heilmeyer, L. M. G., Jr., Haschke, R. H.: Phosphorylase and the control of glycogen degradation. *Curr Top Cell Regul* **4**:211-251, 1971.

84. Larner, J., Villar-Palasi, C.: Glycogen synthase and its control. *Curr Top Cell Regul* **3**:195-236, 1971.
85. Walsh, D. A., Krebs, E. G.: Protein Kinases. *Enzymes* **8**, pt. A: 555-581, 1973.
86. Shea, T. M., Watson, R. M., Piotrowski, S. F., et al.: Anaerobic myocardial metabolism. *Amer J Physiol* **203**:463-469, 1962.
87. Brachfeld, N., Scheuer, J.: Uptake and metabolism of glucose by the ischemic myocardium. *J Clin Invest* **43**:1301-1302, 1964.
88. Neely, J. R., Morgan, H. E.: Relationship between carbohydrate and lipid metabolism and the energy balance of heart muscle. *Ann Rev Physiol* **36**: 413-459, 1974.
89. Brachfeld, N.: Ischemic myocardial metabolism and cell necrosis. *Bull NY Acad Med* **50**:261-293, 1974.
90. Neely, J. R., Rovetto, M. J., Oram, J. F.: Myocardial utilization of carbohydrate and lipids. *Progr Cardiovasc Dis* **15**:289-329, 1972.
91. Rovetto, M. J., Whitner, J. T., Neely, J. R.: Comparison of the effects of anoxia and whole heart ischemia on carbohydrate utilization in isolated, working rat hearts. *Circ Res* **32**:699-711, 1973.
92. Bing, O. H. L., Brooks, W. W., Messer, J. V.: Heart muscle viability following hypoxia: protective effect of acidosis. *Science* **180**:1297-1298, 1973.
93. Kubler, W., Spieckermann, P. G.: Regulation of glycolysis in the ischemic and the anoxic myocardium. *J Mol Cell Cardiol* **1**:351-377, 1970.
94. Scheuer, J., Stezoski, S. W.: Protective role of increased myocardial glycogen stores in cardiac anoxia in the rat. *Cir Res* **27**:835-849, 1970.
95. Muller-Rughholtz, E. R., Lochner, W.: Utilization of glycolytic energy for external heart work. *J Mol Cell Cardiol* **3**:15-29, 1971.
96. Scheuer, J.: The effect of hypoxia on glycolytic ATP production. *J Mol Cell Cardiol* **4**:689-692, 1972.
97. Gudbjarnason, S., Mathes, P., Ravens, K. G.: Functional compartmentation of ATP and creatine phosphate in heart muscle. *J Mol Cell Cardiol* **1**:325-339, 1970.
98. Gudbjarnason, S.: Inhibition of energy transfer in ischemic heart muscle, in *Myocardiology*, Vol. 1, edited by Bajusz, E., Rona, G., University Park Press, Baltimore, 1972, pp. 17-26.
99. Katz, A. M., Hecht, H. H.: The early "pump" failure of the ischemic heart. *Amer J Med* **47**:497-502, 1969.
100. Scheuer, J., Stezoski, S. W.: Effects of high-energy phosphate depletion and repletion on the dynamics and electrocardiograms of isolated rat hearts. *Circ Res* **23**:519-530, 1968.
101. Penney, D. G., Cascarano, J.: Anaerobic rat heart. Effects of glucose and tricarboxylic acid-cycle metabolites on metabolism and physiological performance. *Biochem J* **118**:221-227, 1970.
102. Wood, J. M., Lewis, R. M., Schwartz, A.: Effect of chronic ischemia in canine heart on the activity of carnitine palmityltransferase. *Circulation* **46**: II-237, 1972.
103. Opie, L. H., Lochner, A., Owen, P., et al.: Substrate uptake in experimental myocardial ischemia. Evaluation of role of glucose, fatty acids and glucose-insulin-potassium therapy, in *Effect of Acute Ischemia on Myocardial Function*, edited by Oliver, M. F., Julian, D. G., Donald, K. W., The Williams and Wilkins Co., Baltimore, 1972, pp. 181-199.
104. Opie, L. H., Owen, P., Mansford, K. R. L.: Metabolic adjustments to acute heart work: observations in the isolated perfused rat heart. *Cardiovasc Res* (**suppl 1**): 87-95, 1971.
105. Opie, L. H., Owen, P.: Glycolysis in acute experimental myocardial infarction: Pathways of metabolism and preliminary results, in *Cardiomyopathies:*

Recent Advances in Studies on Cardiac Structure and Metabolism, Vol. 2, edited by Bajusz, E., Rona, G., University Park Press, Baltimore, 1973, pp. 567-579.

106. Opie, L. H.: Acute metabolic response in myocardial infarction. Brit Heart J (suppl) 33:129-137, 1971.

107. Owen, P., Thomas, M., Opie, L.: Relative changes in free-fatty-acid and glucose utilization by ischaemic myocardium after coronary artery occlusion. Lancet 2:1187-1190, 1969.

108. Opie, L. H.: Metabolic response during impending myocardial infarction. I. Relevance of studies of glucose and fatty acid metabolism in animals. Circulation 45:109-116, 1972.

109. Oliver, M. F.: Metabolic response during impending myocardial infarction. II. Clinical implications. Circulation 45:117-126, 1972.

110. Oliver, M. F., Rowe, M. J., Vetter, N.: Metabolic intervention, in Effect of Acute Ischaemia on Myocardial Function, edited by Oliver, M. F., Julian, D. G., Donald, K. W., The Williams and Wilkins Co., Baltimore, 1972, pp. 354-366.

111. Olson, R. E.: Metabolic interventions in the treatment of infarcting myocardium. Circulation 39-40 (suppl 4): 195-201, 1969.

112. Opie, L. H., Thomas, M., Owen, P., et al.: Failure of high concentrations of circulating free fatty acids to provoke arrhythmias in experimental myocardial infarction. Lancet 1:818-822, 1971.

113. Chain, E. B., Mansford, K. R. L., Opie, L. H.: Effects of insulin on the pattern of glucose metabolism in the perfused working and Langendorff heart of normal and insulin-deficient rats. Biochem J (London) 115:537-546, 1969.

114. Editorial: Glucose and the heart. Lancet 2:1295-1296, 1972.

115. Mjos, O. D.: Effect of substrate alteration on myocardial oxygen consumption, in Effect of Acute Ischaemia on Myocardial Function, edited by Oliver, M. F., Julian, D. G., Donald, K. W., The Williams and Wilkins Co., Baltimore, 1972, pp. 261-276.

116. Peterson, M., Sonnenblick, E. H., Lesch, M.: Preservation of cellular viability during anoxia with high levels of glucose. Circulation 45-46:II-121, 1972.

117. Nelson, P. G.: Effect of heparin on serum free-fatty-acids, plasma catecholamines, and the incidence of arrhythmias following acute myocardial infarction. Brit Med J 3:735-737, 1970.

118. Hearse, D. J., Chain, E. B.: Effect of glucose on enzyme release from, and recovery of, the anoxic myocardium, in Myocardial Metabolism—Recent Advances on Studies in Cardiac Structure and Metabolism, Vol. 3, edited by Dhalla, N. S., Rona, G., University Park Press, Baltimore, 1973, pp. 763-772.

119. Willebrands, A. F., Ter Welle, H. F., Tasseron, S. J. A.: The effect of a high molar FFA/albumin ratio in the perfusion medium on rhythm and contractility of the isolated rat heart. J Mol Cell Cardiol 5:259-273, 1973.

120. Opie, L. H.: Effect of fatty acids on contractility and rhythm of the heart. Nature 227:1055-1056, 1970.

121. Henderson, A. H., Craig, R. J., Gorlin, R., et al.: Free fatty acids and myocardial function in perfused rat hearts. Cardiovasc Res 4:466-472, 1970.

122. Carlson, L. A., Lassers, B. W., Wahlqvist, M. L., et al.: The relationship in man between plasma free fatty acids and myocardial metabolism of carbohydrate substances. Cardiology 57:51-54, 1970.

123. Kurien, V. A., Oliver, M. F.: Free fatty acids during acute myocardial infarction. Progr Cardiovasc Dis 13:361-373, 1971.

124. Oliver, M. F.: The metabolic response to acute myocardial infarction, in Textbook of Coronary Care, edited by Meltzer, L. E., Dunning, G. J., The Charles Press, Philadelphia, 1972, pp. 231-241.

125. Mjos, O. D., Kjekshus, J. K., Lekven, J.: Importance of free fatty acids as a determinant of myocardial oxygen consumption and myocardial ischemic injury during norepinephrine infusion in dogs. *J Clin Invest* **53**:1290-1299, 1974.

126. Most, A. S., Lipsky, M. H., Szydlik, P. A., et al.: Failure of free fatty acids to influence myocardial oxygen consumption in the intact, anesthetized dog. *Cardiology* **58**:220-228, 1973.

127. Taylor, S. H., Majid, P. A.: Insulin and the heart. *J Mol Cell Cardiol* **2**:293-317, 1971.

128. Ceremuzynski, L., Staszewski-Barczak, J., Herbacynaska-Cedro, K.: Cardiac rhythm disturbances and the release of catecholamines after acute coronary occlusion in dogs. *Cardiovasc Res* **3**:190-197, 1969.

129. Mathes, P., Cowan, C., Gudbjarnason, S.: Storage and metabolism of norepinephrine after experimental myocardial infarction. *Amer J Physiol* **220**: 27-32, 1971.

130. Prakash, R., Parmley, W. W., Horvat, M., et al.: Serum cortisol, plasma FFA, and urinary catecholamines as indicators of complications of acute myocardial infarction. *Circulation* **45**:736-745, 1972.

131. Jacobs, H. S., Nabarro, J. D. N.: Arrhythmias during acute myocardial hypoxia. *Lancet* **1**:1224, 1970.

132. Opie, L. H., Hartog, M.: Growth hormone in acute myocardial infarction. *Lancet* **1**:1401, 1970.

133. Kurt, T. L., Genton, N., Chidsey, C., III, et al.: Carbohydrate metabolism and acute myocardial infarction, circulating glucose, insulin, cortisol and growth hormone responses and excretion of catecholamines. *Chest* **64**:21-25, 1973.

134. Prakash, R., Chhablani, R.: Immunoreactive serum insulin and growth hormone response in patients with preinfarction angina and acute myocardial infarction. *Chest* **65**:408-414, 1974.

135. Allison, S. P.: Endocrine changes associated with myocardial ischaemia, in *Effect of Acute Ischaemia on Myocardial Function*, edited by Oliver, M. F., Julian, D. G., Donald, K. W., The Williams and Wilkins Co., Baltimore, 1972, pp. 237-248.

136. Opie, L. H.: The glucose hypothesis: relation to acute myocardial ischemia. *J Mol Cell Cardiol* **1**:107-112, 1970.

137. Wildenthal, K.: On glucose and the heart. *J Mol Cell Cardiol* **2**:67-68, 1971.

138. Bihler, I., Sawh, P. C.: Regulation of sugar transport in the perfused left atrium of the rat. *Fed Proc* **33**:252, 1974.

139. Ignarro, L. J., White, L. E., Wilkerson, R. D., et al.: Cardiac guanyl cyclase: stimulation by acetylcholine and calcium. *Circulation* **47-48** (suppl IV): 12, 1973.

140. Rovetto, M. J., Neely, J. R., Whitner, J. T.: The relationship between glycolytic flux and coronary flow in isolated rat hearts. *Fed Proc* **33**:363, 1974.

141. Spitzer, J. J., Archer, L. T., Black, M. R., et al.: Effects of prolonged coronary hypotension on myocardial substrate utilization. *Fed Proc* **33**:317, 1974.

142. Moravec, J., Corsin, A., Owen, P., et al.: Effect of increased aortic perfusion pressure on fluorescent emission of the isolated rat heart. *J Mol Cell Cardiol* **6**:187-200, 1974.

143. Rowe, M. J., Kirby, B. J., Dolder, M. A., et al.: Effect of a nicotinic-acid analogue on raised plasma-free-fatty-acids after acute myocardial infarction. *Lancet* **2**:814-818, 1973.

144. Dobson, J. G., Jr., Rubio, R., Berne, R. M.: Role of adenine nucleotides,

adenosine, and inorganic phosphate in the regulation of skeletal muscle blood flow. *Circ Res* **29**:375-384, 1971.

145. Rubio, R., Berne, R. M., Katori, M.: Release of adenosine in reactive hyperemia of the dog heart. *Amer J Physiol* **216**:56-62, 1969.

146. Imal, S., Riley, A. L., Berne, R. M.: Effect of ischemia on adenine nucleotides in cardiac and skeletal muscles. *Circ Res* **15**:443-450, 1964.

147. Rubio, R., Berne, R. M.: Release of adenosine by the normal myocardium in dogs and its relationship to the regulation of coronary resistance. *Circ Res* **25**:407-415, 1969.

148. Berne, R. M.: Cardiac nucleotides in hypoxia: possible role in regulation of coronary blood flow. *Amer J Physiol* **204**:317-322, 1963.

149. Rubio, R., Berne, R. M., Dobson, J. G., Jr.: Sites of adenosine production in cardiac and skeletal muscle. *Amer J Physiol* **225**:938-952, 1973.

150. Hill, A. V.: The laws of muscular motion. *Proc Roy Soc B* **100**:87-108, 1926.

151. Hill, A. V.: Work and heat in muscle twitch. *Proc Roy Soc B* **136**:220-228, 1949.

152. Hill, A. V.: *First and Last Experiments on Muscle Mechanics*, New York, Cambridge University Press, 1970.

153. Gibbs, C. L., Mommaerts, W. F. H. M., Ricchiuti, N. V.: Energetics of cardiac contractions. *J Physiol* **191**:25-46, 1967.

154. Mommaerts, W. F. H. M.: Energetics of muscular contraction. *Physiol Rev* **49**:427-508, 1969.

155. Brady, A. J.: Active state in cardiac muscle. *Physiol Rev* **48**:570-600, 1968.

156. Homsher, E., Mommaerts, W. F. H. M., Ricchiuti, N., et al.: Activation heat, activation metabolism and tension-related heat in frog semitendinosus muscles. *J Physiol* **220**:601-625, 1972.

157. Homsher, E., Mommaerts, W. F. H. M., Ricchiuti, N.: Energetics of shortening muscles in twitches and tetanic contraction. II. The force-determined shortening heart. *J Gen Physiol*: in press.

158. Gibbs, C. L., Gibson, W. R.: Effect of alterations in the stimulus rate on energy output, tension development and the tension-time integral of cardiac muscle. *Circ Res* **27**:611-618, 1970.

159. Chapman, J. R., Gibbs, C. L., Gibson, W. R.: Effects of calcium and sodium on cardiac contractility and heat production in rabbit papillary muscle. *Circ Res* **27**:601-610, 1970.

160. Gibbs, C. L., Gibson, W. R.: Energy production in cardiac isotonic contractions. *J Gen Physiol* **56**:732, 1970.

161. Dreizen, P., Gershman, L. C.: Molecular basis of muscular contraction. Myosin. *Trans NY Acad Sci* **32**:170-203, 1970.

162. Hill, A. V.: A further challenge to biochemists. *Biochem Z* **345**:1-8, 1966.

163. Davies, R. E., Kushmerick, M. J., Larson, R. E.: (Professor A. V. Hill's further challenge to biochemists) ATP, activation, and the heat of shortening of muscle. *Nature* **214**:148-151, 1967.

164. Banks, B. E. C., Vernon, C. A.: Reassessment of the role of ATP *in vivo*. *J Theor Biol* **29**:301-326, 1970.

165. Kushmerick, M. J., Davis, R. E.: Energetics and efficiency of maximally working muscle, Ph.D. Thesis, University of Pennsylvania, Philadelphia, Pa., 1967.

166. Mommaerts, W. F. H. M.: Current problems in myocardial metabolism. *Circ Res* **34-35** (suppl III): 2-7, 1974.

167. Gibbs, C. L.: Cardiac energetics, in *The Mammalian Myocardium*, edited by Langer, G. A., Brady, A. J., John Wiley and Sons, New York, 1974, pp. 105-133.

168. Fenn, W. D.: A quantitative comparison between the energy liberated and the work performed by the isolated sartorius muscle of frog. *J Physiol* **58**:175-203, 1923.

169. Gibbs, C. L.: Role of catecholamines in heat production in the myocardium. *Circ Res* **21(III)**: 223-230, 1967.
170. Gibbs, C. L.: Changes in cardiac heat, production with agents that alter contractility. *Australian J Esp Biol Med Sci* **45**:379-392, 1967.
171. Gibbs, C. L., Gibson, W. R.: Effect of ouabain on the energy output of rabbit cardiac muscle. *Circ Res* **24**:951-967, 1969.
172. Chapman, J. B.: Quantal energetic theory of muscle contraction. *Proc Aus Physiol Pharmacol Soc* **1**:47-48, 1970.
173. Coleman, H. N., Sonnenblick, E. H., Braunwald, E.: Myocardial oxygen consumption associated with external work: the Fenn effect. *Amer J Physiol* **217**:291-296, 1969.
174. Chapman, J. B., Gibbs, C. L.: Energetics of isometric and isotonic twitches in toad sartorius. *Biophys J* **12**:215-226, 1972.
175. Chapman, J. B., Gibbs, C. L.: An energetic model of muscle contraction. *Biophys J* **12**:227-236, 1972.
176. Saks, V. A., Chernousova, G. B., Voronkow, I. Iu, et al.: Study of energy transport mechanism in myocardial cells. *Circ Res* **34-35** (suppl III): 138-149, 1974.
177. Gellai, M., Norton, J. M., Detar, R.: Evidence for a direct control of coronary vascular tone by oxygen. *Circ Res* **32**:279-289, 1973.
178. McNamara, J. J., Soeter, J. R., Suehiro, G. I., et al.: Surface pH changes during and after myocardial ischemia in primates. *J Thoracic Cardiovas Surg* **67**:191-194, 1974.
179. Mueller, H., Ayres, S. M., Grace, W. J.: Principal defects which account for shock following acute myocardial infarction in man: implications for treatment. *Crit Care Med* **1**:27-38, 1973.
180. Skelton, C. L., Kirk, E. S., Sonnenblick, E. H.: Influence of hypoxia and ischemia on myocardial contractile function. *Bull NY Acad Med* **50**:294-307, 1974.
181. Bishop, R. L., Weisfeldt, M. L., Ross, R. S.: Effects of pH and $pCO_2$ on performance of hypoperfused myocardium. *Fed Proc* **33**:363, 1974.
182. Flaherty, J. T., Khuri, S. F., O'Riordan, J. B., et al.: Quantitation of myocardial ischemia by intramyocardial carbon dioxide, oxygen, and electrograms. *Fed Proc* **33**:395, 1974.
183. Katz, A. M.: Effects of interrupted coronary flow upon myocardial metabolism and contractility. *Progr Cardiovasc Dis* **10**:450-465, 1968.
184. Katz, A. M.: Effects of ischemia on the contractile processes of heart muscle. *Amer J Cardiol* **32**:456-460, 1973.
185. Effros, R. M., Haider, B., Ettinger, P., et al.: In vivo response of myocardial cell pH to changes of plasma pH and ischemia. *Fed Proc* **33**:396, 1974.
186. Mayer, S. E.: Effect of catecholamines on cardiac metabolism. *Circ Res* **34-35** (suppl III): 129-135, 1974.
187. Niki, A., Niki, H., Miwa, I., et al.: Insulin secretion by anomers of D-glucose. *Science* **186**:150-151, 1974.
188. Hearse, D. J., Stewart, D. A., Chain, E. B.: Recovery from cardiac bypass and elective cardiac arrest. The metabolic consequences of various cardioplegic procedures in the isolated rat heart. *Circ Res* **35**:448-457, 1974.
189. Zimmer, H-G., Trendelenburg, C., Kammermeier, H., et al.: De novo synthesis of adenine nucleotides in the rat: acceleration during recovery from oxygen deficiency. *Circ Res* **32**:635-642, 1973.
190. Zimmer, H-G., Gerlach, E.: Effect of beta-adrenergic stimulation on myocardial adenine nucleotide metabolism. *Circ Res* **35**:536-543, 1974.
191. Bihler, I.: Mechanisms regulating the membrane transport of sugars in the myocardium, in *Recent Advances in Studies on Cardiac Structure and Metabolism: Myocardial Biology*, University Park Press, Baltimore, 1974, Vol. 4, pp. 209-216.

# CHAPTER 2

# INSULIN

Since the work of von Mering and Minkowski in 1899 showing that the pancreas was involved in diabetes mellitus, and the discovery of insulin in 1922 by Banting and Best, great interest has been shown in the effects of insulin on the heart. Even before this time, in 1912, Goulston advocated oral glucose for heart disease[1] and in 1914 Budingen detailed its advantages for this purpose.[2] Soon thereafter, several investigators found benefit from insulin therapy in several classes of heart disease.[3-8] To date, while significant advances have been made in the understanding of certain insulin actions, its fundamental and primary mechanism of action—in heart muscle and elsewhere—is unproved. In this chapter the direct and indirect actions of insulin on the heart will be considered.

## I. INSULIN EFFECT ON ORGANS PROVIDING MYOCARDIAL SUBSTRATE

### A. Overview of insulin actions

The integration of metabolic processes effected by insulin begins in the gastrointestinal tract,[9] where the primary stimuli, substrates, elicit neuroendocrine responses to begin a series of synchronous metabolic processes. Among these responses is insulin secretion, leading to co-ordinated anabolism in insulin-sensitive tissues: liver, adipose, heart, and skeletal muscle. Insulin is secreted in response to a glucose load by a rapid release of preformed insulin and a slower response characterized by further insulin synthesis.[10, 11] Since several substrates effect $\beta$-cell release of insulin, it is likely that an increased respiratory rate of the $\beta$-cell plays a part in insulin release.[12-14] Medium chain triglycerides[15] and amino acids[16, 17] also effect insulin release, but the relative physiologic importance and mechanisms of these processes are uncertain. Glucagon, secretin, pancreozymin, and possibly gastrin are insulin secretogogues which play a part in physiological insulin release.[18-21] Glucagon, produced by the $\alpha$-cells of the pancreas, is an important hormone with potent insulin-secreting actions. The metabolic and hormonal interrelations of glucagon[18] in glucose homeostasis and its interesting cardiotropic actions have recently been reviewed and will not be considered here.[9, 22-24] Insulin secretion is also modified by the autonomic nervous system and catecholamines, and will be further discussed in a subsequent section.

The insulin space is not well characterized in patients with heart disease. The insulin plasma disappearance curve is a multiexponential function of time, each component not classically correlating with recognized spaces.[25] Recently the kinetics of insulin in man was better characterized with the use of a SAAM 25 computer program.[25a] A three compartment insulin model was defined: the first was the plasma space (4.5% body weight), the second was small (1.7%) and equilibrated rapidly with plasma, and the third was large (9.5%) and equilibrated slowly with plasma. Insulin in compartment three correlated well with a servo-controlled glucose infusion and therefore compartment three insulin, rather than plasma insulin, was felt to be a more direct determinant of glucose utilization.

Crystalline insulin half-life is on the order of 5 min in man.[26] The insulin excreted by the kidney is less than 1.5 percent of that filtered and is thought to be completely resorbed in the proximal convoluted tubule,[27] a process that may be affected by renal disease.[28]

Significant fluctuations of glucose and insulin arterial plasma concentrations of fasted animals do not occur frequently.[386] However, during a constant infusion of glucose-insulin, there is an initial rise in plasma concentrations of both glucose and insulin, which then settles into a sustained oscillation with frequencies 1 cycle/2-3 hr. for both components. Insulin has an additional frequency peak of 1 cycle/50 min. Hence the performance of the system regulating glucose levels may be characterized as that of a limit cycle oscillator, described by a nonlinear, nonconservative equation of at least second order.

Insulin binding to cell surfaces is specific, selective, reversible, stereochemically sensitive with respect to insulin, and saturable. Insulin need not enter the cell to effect its many actions. In addition to facilitating entry of glucose, amino acid and potassium movement into muscle and adipose, intracellular events—for instance, formation of long-chain fatty acids from 2-carbon moieties, glycogen synthesis, and amino acid incorporation residues into protein—occur in response to insulin action. Insulin reduces plasma amino acid levels, in part through suppression of release from muscle.[306] The signal transferred to the tissue by insulin begins processes for which information is already present within the differentiated cell. The storage and retrieval of this information may be in the form of protein substrates for cyclic AMP-activated protein kinase(s).

During the interprandial periods, circulating insulin concentrations are lowest, but are sufficient to reduce potassium leakage from muscle and slow free fatty acid release from adipose tissue. More insulin is required to translocate glucose than to influence potassium and free fatty acid metabolism.

## B. Insulin binding

The nature of insulin binding has received much attention. The binding constant for the hormone ($K_b = 3\text{-}7$nmol) is higher than the concentration that gives half-maximal activation of glucose utilization ($K = 50$ pmol).[307-311] Only a small number of insulin receptors need interact with the hormone to eventually induce the associated metabolic changes.[308, 312] Alternatively, insulin-sensitive cells may have a small number of high-affinity specific receptor sites and a relatively larger number of nonspecific sites.[313-315] Kono and Barham [308, 312] calculate that an adipose cell has approximately 160,000 insulin receptors and that glucose uptake is maximally stimulated when only 4000 sites are occupied to result in a measurable metabolic response. Crofford [307] estimates that a sufficient signal is generated when 100 insulin sites are occupied to result in a measurable metabolic response. Although the amplification of the insulin signal is great, some metabolic actions of insulin require the generation of stronger signals than others. For instance, the stimulation of protein synthesis or lipolytic activation by insulin requires a much greater amplitude of signal (assuming a single receptor type) than does the enhancement of glucose transport or antilipolysis.

An insulin-binding protein has been separated from extracardiac tissues which is an asymmetrical protein of molecular weight 300,000 amu.[316, 317] However, it is unknown whether this is the physiological insulin receptor. There is also some question about the fate of insulin upon binding to the receptor. Inactivation of insulin after initiation of its metabolic impulse may result,[318, 319] in which case an alteration in the insulin molecule would function as an "on-off" switch for metabolic processes under insulin control (see discussion re the postulate that cyclic adenylate may so function on page 117). There is recent evidence —at least in one tissue—suggesting that the interaction between insulin and its receptor and the degradation of insulin are separate events.[320]

A covalent bond between insulin and its receptor involving disulfide bonds was postulated some time ago.[321-323] This is highly unlikely in view of the failure of sulfhydryl-blocking agents to prevent insulin binding [314, 324, 325] and lack of correlation between such covalent binding and effect of insulin on membrane transport.[313] Moreover, covalent binding by disulfide bonds implies that the bound insulin molecules would be degraded or removed from the receptor, otherwise the receptors would soon become permanently saturated. There is no evidence that such processes occur. In fact, experiments with various analogues of insulin show that the binding strength is unrelated to the biodegradability. Prior presentation of intact cells have no effect on the insulin bound, since biologic activity is unimpaired after release. Finally, experiments with labelled insulin explicitly reflect the kinetics of a simple dissociable interaction between insulin and receptor, largely affected by changes in temperature and concentration.

The effect of proteases on the insulin "receptor" has been used to elucidate its nature, and suggests that at least part of the insulin receptor is a protein or peptide. Protease incubation in low concentrations produces insulin-mediated effects in muscle and other tissues.[308, 326-328] Light exposure to $p$-chloromercuribenzoate also may trigger a signal which results in enhanced glucose transport and inhibition of lipolysis with lowered adenyl cyclate levels.[329] After heavy exposure to trypsin, insulin binding by the receptor may be impaired, with loss of biological activity, an action which may be reversed by soybean trypsin inhibitor.[312, 328, 330] Pretreatment with insulin protects the receptor from proteolytic agents.[331] Light exposure of tissue to N-ethylmaleimide blocks the insulin-mediated acceleration in membrane transport while basal levels of transport continue.[332, 333] It is uncertain whether chemical treatment of the insulin receptor lowers the affinity of the binding site for insulin,[330] or reduces the number of sites without changing the affinity.[312]

Insulin bound to sepharose beads will produce insulin effects without entering the cell.[334] If free insulin is not present in the experimental preparation, then these data are consistent with the view that insulin need not enter the cell to effect metabolic changes. In addition to experiments involving plastic beads the data from insulin action on erythrocyte and adipose support a surface action of the hormone. "Ghost" membranes of fat cells bind insulin in equilibrium with the surrounding medium. After preparing these ghosts in an everted, or "inside out" form, no insulin is bound. If insulin is added to the preparation before the ghosts are everted, it becomes trapped inside the inverted vesicles, as evidenced by an extremely slow release of insulin into the medium.[205] Such studies with everted vesicles show that insulin receptors are located only on the outside surface of the plasma membrane, and that physical inversion of the membrane is not accompanied by a major reorientation of the involved membrane protein components. This is consistent with the fluid mosaic model of membranes, in which lateral motion of proteins—but not "submerging"—may occur, as thermodynamically predicted. There is little doubt at present that insulin action occurs first at the external plasma membrane surface.[361]

The potential clinical importance of a deficiency in the insulin receptor is unknown. In cardiogenic shock or heart disease of long standing an alteration in hormone receptors has been proposed.[335, 336] Obesity may alter the hepatic insulin receptor in mice [337] but there is currently no evidence suggesting that such a mechanism participates in the relative insulin deficiency acompanying low cardiac output states.

In conclusion, it appears that the insulin-receptor (polypeptide component) interaction(s) may result in a conformational change in the membrane, resulting in a signal or a number of signals, depending upon the number of such interactions, to produce insulin's varied metabolic actions. Further remarks about the mechanism of this process will be made in the appropriate sections.

## II. INSULIN AND SUBSTRATE TRANSPORT

### A. Facilitated diffusion

Insulin facilitates the entry of substrate into the myocardial cell by the stimulation of transport systems that will be considered in this section (Fig. 1). A number of subsances—glucose, amino acids, and vitamins—permeate membranes at a much faster rate than would be expected from their molecular size and lipid solubility.[29] These specialized transport systems which are mediated by constituents of the membrane are called facilitated diffusion.[30] The properties of this type of transport are:

1. They operate on the existing electrochemical gradient of the permeant and lead to the disappearance of the gradient. No additional energy input is required other than that necessary to maintain the integrity of the membrane and the existing electrochemical gradient. Active transport systems are excluded by definition, but facilitated diffusion may occur against an electrochemical gradient if they are coupled to another transport mechanism.

2. The unidirectional flux as measured with the use of an isotopic label is larger than the rate of net diffusion of the permeant.

3. The rate of permeation is not directly proportional to the concentration of the solute, and hence does not obey Fick's law of diffu-

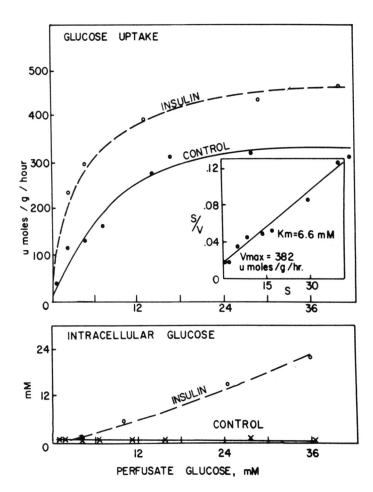

**Figure 1** Effect of glucose concentration in perfusate and insulin on glucose uptake and intracellular glucose levels in the perfused rat heart. Results are expressed per gram of dry heart. Inset in upper panel is a Lineweaver Burk plot of the glucose uptake of control hearts. S, sugar concentration (mM); V, rate of uptake ($\mu$moles/g per hr); x, intracellular glucose not detected. From Morgan et al.[45]

sion but reaches a limiting (saturation) value as concentration is increased.

4. The rate of permeation is highly stereospecific: optical enantiomorphs and isomers will diffuse at different rates.

5. The rate of penetration is greater than would be expected from the number of hydrogen-bonding groups present on the permeant,

while the temperature coefficient is less than that predicted from the number of hydrogen-bonding groups present. However, the temperature coefficients are also on the order of magnitude of those characteristic of chemical reactions.

6. The rate of permeation may be considerably reduced in the presence of structurally-similar solutes, which compete with the permeant. The saturation kinetics observed in the absence of a second solute may be explained by considering competition between identical molecules.

7. Substances that are inhibitors of enzyme systems may retard solute permeation.

### B. Kinetics of facilitated transport

For systems obeying the above criteria the unidirectional flux, $J$, of permeant is given by

$$J = \frac{SV_{max}}{K_m + S},$$
(equation 1)

where $S$ is the concentration of permeant at the face of the membrane from which flow is occurring and $V_{max}$, $K_m$ are constants differing with the cell and solute considered. The validity of equation 1 has been confirmed in heart muscle,[31-33] as well as in a number of mammalian tissues. The resemblance of this equation to the Michaelis-Menton expression, rather than Fick's law, will be noted. $V_{max}$ is then the maximum flow of the permeant, and $K_m$ is the solute (permeant) concentration at which the flux is $V_{max}/2$. Net flux, the difference between an inward flux $J_{in}$ and an outward flux $J_{out}$ is given by

$$J_{net} = J_{in} - J_{out} = \frac{S_o V_{max}}{K_m + S_o} - \frac{S_i V_{max}}{K_m + S_i}, \text{ or}$$
(equation 2)

$$J_{net} = \frac{(S_o - S_i)K_m V_{max}}{(K_m + S_o)(K_m + S_i)},$$
(equation 3)

where $S_o$ and $S_i$ are the concentrations of permeants at the outer and inner faces of the membrane respectively, assuming that $V_{max}$ and $K_m$ are the same for both $J_{in}$ and $J_{out}$.[34] When $S_o$ and $S_i$ are small compared to $K_m$, equation 3 reduces to a form analogous to the Fick equation:

$$J_{net} = \frac{(S_o - S_i)V_{max}}{K_m}.$$
(equation 4)

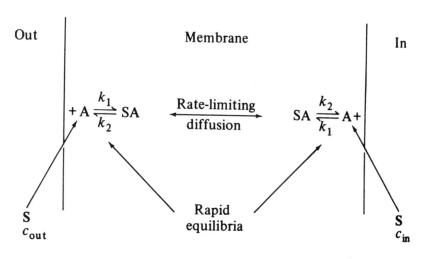

**Figure 2** A diagram illustrating the hypothetical carrier mechanism for facilitated diffusion. The solute combines with a carrier at the membrane interface. The reaction leading to the formation of a complex is judged to be rapid compared with the rate of diffusion of the complex across the membrane. Reproduced with permission from Dowben: *General Physiology*, Harper and Row, 1969.

Integration of the expressions of instantaneous rate, equations 1 and 2, with respect to time gives

$$\frac{dS_i}{dt} = \left( \frac{S_o}{S_o + K_m} - \frac{S_i}{S_i + K_m} \right). \qquad \text{(equation 5)}$$

## C. The "carrier hypothesis": further remarks

A molecular model of facilitated diffusion has gained wide acceptance, the so-called "carrier hypothesis."[34] The permeant is thought to combine with a hypothetical element, the "carrier," [*] which facilitates the translocation of permeant and "carrier" (Fig 2). The carrier is defined by its properties as follows: it may combine with the permeant to form a transient complex; it may or may not cross the membrane itself; and the substrate permeates at a negligible rate when uncombined.[35, 36] Whether the "carrier-solute moiety" physically moves through the membrane or not remains unsettled. The evidence that

---

[*] The word carrier is used in this discussion to refer to any mechanism with certain kinetic properties: primarily that the number of transport sites is restricted and that fluxes of the carried species in the two directions interact.

the carrier-substrate complex is mobile in certain cases has recently been reviewed.[387, 388] Some features of the observed kinetics may be simulated by alternate models, for example, stereospecific channels, which will be discussed.

The kinetic analysis of facilitated transport has revealed the following properties: [37]

(a) "carriers" are present in limited numbers within the membrane,
(b) the strength of the bond(s) between permeant and "carrier" is a function of the properties of both substances, and
(c) the "carrier-permeant complex" can translocate through the membrane and may be physically moveable for permeation to occur.

Another phenomenon that is a consequence of the saturation equations 1 and 2 is termed counterflow, during which a permeant may be transported against its concentration gradient using the free energy of a coupled transport of related substance in the opposite direction (Fig. 3). For this to occur the two substrates must share a common "carrier system," a concentration gradient of one substance must be maintained and be high in relation to its $K_m$, and the influx and efflux pathways must not interfere with each other.[31, 34, 36] Although, as mentioned, the mobile carrier model has been preferred,[36] the phenomenon of countertransport may be observed within a system comprised of unidirectional pores reserved for either entry or exit of the substrate or complex.[38] Further discussion of the physical chemistry of reversible coupling between transport and chemical reactions appears elsewhere.[37, 39, 40]

## 1. Protein folding, a digression

In order to discuss these carrier models, it is first necessary to digress and introduce some newer concepts of protein structure. Recently, models of membrane architecture and topography have been proposed, strongly supporting the existence of channels rather than carriers.[37a, 37b] Protein molecules comprising a membrane have ionic and polar amino acid residues, in addition to other moieties which are nonpolar. As a result, two important noncovalent interactions may occur: *hydrophobic* and *hydrophilic*. The thermodynamic constraints imposed on these interactions are no different from those which apply to any macromolecular system in aqueous solution. A *hydrophobic* interaction is one which results in sequestration of nonpolar (hydro-

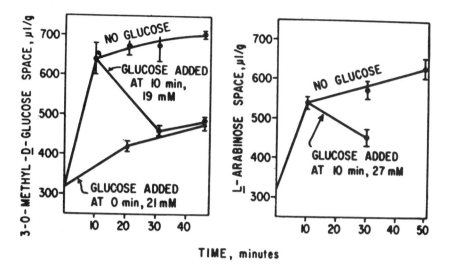

TIME, minutes

**Figure 3** Countertransport of 3-*O*-methyl-D-glucose and L-arabinose in the isolated perfused rat heart on addition of D-glucose to the perfusate. Hearts were perfused for the times indicated with oxygenated buffer containing 3-*O*-methyl-[14C]-D-glucose (0.75 mM) or L-arabinose (13 mM) (open circles). In two groups of hearts perfused with 3-*O*-methylglucose, perfusion was switched after 10 min to buffer containing an additional 21 mM D-glucose, and perfusion was continued for either 20 or 35 min, (closed circles). Additional groups were perfused with 0.75 mM 3-*O*-methylglucose and 21 mM glucose from zero time (closed triangles). One group of hearts perfused with L-arabinose for 10 min was perfused for an additional 20 min with buffer containing L-arabinose (13 mM) and D-glucose (27 mM) (closed circles). Distribution of 3-*O*-methylglucose and L-arabinose is expressed as the sugar "space." Space is the volume of tissue water required to dissolve the sugar found in the heart at the concentration of sugar in the perfusate. At least six hearts were perfused for each point. The vertical line through each point indicates 2 SEM. From Morgan et al [31] with permission.

phobic) groups away from water, the solvent. The nonpolar residues tend to cluster together to minimize exposure to the aqueous environment.

Considering the folding of a protein represented in Figure 4, panel a, it is suggested that the sum of all interaction energies between moieties such as A and B, C and D, should reflect the decreased energy of the product (folded protein) as compared with the reactant (unfolded protein). In forms of free energy, for the interaction A-B we may write (see appendix):

$$\Delta G_{A\text{-}B} = G_{A\text{-}B} - (G_A + G_B)$$

However, in panel b of Figure 4, the truer situation is shown in which groups A-D are interacting with the solvent in the unfolded form. The actual change in free energy must consider the difference in free energies between the interactions of the groups with each other (in the folded state) and of the groups with water (unfolded state). Formally, this statement becomes

$$\Delta G_{A-B} = (G_{A-B} + G_{H_2O-H_2O}) - (G_{A-H_2O} + G_{B-H_2O}).$$

Assume that groups A and B are nonpolar for the purpose of discussing hydrophobic interactions. In the unfolded form A and B exhibit van der Waals interactions with water molecules. If the distances between moieties are comparable in the unfolded and folded

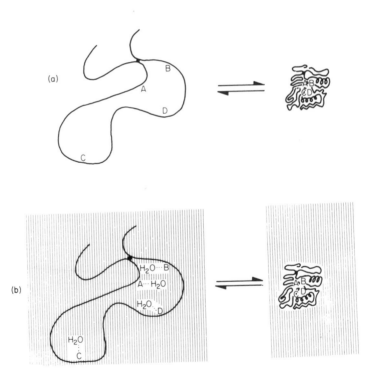

**Figure 4** Schematic distinction between the processes of folding a polypeptide chain in (a) a vacuum and (b) in the solvent water. A, B, C, and D represent amino acid residues on the polypeptide chain (see text). Reproduced with permission.[37b]

forms, these van der Waals interactions with water will be of similar strength as those between A and B. Thus the clustering of nonpolar groups cannot be explained by their van der Waals attractions for one another. For a nonpolar moiety A in a polar and nonpolar solvent

$$A_{(\text{nonpolar solvent})} \rightleftharpoons A_{(\text{polar solvent})}$$

there is a $\Delta G > 0$ associated with the transfer of this nonpolar moiety to a polar solvent, *i.e.*, work must be expended to effect this change. Remembering that

$$\Delta G = \Delta H - T\Delta S \qquad \text{(see appendix)}$$

and with the knowledge that $\Delta H < 0$ for the transfer under consideration—the reaction is exothermic—it follows that $\Delta S < 0$. This decrease in entropy of solvation renders such a process thermodynamically unfavorable. Such an entropy decrease may be due to an ordering of polar solvent molecules around the nonpolar moiety. In the model depicted in Figure 4, panel b, the nonpolar groups are sequestered from water, and the values of $\Delta G$, $\Delta H$, and $\Delta S$ are opposite in sign to the situation just discussed. During folding, $\Delta G < 0$ for each buried nonpolar group, contributed by a $\Delta S > 0$, as ordered water molecules are "released" from surrounding each of the nonpolar groups in the unfolded form. X-ray crystallographic studies of proteins have confirmed this thermodynamic prediction regarding clustering of nonpolar groups.

X-ray crystallography also reveals the exclusion of ionic residues from the interior areas of folded proteins—the fixed polar groups are all on the exterior portions of the molecule in contact with water. Translocation or "burying" a charged group in the nonpolar interior of a polypeptide chain with a low dielectric constant would require a large expenditure of energy. Charge neutralization by ion pairing and/or proton binding or dissociation to remove charges are two mechanisms available. The electrostatic free energy of an ion pair is inversely proportional to the dielectric constant of the medium, because an ion pair may interact more strongly with molecules of polar solvents. For an ion pair, $P^{\pm}$ undergoing the transfer:

$$P^{\pm}_{(\text{polar solvent})} \rightleftharpoons P^{\pm}_{(\text{nonpolar solvent})}$$

$$\Delta G \approx RT \ln \left( \frac{\text{mole fraction of P in saturated solution in polar solvent}}{\text{mole fraction of P in saturated solution in nonpolar solvent}} \right)$$

$\Delta G \gg 0$ for all nonaqueous solvents, *i.e.*, the ion pair is at a lower free energy state in the polar solvent.

A charged moiety may also be discharged and "buried" as a polar rather than ionic group. The free energy required for this process is also large. To discharge the group would require:

$$\Delta G = 2.303 RT |(pH - pK)|$$

where pK is the negative logarithm of the acid dissociation constant of the group involved.

## 2. *Relevance to membrane structure*

Remembering that a membrane consists predominantly of proteins, lipids, and oligosaccharides, these considerations place the following overall thermodynamic constraints upon a membrane, assuming that at the level of a *domain* ° in a membrane the steady-state structure attained is one of lowest free energy:

(a) all ionic, zwitter ionic, and polar groups (*e.g.*, sugars) should be in contact with the water phase in order to maximize hydrophilic interaction;

(b) all nonpolar groups—lipids and nonpolar areas of proteins, should be sequestered within the interior of the membrane in order to maximize hydrophobic interactions;

(c) potential hydrogen bond donor and acceptor groups of the protein not in contact with water should form hydrogen bonds with each other maximally.

A phospholipid bilayer satisfies the first two of these constraints simply: the nonpolar fatty acid chains of the phospholipids are sequestered together away from water, maximizing hydrophobic interactions (Fig. 5 left). Polar groups are in maximal contact with the water phase at both interphases.

The classic Davson-Danielli model of a membrane consisted of a lipid bilayer covered on both sides with unfolded protein; hydrophobic amino acid residues interacted with similar lipid chains, and hydrophilic residues formed pores for transport. This model, however, did not conform to the thermodynamic constraints mentioned above, since an unfolded protein would have many nonpolar residues exposed to water, and the protein layer would cover the hydrophilic heads of the

---

° A domain is a limited region of interest containing a small number of protein molecules and associated lipids within the solvent and water.

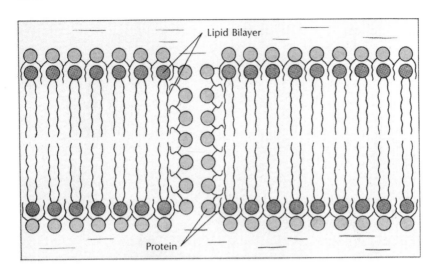

**Figure 5** A phospholipid bilayer: schematic cross-sectional view. The circles represent the ionic and polar head groups of the phospholipid molecules, which make contact with water; the lines represent two fatty acid chains.

lipid molecules. In addition, there is direct evidence from optical measurements that membrane proteins are globular rather than unfolded, and are not exclusively exterior, but are "floating" in the membrane.

According to Singer and co-workers,[37a, 37b, 37c] the thermodynamic and experimental data are satisfied by a mosaic membrane model in which globular integral proteins alternate with areas of phospholipid bilayer (Figs. 5, right panel, 6, and 7). The globular proteins are postulated to be *amphipathic* (as are the phospholipids)—asymmetric, with one polar end and one nonpolar end. The hydrophobic end would be located in the interior of the lipid bilayer, in touch with the hydrophobic lipid tails, and the hydrophilic end would be nearly contiguous with the hydrophilic lipid heads exposed to the aqueous environment. If such proteins were large, they would extend across the entire membrane,

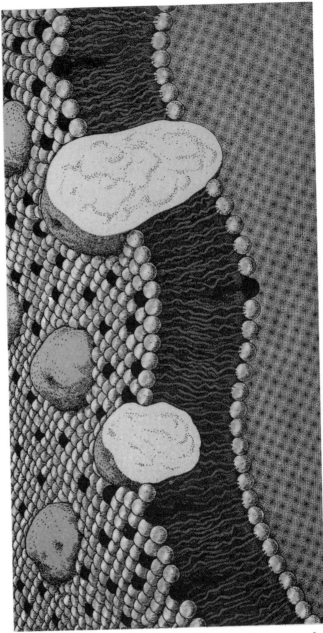

**Figure 6**  Current (Singer) membrane model sees proteins as predominantly globular and amphipathic, with their hydrophilic ends protruding from the membrane and their hydrophobic ends embedded in the bilayer of lipids (gray) and cholesterol (black). The proteins make up the membrane's "active sites"; some are simply embedded on one or the other side, others pass entirely through the bilayer. Some of the latter presumably contain transport pores. Reproduced with permission.[37a]

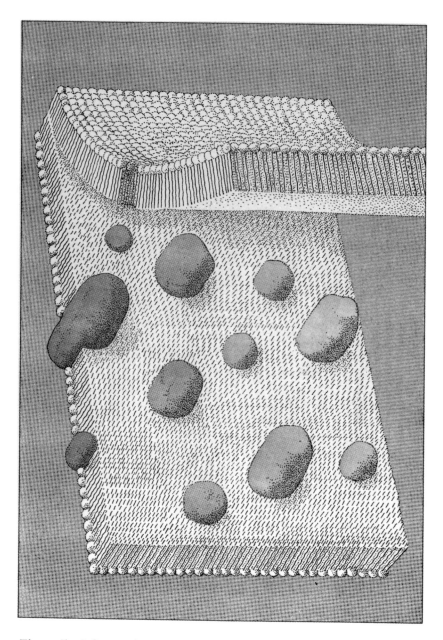

**Figure 7** Splitting of membrane shows interior of model depicted in Figure 6. Reproduced with permission.[37a]

and could have two protruding hydrophilic ends with a hydrophilic center. The amphipathic structure assumed by a globular protein, and the extent to which it is buried in the membrane, are under thermodynamic control in such a way to minimize the free energy of the system.

The available evidence also supports the contention that the matrix of the mosaic membrane is lipid and the proteins are in a fluid state in the intact membrane. As a result, this model has been likened to icebergs (proteins) floating in a lipid sea. While translational (lateral) motion would be possible, relocations of the depth of the protein in the lipid bilayer would not be possible because of the thermodynamic principles discussed. Rotational diffusion is restricted to these same axes perpendicular to the plane of the membrane. These same constraints, therefore, ensure the asymmetry of the membrane between inside and outside surfaces.

### 3. Application to the "carrier hypothesis"

The fluid mosaic model of a membrane as an oriented, two-dimensional, discontinuous, viscous solution of amphipathic proteins and lipids in instantaneous themodynamic equilibrium leads to some predictions about ion and substrate transport. The model of carrier transport which postulates the existence of free carrier proteins capable of binding to substrate and moving through the membrane is clearly in violation of the thermodynamic constraints mentioned. A transport protein would have to submerge its hydrophilic exterior while passing through the hydrophobic interior of the membrane, a process which would require a large expenditure of energy.

Of interest with relation to this discussion of channels is the effect of cations upon insulin-induced enhancement of glucose transport. Stimulation of glucose uptake by insulin is not a function of the presence of monovalent (oxidation state "+1") cations in the incubation medium.[350, 351] However, EDTA pretreatment of muscle, depleting $Ca^{++}$ and $Mg^{++}$ renders muscle glucose uptake insensitive to insulin, which may be reversed by the subsequent addition of $Mg^{++}$ or $Ca^{++}$ to the medium. It is now postulated that $Mg^{++}$ is necessary for the enhanced interaction between glucose and transport system in the presence of insulin.

Grouping of proteins which span the entire width of the membrane, with two hydrophilic ends and a hydrophobic center would be consistent with the mosaic fluid model of membranes and also exhibit carrier kinetics. Such a grouping is shown in Figure 8, with a central water-filled pore. Transport proteins would then be relatively fixed

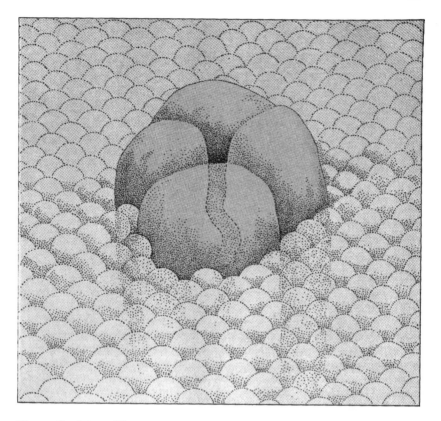

**Figure 8** Water-filled channels for transport of specific ions and hydrophilic molecules through membrane may be formed by groupings of four (or more) protein subunits, as schematized above. Reproduced with permission.[37a]

embedded subunits with a central channel lined with polar groups. A polar moiety, such as an ion or sugar, could pass through such a channel by diffusion. Or, a conformational change in the channel could occur once the substrate associated with the interior surface, realigning the channel in such a way to allow egress of the substrate on the other side of the membrane (Fig 9). This model of transport is presently the one most widely accepted, although a defense of the mobile "carrier-substrate complex" has recently appeared.[387]

## D. Insulin and glucose transport

The affinity of a particular sugar for the "carrier" affects its transport in insulin sensitive tissues.[31, 41-43] Glucose uptake follows Michaelis-

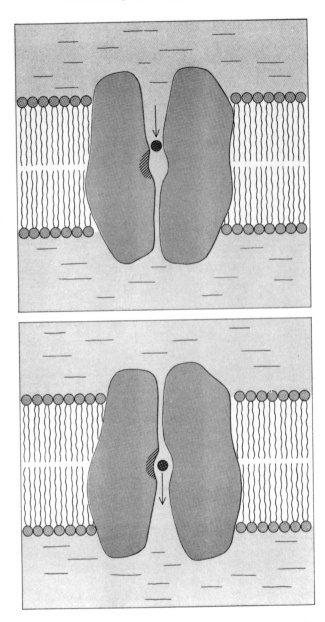

**Figure 9** Active or facilitated transport of molecule through membrane protein channel is visualized two-dimensionally. Molecule impinges (top) on active site (shaded) of protein, following which some energy-yielding enzyme reaction triggers shift in subunit configuration (bottom) that "squeezes" the molecule through the membrane. Reproduced with permission.[37a]

Menton kinetics, where $V_{max} = 382$ $\mu$mole/g/hr and $K_m = 6.6$ mM, indicating that transport rate differences may occur within physiological ranges of glucose concentrations. While insulin markedly accelerates the transport of D-glucose, it has no effect on L-glucose transport,[31] supporting the contention that insulin acts on facilitated channel transport. Insulin increases the maximal rate of glucose transport in the perfused heart and decreases the affinity slightly. Phlorizin and its aglycone, phloretin, and stilbesterol act as reversible competitive inhibitors of the glucose transport system [35] while sulfhydryl group binding causes *p*-chloromercuribenzoate, gold and mercury to act as nonpenetrating noncompetitive inhibitors. The rapidity of insulin effects argues that no new synthesis of "carrier" or molecule is involved.

Sugars are composed of pyranose rings, similar to that of cyclohexane, containing five carbon atoms and one oxygen atom, and may exist in two conformations: chair and boat. Under prevailing conditions, chair conformations predominate, and the affinity of the transport carrier for the sugar parallels the relative frequency of the C-1 conformation—that with the greatest number of hydroxyl groups in the equatorial position (Fig 10).

It is important to note that since sugar transport is passive, the carrier-facilitated mechanism leads only to equilibration of intracellular and extracellular glucose concentrations. Selective accumulation within the cell against a concentration gradient does not occur, with or without insulin present. However, if glucose immediately disappears and participates in one of several intracellular metabolic pathways, "equilibration" would constantly effect net glucose influx.

Insulin bound to LMW dextran (40,000 amu molecular weight) stimulates glycogen formation in proportion to the increase in glucose transport as observed with free insulin.[352] Apparently, insulin need not enter the cell to effect the changes in glucose transport and glycogen synthesis. However, under certain experimental conditions, insulin may enhance glycogen formation in the absence of accelerated glucose transport.[353] Other studies in the perfused rat heart indicate that the pattern in change of glucose metabolism brought about by the addition of insulin and by the increase in concentration of glucose in the perfusate are quite different.[354] This same conclusion is reached when muscle is subjected to an acute increase in work load.[355, 356]

When intracellular glucose concentration is below that required to saturate phosphorylation, stimulation of glucose transport by insulin may accelerate glycolysis. In heart muscle as well as in other insulin sensitive tissues, glucose transport is a rate-limiting step for glucose

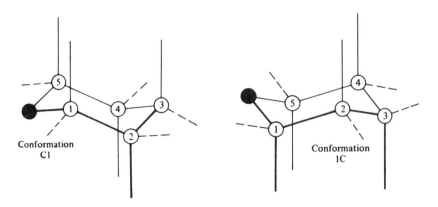

**Figure 10**   A diagram of the two chair conformations of the pyranose ring of simple sugars. The filled circle represents the oxygen atom while the numbered circles represent the corresponding carbon atoms. The side of the ring facing the observer is heavier, equatorial bonds are shown by broken lines, and axial bonds are depicted by vertical solid lines. From Le Fevre, P. G. and Marshall, J. K.: *Am J Physiol* **194**:335, 1958.

uptake under certain circumstances.[44-46] Thus, the rate of glucose uptake is not a linear function of glucose concentration in the perfusate but saturates at higher concentrations. Since no free glucose exists in myocytes, these kinetics may be attributed to the transport process. In the perfused rat heart, insulin may double or triple glucose uptake at low glucose concentrations. At higher glucose concentrations, the insulin effect is diminished as intracellular glucose concentration rises.[45] These data are consistent with the view that insulin stimulates glucose transport, but then phosphorylation becomes rate-limiting as glucose is made available for oxidation. This view is further supported by much related experimental evidence. For instance, entry of a variety of nonmetabolized sugars into the cell is also accelerated,[47, 48] efflux of sugar from the heart is also increased,[49] $K_m$ and $V_{max}$ are changed by insulin,[50, 51] and similar actions are well-documented in a variety of other tissues. Tissues from diabetic animals are less sensitive to insulin, whereas tissues from adrenalectomized and hypophysectomized animals are more sensitive to insulin's actions, which may be reversed in the latter instances by corticosteroids and growth hormone respectively.[52-54] Of especial importance is the fact that myocardial insulin sensitivity is also increased during a shift to anaerobic metabolism or by experimental conditions leading to an increased peak left ventricular pressure.[55] However, glucose transport is also accelerated by these conditions in the absence of insulin.[45, 56-59]

Normally, inhibition of glucose transport by free fatty acids plays a part in the preferential use of free fatty acids by the myocardium.[60] However during hypoxia and ischemia the accompanying metabolic changes, insulin, and mechanical activity may act in concert to increase needed glucose transport.

In summary, insulin accelerates glucose transport by a saturable and chemically specific process. In addition, glucose transport is also enhanced by anoxia, inhibition of the $Na^+$, $K^+$-pump by ouabain, hyperosmolarity and by enhanced muscle work, a function of both beat frequency and contractility. Apart from the action of epinephrine on heart rate and contractility, part of the enhanced glucose transport observed after incubation with this agent is also "metabolic." Glucose transport is depressed in the isolated muscle preparations by the absence of insulin, by hypoosmolarity, and by maneuvers increasing $Na^+$ and $K^+$ gradients such as high-$K^+$ medium, diphenylhydantoin, and very low concentrations of ouabain.

## III. INSULIN AND AMINO ACID ANABOLISM

### A. Myocardial protein synthesis

The prompt and substantial capacity of heart muscle to synthesize cell constituents is now appreciated.[79-81] This is reflected in a considerable physiologic turnover of components: the half-life of the contractile proteins is approximately 8 to 11 days,[80, 82, 83, 83a] and that of mitochondrial proteins is 5 to 6 days.[84] This rapid turnover allows structural flexibility to meet the mechanical demands imposed upon the heart, during which myocardial mass may reversibly increase as much as 30 to 50 percent in 36 to 48 hours (after experimental constriction of the ascending aorta).[85-87] However, unlike the skeletal muscle cell, the adult heart myocyte is unable to regenerate but is normally able to survive as long as the organism.

Stimuli leading to myocardial protein synthesis—via augmented amino acid transport, and increased DNA and RNA synthesis—include pressure and volume overload, hormonal influence (insulin, growth hormone, catecholamines, thyroid hormones) and muscle infarction, among others. Protein synthesis in the heart is thought to be roughly similar to protein synthesis in other tissues (Figs. 11A and 11B).[262] Two initial stimuli are currently under consideration as the initiating event for myocardial RNA and protein synthesis. One hypothesis suggests that transient ATP depletion triggers the biochemical events leading to protein synthesis. A variation on this theme is the hypothesis of Badeer [263] who postulates that a sustained increase in stroke energy

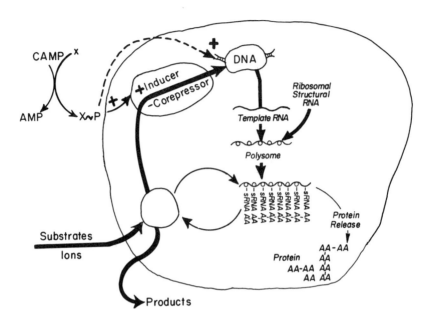

**Figure 11A** Protein synthesis within a cell. Messenger or template RNA carries genetic information from DNA in the nucleus to protein-synthesizing cytoplasmic sites. Template RNA has a base sequence which is complementary to DNA, from which it is synthesized during transcription. The sequence of bases provides the coded information for polypeptide synthesis. Ribosomes attach to messenger RNA to form a polyribosome from which protein synthesis occurs from the single active ribosomal site sequentially from free amino acid to the free carboxyl end as messenger RNA moves over the ribosome. For each amino acid there is a specific soluble RNA which binds the amino acid using energy in the presence of a specific enzyme, the amino acyl synthetases. Activated amino acids are then transferred to the appropriate spot on the polypeptide chain which is subsequently released enzymatically. In some mammalian cells in culture, agents which depress cyclic AMP levels stimulate growth, and an increase in cyclic AMP levels suppresses growth. However, the precise role of cyclic AMP, high energy substrates and inducers, repressors is not yet fully understood.

expenditure per unit mass of myocardium is the initiating event, as outlined in Figure 12. In order to account for the increase in protein synthesis effected by hormones, Cohen [264] has further suggested that a very early event initiating protein synthesis is the acceleration of state 4 (basal) mitochondrial respiration (Fig. 13) which is in agreement with Badeer's hypothesis.

A second possible trigger for myocardial protein synthesis is an

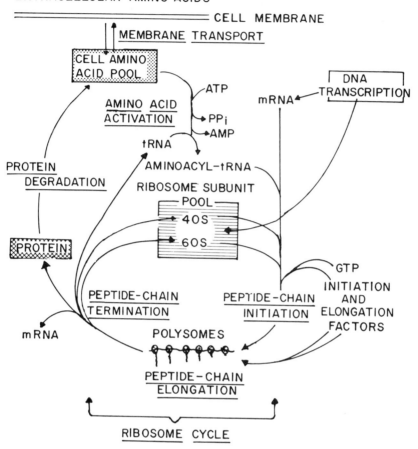

EXTRACELLULAR AMINO ACIDS

CELL MEMBRANE

MEMBRANE TRANSPORT

CELL AMINO ACID POOL

AMINO ACID ACTIVATION

ATP

PPᵢ

AMP

mRNA

DNA TRANSCRIPTION

tRNA

PROTEIN DEGRADATION

AMINOACYL–tRNA

RIBOSOME SUBUNIT POOL

40S

60S

PROTEIN

mRNA

PEPTIDE–CHAIN TERMINATION

PEPTIDE–CHAIN INITIATION

GTP

INITIATION AND ELONGATION FACTORS

POLYSOMES

PEPTIDE–CHAIN ELONGATION

RIBOSOME CYCLE

**Figure 11B**  Pathway of protein turnover in myocardium. Amino acids are supplied to the intracellular pool by either membrane transport or protein degradation. Intracellular amino acids are activated to form aminoacyl derivatives by combination with transfer RNA (tRNA). Polymerization of activated amino acids into protein is catalyzed by a series of ribosome-catalyzed reactions that make up the ribosome cycle. These reactions include initiation of peptide chains on the ribosomes and elongation and termination of chains. Peptide-chain initiation involves binding of messenger RNA (mRNA) and the initiator tRNA, probably a methionyl-tRNA, to the small ribosomal subunit (40S) and is dependent upon initiation factors. Binding of the large subunit (60S) follows and requires guanosine triphosphate (GTP). Chain elongation involves successive addition of activated amino acids determined by the code contained within mRNA and is dependent upon transfer factors. When the protein is complete, the peptide chain and ribosomal subunits are released into the cytoplasm. Protein degradation involves reactions catalyzed by proteases and releases free amino acids into the intracellular pool. Reproduced by permission of the American Heart Association, Inc.[383]

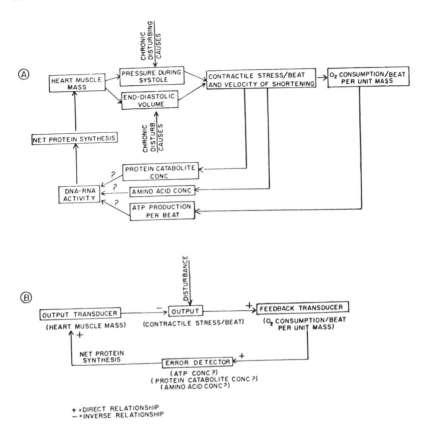

**Figure 12A** Slow-acting feedback loop regulating the stroke energy expenditure of the myocardium by altering the mass of cardiac muscle in pathologic conditions that induce a sustained disturbance of energy expenditure. **12B** Simplified scheme of the above using the terminology of systems engineers. Reproduced with permission.[263]

increased muscle fiber length itself, or a "stretch." Translation of this event into protein synthesis could be accomplished through primary alterations in membranes and resultant changes in substrate transport. Indeed, passive stretch does augment the uptake of α-amino-isobutyric acid into papillary muscle.[265] In 1969, Meerson [266] suggested that increased intramyocardial (wall) tension may stimulate protein synthesis through the accumulation of small structured breakdown products of macromolecules. More recently, Meerson [267] proposed that an increased ratio of $\dfrac{(ADP)\,(P_i)}{ATP}$ is the responsible initiating event for polypeptide synthesis (Fig. 14).

SEQUENCE OF EVENTS IN THE
DEVELOPMENT OF CARDIAC HYPERTROPHY

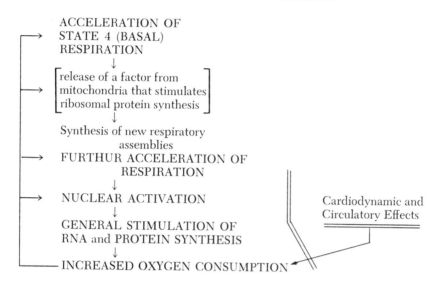

**Figure 13** Hypothetical scheme of events in the pathogenesis of cardiac hypertrophy according to Cohen.[264] Reproduced with permission of American Heart Association, Inc.

## B. Amino acid transport during myocardial protein synthesis

In contrast with glucose, amino acids are transported against an electrochemical gradient and the process requires the expenditure of energy.[61] No less than three facilitated diffusion systems exist for amino acid transport: one for L-methionine and related amino acids, one for L-glycine and relatives, and one for L-valine and congeners, each with overlapping specificity.[62-65] The transport of neutral amino acids is in some way linked to the cotransport of $Na^+$ on a single carrier.[65-67] When $Na^+$ is bound to the "carrier," affinity for the amino acid increases, and amino acid flux is accelerated in a parallel direction. Energy from intermediary metabolism is necessary to fuel the $Na^+$, $K^+$-ATPase pump and thus assure a low intracellular $Na^+$ concentration. Coupling of $Na^+$ with amino acid transport provides the necessary energy to drive amino acids into the cell against their concentration gradients. The maintenance of a high extracellular-intracellular $Na^+$ gradient also insures that the affinity of the "carrier" for amino acid is greater outside the cell, such that the influx of the $Na^+$-carrier-amino acid complex is greater than its efflux.

The nature of the chemical bond between $Na^+$ and "carrier" is not

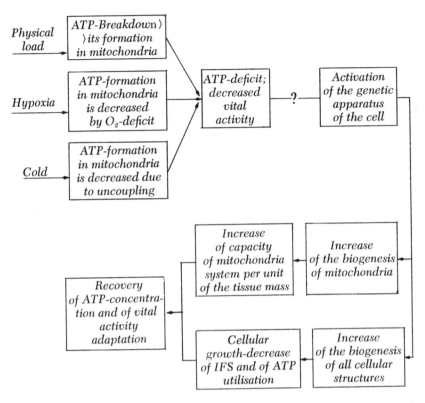

**Figure 14** Scheme of the cell link of adapation to the prolonged action of intensive load, hypoxia, and cold. Reproduced with permission.[266] Copyright 1974, American Heart Association, Inc.

understood. Also unknown is the mechanism of energy supply to systems of amino acid transport in which Na⁺ is uninvolved. In one instance, coupling of transport between two amino acids (methionine Na⁺-linked, and leucine unlinked) has been proposed[68] (Fig. 15). Recently it has been suggested that the side chains of various neutral amino acids may complete a reactive binding site for Na⁺. For a number of polypeptide chains, a sequence of transport sites for alkali-metal cations might thus be generated in a region of low dielectric properties.[67, 69, 70]

Investigation of the role of amino acid transport in the regulation of polypeptide synthesis has been facilitated by the use of two amino acid derivatives: α-aminoisobutyric acid and L-amino-cyclopentane-2-carboxylic acid, or cycloleucine. These substances share the same transport systems with naturally-occurring amino acids but are not utilized

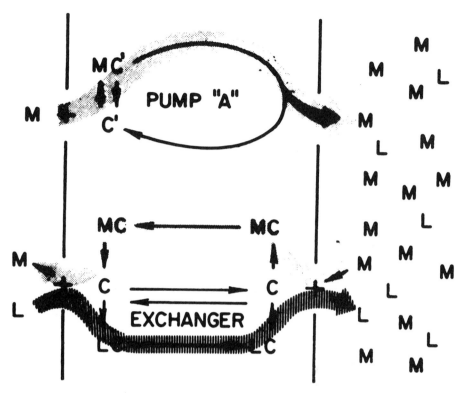

**Figure 15** Visualization of way an amino acid entering cell by uphill transport may drive uphill transport of an amino acid entering by a passive exchange diffusion. M, molecules of methionine, entering by the "uphill" system A; and L, molecules of leucine, concentrated into the cell (to the right) by exchange for accumulated methionine molecules. From Christensen.[68]

within the cell. Under these circumstances, uptake is largely a function of membrane transport.

Although the connection between enhanced amino acid transport and tissue growth was suggested by the studies of Christensen,[268] it is now appreciated that the membrane protein apparatus involved with amino acid transport is affected by a number of inducers, repressors, and other experimental conditions unrelated to amino acid incorporation into polypeptides. In the best studied models of increased myocardial protein synthesis—activation of synthetic processes in response to pressure overload leading to hypertrophy—augmented heart work is associated with enhanced α-aminoisobutyric acid [269-271] and cycloleucine [272] uptake.

However, some investigators have not found any such increase in lysine transport in hearts working against elevated afterloads.[273] In addition, there is evidence that the intracellular concentration of some amino acids remains nearly unchanged at a time when active protein synthesis is taking place.[75, 77] Moreover, increased $\alpha$-aminoisobutyric acid,[276] lysine [277] and proline [278] transport in response to work-induced protein synthesis occurs at a much later time after the cardiac work load is increased.

The relationship between amino acid transport and intracellular synthetic events are obscured by issues which remain unproved. Compartmentalization of amino acids within the cell may result in a sequestered intracellular pool from which polypeptide synthesis proceeds.[279, 280] Measurement of levels of one or two amino acids might not reflect changes in the transport of other amino acids. Finally, the transport of some amino acids may be more important, or even rate-limiting, with respect to other amino acids. From these data presently available, no definitive statement regarding the role of amino acid transport in protein synthesis may be made. However, in some experimental preparations an increase in amino acid transport may be related to polypeptide synthesis in a manner which is yet to be clarified. Some unanswered questions regarding protein synthesis in the heart have recently been outlined by Rabinowitz: [281]

1. Initiating stimulus to protein synthesis
2. Mediators and mechanisms of regulation
3. Role of hormones and cyclic adenylate
4. Independent control of different myocardial constituents and significance
5. Mechanisms and control of biological turnover
6. Mechanisms and controls of contractility in relation to synthetic processes
7. Constraints responsible for hypertrophy rather than hyperplasia

## C. Effect of insulin on amino acid transport and protein synthesis

Insulin increases the incorporation of radioactive amino acids into the rat diaphragm [71] and perfused rat heart independent of its action on glucose transport.[338] The synthesis of all proteins in muscle is increased by insulin, but it is now apparent that the transport of only some amino acids can be enhanced by insulin *in vitro*.[72, 73] Insulin effects incorporation of many amino acids into protein, and intracellular amino acid concentrations are enhanced by insulin in the presence of puromycin which blocks protein synthesis.[74] *In vivo*, insulin stimulates the incorporation of all amino acids—including those formed intracellularly—into protein.[310] Therefore, the important action of insulin on protein synthesis may not be at the transport level, and need not be rate-limiting either. The possibility also exists that amino acids entering the cell are sequestered in a special compartment rather than be introduced to the free intracellular amino acid pool,[341] from which amino acids for protein synthesis are preferentially removed.

Some insight into the effects of insulin upon protein synthesis comes from studies in insulin-deficient animals. A significant decrease in hepatic ribosomal protein synthesis accompanies acute diabetes mellitus, which appears to occur at the level of membrane-bound polyribosomes. Bound ribosomes from acutely diabetic rats synthesize less protein, probably because of disruption and disaggregation of rough endoplasmic reticulum with production of smaller ribosomal messenger RNA aggregates, which incorporate less amino acids into protein.[274] Ribosomes from hearts of diabetic animals also do not synthesize protein as well as do hearts from normal animals.[338, 342] Insulin administration to the diabetic animal enhances polysome assembly and protein synthesis without increasing RNA synthesis,[343] pointing to an effect of insulin on translation of mRNA. Indirect evidence supports the contention that the reduction in peptidyl-tRNA bound to ribosomes occurring during insulin-deprivation is explained by decreased initiation of endogenous protein synthesis.[344-346] However, there is some question about this mechanism in myocardium as compared with skeletal muscle.[348] In streptozotocin-induced diabetes in particular, polysome profiles and amino acid incorporation by ribosomal preparations are unhampered, in disagreement with the data presented above.[349]

Wool and co-workers [346] reported that the translation of polyuridylic acid and a viral mRNA by ribosomes from diabetic animals were poor in relation to the same processes in ribosomes from normal animals. This adds still more data buttressing the idea that insulin is necessary for maximum efficiency during initiation of peptide chain synthesis.

The major substrate used by the well-oxygenated postabsorptive myocardium is free fatty acid, as previously discussed. When hearts are removed from diabetic rats, protein synthesis declines after 1 hr., perhaps due to a lower RNA content.[285] These data also suggest that protein synthesis in hearts of diabetic animals may be in part protected from the effects of insulin deficiency *in vivo* by higher levels of plasma free fatty acids. In alloxan-diabetic dogs it has recently been shown that ketone bodies, such as beta-hydroxybutyrate, may replace free fatty acids as the major myocardial fuel.[275] While this experimental situation is quite different from the clinical one in which the suppression of insulin secretion results from depressed cardiac output, it will certainly be of further interest to determine if myocardial protein synthesis is altered by a change in predominant substrate.

In the perfused rat heart, the *in vitro* rate of protein synthesis is supported by *in vivo* concentrations of amino acids for thirty minutes. A decline in rate of protein synthesis is then observed, which may be tempered by exogenous supplementary amino acids in the perfusate.[75] The biochemical defect is thought to be due to a block in formation of peptide chains on ribosomes, and not to diminished intracellular amino acid levels. Polypeptide synthesis can be restored with insulin, presumably by releasing the block. Levels of subunits decrease and polysome levels rise, showing that insulin has stimulated peptide chain initiation.[339, 347] Since this action of insulin occurs equally well when both normal and five times normal levels of amino acids are present in the perfusate, it is unlikely that insulin's effect is primarily on amino acid transport; more probably the effect is at the level of the initiation of peptide chain formation in this system.[76, 77] It is currently believed that the acceleration of polypeptide synthesis that results from 5-fold increases in amino acid concentration is due to their oxidation and not to a primary effect. Therefore, a decrease in the ability of muscle ribosomes to initiate protein synthesis during insulin-lack has been postulated.[78] A lack of primary change in amino acid transport and intracellular levels of amino acids was recently reported in rapid myocardial protein turnover stimulated by mechanical stress.[261]

The block in polypeptide synthesis induced by insulin-lack is also a function of substrate availability. As noted, raising the concentration of amino acids in the solution perfusing a rat heart will increase ribosome aggregation and enhance incorporation into protein.[339] The development of the block in protein synthesis in the preparation discussed corresponds to the time required to wash insulin from the heart, and to the depletion of triglyceride stores.[282, 283] Oxidizable noncarbohydrate substances, including fatty acids, ketone bodies, pyruvate, lactate, and acetate, maintain protein synthesis during *in vitro* perfusion of isolated rat hearts,[284] although evidence has also been presented to the contrary.[291] The mechanism of reversal of the block in polypeptide synthesis by such compounds, for instance, palmitate, is uncertain. This action is not due to a change in membrane amino acid transport, since the accumulation of α-aminoisobutyric acid is inhibited, but rather appears to be mediated by changes in a metabolite of the compounds mentioned.

Upon considering that intracellular availability of high energy phosphates may play a role in the dependence of myocardial protein synthesis upon free fatty acid oxidation, it is noteworthy that creatine phosphate levels are lower in hearts provided with glucose as compared with palmitate as substrate. Palmitate-supported hearts maintain higher rates of protein synthesis than those provided only glucose.[284] Also, higher levels of creatine phosphate and lower intracellular levels of inorganic phosphate are measured in hearts provided palmitate.[254] The role of the higher energy charge of the adenylate system [284, 286] and higher levels of creatine phosphate in fatty acid-induced polypeptide synthesis is uncertain. Intracellular levels of GTP and ATP are above the $K_m$ for the aminoacyl-tRNA synthetases and enzymes catalyzing polypeptide chain synthesis in these experiments.[287-290] The understanding of the relationship between energy availability and protein synthesis must await the elucidation of effects of many other metabolites on peptide-chain initiation. In conclusion, the precise role of insulin action in the transport and metabolism of amino acids into the normal myocardium is unknown, and is even less understood in ischemic heart muscle.

## D. Effect of insulin on changes in protein metabolism induced by hypoxia and ischemia

Following experimental myocardial infarction, Gudbjarnason and co-workers [88] reported that the incorporation of amino acids in regions surrounding the area of necrosis is substantially increased and reparative processes are promptly and maximally stimulated in response to the insult. Repair begins in the injured tissue and the surrounding muscle may hypertrophy in "compensation" for the deficiency.

Takahashi and co-workers [292] also reported protein anabolism following coronary occlusion. Lochner and colleagues,[89] using the technique of Bajusz [293] to produce a homogeneous area of myocardial infarction, studied *in vitro* and *in vivo* isotopic amino acid incorporation into myocardium. These investigators found that the *in vitro* and *in vivo* incorporation of L-[4,5-³H]-leucine and *in vitro* incorporation of L[U-¹⁴C]-lysine into soluble protein and actomyosin fractions of heart muscle slices was normal up to six hours after the onset of ischemia, but remained high from twelve hours to two months after the coronary occlusion. Protein synthesis was stimulated in both the noninfarcted and infarcted areas of myocardium. When collateral circulation developed in damaged areas, repair occurred as active protein synthesis proceeded.[294]

An area of myocardial infarction consists of necrotic, blighted, and jeopardized zones of muscle, inflammatory cells, connective tissue, and myocytes undergoing hypertrophy. Protein synthesis by fibroblasts and angioblasts [295] as well as hypertrophying cells,[88, 296, 297] may account for the increase in amino acid incorporation observed.[298] In addition, it is known that an increase in DNA concentration in myocardial infarction coincides with the appearance of fibroblasts,[88, 299] and that the incorporation of [³H]-thymidine in myocardial hypertrophy is in great part associated with the nuclei of connective tissue.[300]

Extending their work, Lochner and associates [89a] also noted the delay in stimulation of RNA synthesis after experimental coronary occlusion. Protein synthesis in this model preceded the increase in RNA concentration by as much as eighteen hours, and continued for two months as compared with RNA synthesis, which returned to normal values after fourteen days.

Hypoxia as well as ischemia is said to stimulate reparative protein synthesis.[90, 91] Exposure of rats to a six hour period of 4 percent oxygen results in selective destruction of mitochondria within the muscle cell. Restoration of normal oxygenation is accompanied by a rapid resynthesis of the mitochondrial defects. Myosin and membrane proteins are less sensitive to hypoxia than are the mitochondria. The incorporation of [¹⁴C]-amino acids and [2-¹⁴C]-uridine into myocytes in culture increase as the degree of hypoxia is increased.[302] However, it is probable that the primary stimulus to myocardial protein synthesis is not hypoxia, and that oxygen availability is but one of the conditioning factors in processes mediating protein synthesis. Cohen and associates [301] showed that lack of energy supply could impair protein synthesis in beating atria. The incorporation rate of leucine into myocardium *in vitro* is directly proportional to the availability of oxygen.

In the papillary muscle preparation, Peterson and associates [303, 304] recently affirmed the inhibition of protein synthesis by hypoxia. This inhibition was reversible with 5-15 mM glucose, but could not be reversed with insulin alone. Kao and co-workers [378] perfused hearts by the Langendorff technique with buffer containing 15mM glucose and normal (plasma) levels of amino acids, and progressively reduced the $O_2$ content in the perfusate. Again, loss of polysomes and accumulation of ribosomal subunits suggested that diminished peptide-chain initiation restricted protein synthesis. Addition of insulin to "aerobic" or "anaerobic hearts" prevented this initiation block, but did not result in increased protein synthesis. Ischemia also inhibited protein synthesis which could not be overcome with insulin. These data suggest that in both hypoxic and ischemic hearts protein synthesis is inhibited by a restricted rate of peptide chain elongation. Although insulin may stimulate initiation of peptide chains, it does not increase the rate of protein synthesis in the experimental models studied.[378] More recently, Morgan and associates [383] further reviewed their data concerning release of [¹⁴C]-phenylalanine during heart perfusion. Net release of phenylalanine showed that the rate of protein degradation exceeded that of synthesis in control hearts. The addition of insulin completely prevented or reversed this imbalance, and provision of palmitate was only partially effective. Insulin was effective in stimulating peptide-chain initiation in anoxic myocardium, but could not overcome the depressed peptide-chain elongation accompanying reduced high-energy phosphate stores.

Cathepsin-D activity was estimated, since increased phenylalanine release was accompanied by larger numbers of autophagic vacuoles. "Available" activity was increased 20-33 percent of total during three hours of perfusion, which was prevented or reversed by insulin. Such restraint of protein degradation by insulin was associated with the presence of fewer autophagic vacuoles within the myocyte. This raises the important—but as yet unexplored—possibility that insulin may impede destructive or catabolic processes in the heart during metabolic stress.

In view of the physiologic importance of high protein turnover in the normal myocardium, its rapid and extensive alteration by ischemia, and the significant role of insulin in the initiation of peptide synthesis, it is not unreasonable to suspect that insulin may play a supportive part in the maintenance of myocardial synthetic processes. However, the details of such a role have not yet been precisely characterized.

Lochner and associates [89] suggested that increases in cyclic adenylate might be involved in ischemia-induced myocardial protein synthesis, perhaps by acting upon histone repressors of DNA, thereby increasing synthesis of messenger and ribosomal RNA. Cyclic AMP is but one of the intermediary compounds which may regulate protein synthesis and be influenced by insulin. However, confirmatory evidence here is lacking and certainly another possible mechanism for increased protein synthesis after ischemia is augmented hexose monophosphate shunt activity since more pentose would be available for nucleic acid and protein synthesis.[305] The possible importance of hormonal control of this pathway remains to be elucidated as well.

## IV. INSULIN, RESTING MEMBRANE POTENTIAL AND MECHANISM OF ACTION

Although insulin may change the intracellular concentrations of several ions and molecules, attention has focused on its effect on $Na^+$ and $K^+$ distribution and the resting membrane potential. If one accepts the contention that these actions of insulin result from a membrane interaction—and indeed much evidence so indicates—then one may make certain inferences about the primary action of insulin as well.

## A. Insulin and potassium influx

Insulin effects net and rapid $K^+$ uptake by the heart [9, 92] and other insulin-sensitive tissues. In addition, insulin leads to hyperpolarization of the muscle cells, i.e., increases the absolute value of the resting membrane potential (increasing $|\mathcal{E}_m|$).[93-95] Both the net $K^+$ influx and hyperpolarization occur in the absence of glucose uptake by the cell.[96] To determine whether the change in membrane potential is secondary to a redistribution in $[K^+]_i/[K^+]_o$, let us first assume that $Cl^-$ movement is passive. The Goldman equation states that [29]

$$\mathcal{E}_m = \frac{RT}{F} \ln \frac{P_K[K^+]_i + P_{Na^+}[Na^+]_i + P_{Cl}Cl^-_o}{P_{K^+}[K^+]_o + P_{Na^+}[Na^+]_o + P_{Cl}Cl^-_i}.$$

But under these circumstances $\mathcal{E}_{Cl^-} = \mathcal{E}_m$, and rearranging,

$$\mathcal{E}_{m'} - \mathcal{E}_m = \frac{RT}{F} \ln \frac{[K^+]_{i'} + b_{Na^+}[Na^+]_i}{[K^+]_i + b_{Na^+}[Na^+]_i}$$

where primed values refer to the values recorded in the presence of insulin. Substitution of data from Zierler and co-workers [93, 97] leads to the absurd conclusion that $b_{Na^+} \equiv P_{Na^+}/P_{K^+} < 0$, indicating that either boundary $Na^+$ condition, that $\mathcal{E}_{Cl^-} = \mathcal{E}_m$ or $b_{Na^+}$ was unchanged by insulin, is incorrect. Thus, the hyperpolarization effected by insulin is not due to a change in steady state ion activities.

From the Goldman equation we note the important relation between $P_{K^+}$ and $\mathcal{E}_m$, namely that there is a decrease in $\mathcal{E}_m$ if $P_{K^+}$ decreases—an effect opposite to that observed with insulin.

## B. Hyperpolarization precedes potassium influx

If the increase in $|\mathcal{E}_m|$ associated with insulin action were a result of $\uparrow[K^+]_i/[K^+]_o$, considering the data cited above and the condition that $[K^+]_o$ is constant (experimentally), one must conclude that $[K^+]_i$ would have to increase by 38 percent if hyperpolarization were in fact due to augmented $[K^+]_i$. Since the conclusion contradicts the observations that (a)$[K^+]_i$ may not increase immediately at all when hyperpolarization is apparent; and (b) even when $[K^+]_i$ does increase three hours after insulin treatment, it does so to approximately $+10$ percent, far short of that predicted above.[94] Therefore, the change in $[K^+]_i/[K^+]_o$ cannot be the primary action of insulin leading to hyperpolarization.

## C. Insulin reduces potassium permeability

The Ussing equation [98] discussed in detail elsewhere [26] describes

$$\frac{J_o}{J_i} = \frac{A_i}{A_o} \exp\left(-\frac{z\mathcal{E}_m\mathcal{F}}{RT}\right), \text{ where}$$

$J_o$, $J_i$ are passive diffusion fluxes, $A_o$, $A_i$ are the activities of an ion, $z$ its oxidation state and $\mathcal{E}_m$ the membrane potential. It is generally accepted that $J_o/J_i$ for $Na^+$ is $\ll 1$, and none of the efflux—but all of the influx—is due to diffusion.[99, 100] Keynes[101] has used a rearranged form of the Goldman equation:

$$b_{Na^+} = \frac{P_{Na^+}}{P_{K^+}} = \frac{[K^+]_i - [K^+]_o \exp(\mathcal{E}_m\mathcal{F}/RT)}{[Na^+]_o \exp(\mathcal{E}_m\mathcal{F}/RT - [Na^+]_i)}, \text{ when } \mathcal{E}_{Cl} = \mathcal{E}_m,$$

to express total flux, $\phi_o$, per unit surface area S as:

$$\frac{(\phi_i)_{Na^+}}{S} = \left[\frac{P_{Na^+}\mathcal{E}_m\mathcal{F}}{RT}\right]\left[\frac{[Na^+]_o}{1 - \exp(-\mathcal{E}_m\mathcal{F}/RT)}\right]$$

if

$$(\phi_i)_{Na^+} = (J_i)_{Na^+}$$

and

$$\frac{(\phi_o)_{K^+}}{S} = P_{K^+}\left[\frac{\mathcal{E}_m\mathcal{F}}{RT}\right]\left[\frac{[K^+]_i \exp(-\mathcal{E}_m\mathcal{F}/RT)}{1 - \exp(-\mathcal{E}_m\mathcal{F}/RT)}\right]$$

if

$$(\phi_o)_{K^+} = (J_o)_{K^+}.$$

Thus $P_{Na^+}/P_{K^+}$ can be calculated from the membrane potential, as can be the activities of $Na^+$ and $K^+$. Rearranging the above, and substituting $\lambda K_1$ for $(\phi_o)_{K^+}/S$, we have

$$P_{K^+} = \lambda\frac{RT}{\mathcal{E}_m\mathcal{F}}\left[(\exp \mathcal{E}_m\mathcal{F}/RT) - 1\right],$$

where $\lambda = (r/2)(V_1/V_f)k$, k is the rate constant for K-efflux, $V_1$ is the volume of sarcoplasm, $V_f$ is fiber volume, V is muscle fiber radius, and $K_1$ is the $K^+$ leaving the sarcoplasm per unit time per unit area of membrane.

By using $^{42}K^+$, it was found that insulin decreases the rate constant for K-efflux in muscle, independent of the presence of glucose.[102] This action is very rapid and is time-dependent.[82] According to the above equation, the calculated $P_{K^+}$ at 0 time exposure is also decreased by insulin.

To determine the consequences of decreased $P_{K^+}$ or reduced diffusion of $K^+$ per unit electrochemical gradient in both directions, we again look to the Ussing relation, which relates passive fluxes to ion activities

$$\frac{(J_o)_{K^+}}{(J_i)_{K^+}} = \frac{(\phi_o)_{K^+}}{(J_i)_{K^+}} = \frac{[K^+]_i}{[K^+]_o} \exp\left[ -\frac{\mathcal{E}_m \mathcal{F}}{RT} \right]$$

and note that the ratio of passive efflux to passive influx is reduced by insulin. By measuring $K_i$, $K_o$, $\mathcal{E}_m$, and calculating $(\phi_o)_{K^+}$ (total $K^+$ efflux), passive K influx, $(J_i)_{K^+}$, is calculated. Arguing that $(\phi_o)_{K^+} - (J_i)_{K^+}$ must be the active $K^+$ influx, Zierler [97, 102] has maintained that his data show that insulin produces no increase in active $K^+$ influx and that which does occur need not be linked to Na efflux. On the other hand, Gourley [103] interprets his data and concludes that insulin in fact does increase $K^+$ influx via a primary increase in $g_{K^+}$ through existing K-channels.

## D. Insulin reduces sodium permeability ($P_{Na^+}$)

The effect of insulin on $P_{Na^+}$ has also attracted attention. Creese [104, 105] reported that insulin decreased the rate constant for Na efflux. From the Nernst equation for Na only, we have

$$\mathcal{E}_{Na^+} = \frac{RT}{F} \ln \frac{[Na^+]_i}{[Na^+]_o}$$

Substitution of physiologic values shows that $\mathcal{E}_{Na^+}$ is approximately $+20$ mV and, therefore a decrease in $P_{Na^+}$ will cause $\mathcal{E}_m$ to approach $\mathcal{E}_{K^+}$, i.e., hyperpolarize the membrane.[97]

## E. Active sodium efflux and insulin

Considerable evidence suggests that insulin stimulates active $Na^+$ efflux, as first suggested by Herman [106] and confirmed by others.[107, 108] With the use of short-circuit current techniques,[109] evidence was presented in several extracardiac tissues that insulin increased the short-circuit current, believed to be proportional to active $Na^+$ transport.[110-112] However, $K^+$ distribution and hyperpolarization cannot be readily explained by a primary action of insulin on $Na^+$ efflux. Zierler [97] postulated that insulin might deform the plasma membrane, thereby changing $P_{Na^+}$ and $P_{K^+}$, to effect $Na^+$ efflux in an unknown fashion. Bittar [113] mentions that this insulin action is "homeostatic" in the sense that "free" $[Na^+]_i$ is maintained at a constant level. Mobilization of "secluded" $[Na^+]_i$ by insulin would lead to overall rate constants showing no decline.[114] Unfortunately, however, there is no evidence supporting an effect of insulin on the $Na^+$, $K^+$-stimulated- and ouabain-inhibited membrane ATPase in myocardium,[115] although insulin stimulates membrane ATPase activity in human lymphocytes.[115a] Very recently, it was reported that $Na^+$, $K^+$-ATPase is not directly stimulated by insulin in rat leg muscle sarcolemma.[115b] Since insulin may inhibit adenyl cyclase in extracardiac tissues (Table I), conserved ATP could stimulate $Na^+$, $K^+$-pumping.[116] The problem is even further complicated by the fact that cyclic AMP itself may direct ion changes of its own (Table II). Yet, rough calculations indicate that in order to exert its action, less than 10 insulin molecules may be bound to a sarcomere surface or one insulin molecule may change a fiber surface of 400 $\mu^2$.[117] Therefore, some system of information transfer involving amplification of insulin's signal must occur at or near its specific receptor site. For instance, one molecule of insulin may translocate $10^7$ molecules of glucose.

## V. INSULIN AND CYCLIC ADENYLATE

### A. Cyclic adenylate system

Many hormones, including insulin, are thought to effect all or some of their actions on the heart through variations in the intracellular level

**Table I** The reactions of cyclic AMP formation and degradation. Since alternate pathways are thought not to exist, the level of cyclic adenylate is determined by the balance in activities of the enzymes, adenyl cyclase and phosphodiesterase. The sensitivities of these two enzymes to substances that alter their activity is tissue-specific.

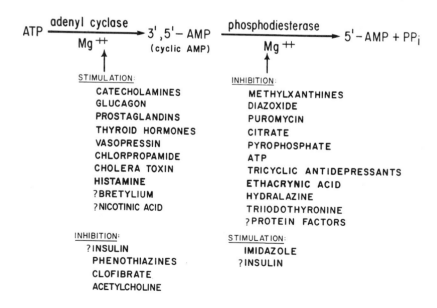

| STIMULATION: | INHIBITION: |
|---|---|
| CATECHOLAMINES | METHYLXANTHINES |
| GLUCAGON | DIAZOXIDE |
| PROSTAGLANDINS | PUROMYCIN |
| THYROID HORMONES | CITRATE |
| VASOPRESSIN | PYROPHOSPHATE |
| CHLORPROPAMIDE | ATP |
| CHOLERA TOXIN | TRICYCLIC ANTIDEPRESSANTS |
| HISTAMINE | ETHACRYNIC ACID |
| ?BRETYLIUM | HYDRALAZINE |
| ?NICOTINIC ACID | TRIIODOTHYRONINE |
| | ?PROTEIN FACTORS |
| INHIBITION: | STIMULATION: |
| ?INSULIN | IMIDAZOLE |
| PHENOTHIAZINES | ?INSULIN |
| CLOFIBRATE | |
| ACETYLCHOLINE | |

**Table II**   Many electrical actions of cyclic adenylate have been proposed. $P_{Na^+}$, $P_{K^+}$ = membrane permeability coefficients of the respective ion; $i,o$ = inside and outside the membrane respectively; $E_m$ = membrane potential; $E_{K^+}$, $E_{Na^+}$ = membrane potential as determined by Nernst equation for single ion alone; $R_m$ = membrane resistance.

### PROPOSED ELECTRICAL EFFECTS OF CYCLIC AMP ON THE CELL

I   **Excitation** (? $^{beta}_{alpha}$ agonism, ? ↑ cyclic AMP)

     A.   Depolarization

         1)   diminished $Na^+$, $K^+$-pump activity

             ($Na^+_i$↑, $K^+_i$↓)

         2)   increased membrane permeability to $Na^+$

             ($P_{Na^+}$↑, $E_m$ → $E_{Na^+}$, $Na^+_i$↑, $K^+_i$↓, $R_m$↓)

         3)   decreased membrane permeability to $K^+$

             ($K^+_i$↓, $R_m$↑)

     B.   No depolarization (e. g., ↑ contractility)

         1)   decreased membrane $Ca^{++}$ binding during depolarization

         2)   increased membrane permeability to $Ca^{++}$

         3)   altered competition between intracellular $Ca^{++}$ pools

II.   **Inhibition** (? $^{alpha}_{beta}$ agonism, ? ↓ cyclic AMP)

     A.   Hyperpolarization

         1)   increased membrane permeability to $K^+$

             ($P_{K^+}$↑, $E_m$ → $E_{K^+}$, $K^+_i$↑)

         2)   increased $Na^+$, $K^+$-pump activity

             ($Na^+_i$↓, $K^+_i$↑)

     B.   No hyperpolarization (e. g., ↓ contractility)

         1)   increased membrane $Ca^{++}$ binding

         2)   decreased membrane permeability to $Ca^{++}$

         3)   altered competition between intracellular $Ca^{++}$ pools

of adenosine 3′,5′-monophosphate, also called cyclic adenylate or cyclic AMP (Table III).[119,2] Cyclic adenylate is formed from ATP, catalyzed by the enzyme adenyl cyclase. Degradation of cyclic adenylate is catalyzed by the enzyme phosphodiesterase (Table I). Since alternate pathways are not believed to exist, the concentration of cyclic AMP is determined by the balance in activities of the synthetic and hydrolytic reactions, the extent of intracellular binding or compartmentalization, and the rate of leakage out of the cell.

**Table III**  Cyclic AMP is thought to mediate many reactions and processes in different organs.

## POSSIBLE ROLES OF CYCLIC AMP

### RELEASE OF HORMONES AND ENZYMES

insulin
thyroid
renin
somatotropic (STH, GH)
thyrocalcitonin
pancreozymin
adrenocorticotropic (ACTH)
follicle-stimulating (FSH)

thyrotropin
amylase
secretin
catecholamines
histamine
serotonin
luteinizing (LH)
?parathormone
?vasopressin

### END ORGAN FUNCTION

parathormone
glucagon
insulin
thyroid
vasopressin (ADH)
catecholamines
adrenocorticotropic (ACTH)
acetylcholine
synapse
neuromuscular junction
erythropoietin
thyrocalcitonin

angiotensin
melanocyte-stimulating (MSH)
luteinizing (LH)
estrogens
prolactin
gastrin
serotonin
histamine
long acting thyroid stimulator (LATS)
testosterone
aldosterone

### PHARMACOLOGIC

alpha/beta stimulants
alpha/beta blocking agents
diazoxide
methylxanthines
l-DOPA/lithium
imidazole
puromycin
phenothiazines
prostaglandins

tricyclic antidepressants
bretylium
clofibrate
cholera toxin
acetylsalicylic acid
chlorpropamide
slow-reacting substance (SRS-A)
phytohemagglutinin

### INTERMEDIARY METABOLISM

lipolysis
glycogenolysis
protein synthesis

DNA synthesis
FFA metabolism
polyribosome synthesis

### INTEGRATED CELLULAR EVENTS

fertilization
platelet aggregation
developmental aggregation
phagocytosis
secretion
lymphocyte transformation
chemotaxis

permeability changes
contractility
growth
transcription
acute hypersensitivity

Adenyl cyclase is located within the cell membrane "beneath" a receptor and is thus in an advantageous position to effect hormone-mediated changes within the cell (Fig 16).[120, 120a] Details of the coupling mechanism between the hormone receptor and adenyl cyclase

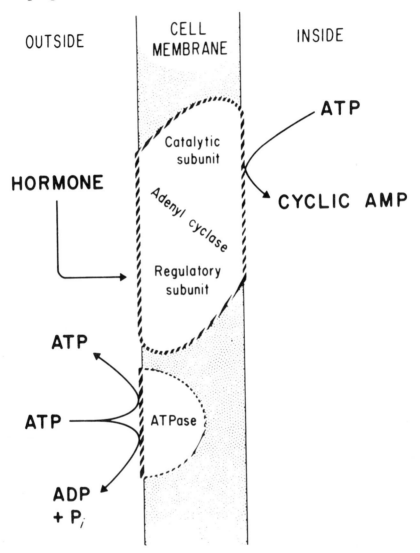

**Figure 16**    The relationships among hormones, extracellular and intracellular ATP, and cyclic AMP in intact cells. Reproduced with permission from Butcher, Robison and Sutherland.[120]

remain unknown (Fig 17) [121] but binding of a hormone to the sarcolemma activates the enzyme, probably by allosteric transformation. The hormone binding to an end organ receptor, in this case insulin to the heart, has been termed a "first messenger." Control and amplification of the message is then mediated by variation in the level of cyclic adenylate, or the "second messenger" (Fig 18).[122]

Considerable specificity is apparent in the hormone receptor-cyclic AMP-system. For instance, ACTH activates adrenal adenyl cyclase, but fails to affect liver or heart cells.[123] Parathormone increases adenyl cyclase solely in the renal cortex, while vasopressin does so solely in the renal medulla.[124] Human leukocyte adenyl cyclase is sensitive to catecholamines and prostaglandin-E₁ but not to either glucagon or ACTH.[125] Loss in specificity of receptors has been reported in a number of tissues.[23, 126-129]

In adipose tissue, adenyl cyclase activity is altered by insulin, ACTH, thyroid stimulating hormone, epinephrine, and glucagon, each hormone being received by a specific receptor, but influencing a single

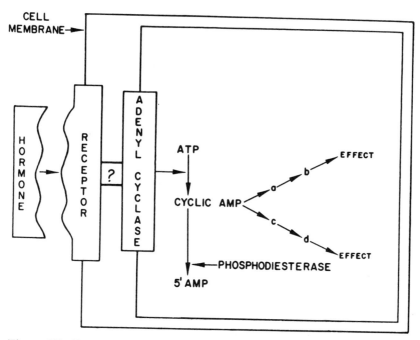

**Figure 17**  Diagram indicating the separate identity of receptor, coupler, and adenyl cyclase system. Reproduced from Epstein et al.[121] with permission.

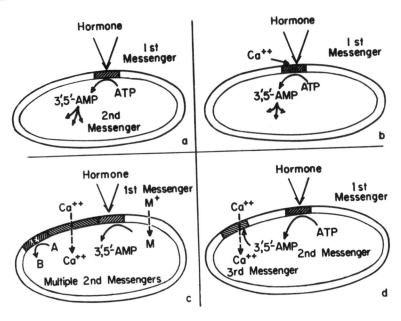

**Figure 18** Possible relationships between hormone-receptor interactions and calcium in effecting an end-organ response: (a) a hormone (1st messenger) interacts with the cell membrane to alter intracellular cyclic AMP concentrations (2nd messenger); (b) requirement for calcium ion in binding or coupling of the 1st messenger; (c) simultaneous increase in membrane calcium permeability with adenyl cyclase activation (both calcium and cyclic AMP function as 2nd messengers); (d) increased calcium permeability results from cyclic AMP action (calcium thus serves as a 3rd messenger). Reproduced from Rasmussen et al.[122] with permission, copyright, 1970, Academic Press.

adenyl cyclase system.[130] However, in the liver, two separate adenyl cyclase systems exist for glucagon and epinephrine.[131, 132] It is apparent that discrimination in the messenger system is derived from the *receptor specificity* and *intracellular enzyme complement* of the tissue in question. Given a hormone-sensitive tissue—myocardium, for instance—raising or lowering cyclic AMP levels by that hormone changes the rates at which processes occur, but cannot of course change the nature of the processes themselves.

Recently the molecular mechanism of action of cyclic AMP has attracted much interest. In the best studied system, glycogenolysis, cyclic AMP is thought to activate phosphorylase kinase kinase (Fig 19). Phosphorylase kinase is in turn phosphorylated in a cascade fashion,

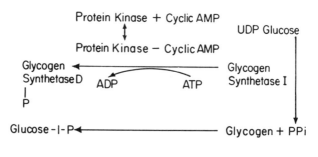

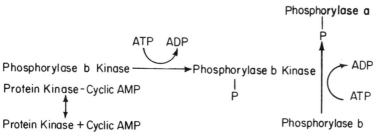

**Figure 19** The reactions involved in the hormonal activation of phospho-rylase in cardiac muscle, resulting in glycogenolysis. Cyclic AMP affects a protein kinase, which activates phosphorylase-*b*-kinase. In turn, phosphoryl-ase *b* is converted to phosphorylase *a*, leading to glycogen cleavage.

leading to the conversion of phosphorylase *b* to the *a* form.[133, 134] Phos-phorylase *a* catalyzes the breakdown of glycogen and is reconverted to the *b* form by phosphorylase phosphatase. A parallel effect of cyclic AMP on enzymes leading to lowered glycogen synthetase activity is also manifest.[135] In these systems, cyclic adenylate activates enzymes by protein phosphorylation. There is evidence that other processes within the myocyte are activated by phosphorylation of cyclic AMP dependent protein kinases.[136-140] In a fascinating discussion, Cheung [140] proposes that cyclic AMP acts as an allosteric effector, and that the high energy content of this molecule endows it with a built-in regula-tory device in the sense that the thermodynamic barrier thus imposed functions as a metabolic all-or-nothing switch (Fig 20). For a further discussion of the unique conformational energy barrier in cyclic AMP, the reader is referred to Jordan.[381] The postulate that cyclic AMP's function is to switch off irreversibly the actions of various hormones is consistent with the hypothesis that the many different effects of cyclic AMP are explained by the kinds of proteins with binding sites specific for the nucleotide.

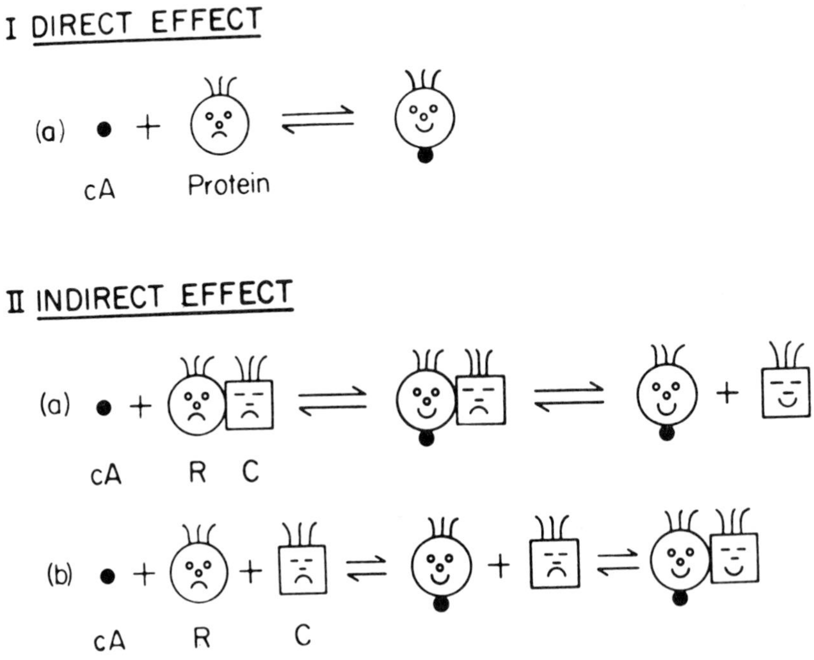

## I DIRECT EFFECT

## II INDIRECT EFFECT

Figure 20   The mechanism of action of cyclic AMP is presented schematically. A protein is depicted with hydrophilic groups extending into its environment. The regulatory subunit of an allosteric enzyme is designated as R, the catalytic subunit as C, and cyclic AMP as cA. The illustration does not specify that the proteins necessarily possess enzymic activity. In fact, a similar representation may also be valid for proteins without enzymic activity. Reproduced with permission from Cheung.[140]

### B. Insulin, cyclic adenylate and cell metabolism

Early studies suggested that lipolysis might be controlled by cyclic AMP,[111] later confirmed by Butcher and associates [142, 143] who specifically showed that insulin lowered intracellular cyclic AMP levels. This was buttressed by a variety of experimental data from different laboratories.[144, 144a, 374] An inhibitory action of insulin on adenyl cyclase [145] and a stimulatory effect on phosphodiesterase could account for the fall in cyclic AMP levels, although these have not been confirmed.[146, 147]

In the liver, insulin directly effects glucose uptake by a reduction in the rate of glycogenolysis, an increase in the rate of glycogen synthesis, and a reduction in the rate of gluconeogenesis. These are related in part to the lowering of cyclic AMP levels and may be attenuated by glucagon or epinephrine, agents that stimulate adenyl cyclase.[148-150] In fact, when insulin antibody is injected into intact animals, hepatic cyclic AMP levels rise and glycogenolysis ensues.[148] This suggests that physiologic levels of insulin normally hold down hepatic cyclic AMP concentrations and restrain glucose and amino acid output. However, the liver is exposed to higher insulin levels than the heart because of the drainage of the portal vein.

Release of gluconeogenic substances—lactate, pyruvate, amino acids and glycerol—from insulin sensitive, nonhepatic tissues is reduced by insulin. Since the plasma levels of these molecules do not saturate the hepatic gluconeogenic pathways, this contributes to the slowing of gluconeogenesis.[150]

Insulin increases, and glucagon decreases, glycogen synthetase activity, both of which actions are mediated by cyclic adenylate (Fig 21).[151] The conversion of glycogen synthetase $I$ (active form) to synthetase $D$ (inactive) occurs when the $I$ form is phosphorylated by ATP in the presence of the catalyst glycogen synthetase $I$ kinase.[135] This kinase is activated by cyclic AMP, and is probably identical with phosphorylase kinase kinase. In both muscle [135] and liver [152, 153] an insulin-induced increase in glycogen synthetase activity may be mediated by a decrease in cyclic AMP level. However, it has recently been postulated that the epinephrine effect on phosphorylase $b$ kinase and on glycogen synthetase may entail a conversion of a cyclic AMP-dependent, associated, protein kinase into a dissociated, cyclic AMP-independent kinase.[154, 155] Insulin's effect would be the reverse, or the induction of an association; or prevention of dissociation, of the allosteric and active parts of the enzyme.° The net effect would be that insulin reduces the sensitivity of glycogen synthetase to cyclic AMP, so its catalytic effectiveness is reduced, even if its level is unchanged.

Agents that raise intracellular cyclic AMP levels (glucagon, epinephrine, and exogenous cyclic AMP) effect net $K^+$ loss from the cell, while insulin opposes this action. However, only a part of the $K^+$-conserving property of insulin may be mediated by a reduction in cyclic AMP levels in nonmuscular tissues. Recently it was shown that high concentrations of dibutyryl cyclic AMP could enhance $K^+$ uptake in Purkinje fibers, but the opposite effect was observed at low concentrations of this cyclic AMP derivative.[380] These authors postulated that beta- and alpha-receptors could be involved, but secondary re-

---

° A number of cyclic AMP-dependent protein kinases may be dissociated into a cyclic AMP-binding protein and a cyclic AMP-independent protein kinase.

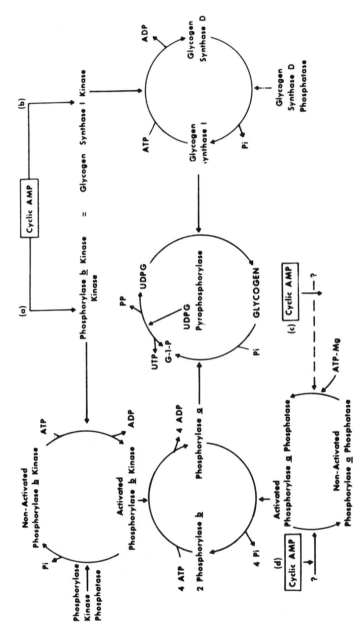

**Figure 21** Mechanisms of control of glycogen synthesis and degradation affected by cyclic AMP. Reproduced with permission from Villar-Palasi et al.[155]

lease of catecholamines might also play a part. One may conclude that the relationship among the substances insulin, cyclic AMP, and K⁺ ion is certainly not simple and is far from clear in any tissue, especially in myocardium.

Evidence indicating that insulin decreases cyclic adenylate levels via a reduction in adenyl cyclase activity largely comes from work in adipose tissue.[144a] In this situation, the rise in adenyl cyclase activity expected from treatment with other hormones (*e.g.*, the catecholamines) is blocked or inhibited by insulin. There are investigators who cannot confirm these data as well.[357] The effect of insulin in muscle is even less certain. Insulin injection into rats effects a slight increase in skeletal muscle cyclic AMP levels.[358] In other studies, insulin has no effect on cyclic AMP content in rat diaphragm.[359, 360] Insulin may stimulate glycogen synthetase *I* activity when no alteration in cyclic adenylate levels occurs, although a change in experimental conditions may result in a lowering of cyclic AMP levels.[135] Keely and co-workers [361] report that insulin elevates cyclic AMP levels in myocardium with epinephrine present.[361]

In muscle, insulin may profoundly affect K⁺ uptake, as discussed, in the absence of detectable changes in level of cyclic AMP.[156, 157] Similarly, the important insulin effect on glucose transport [158] does not appear to be mediated by cyclic AMP, since no decrease in cyclic AMP level occurs at a time when glucose transport is quite accelerated.[362] In addition, substances which activate adenyl cyclase and elevate cyclic AMP levels do not inhibit glucose transport.

Assuming insulin decreases muscle and heart cyclic adenylate levels in a given instance, the reason for the change—decrease in adenyl cyclase activity, or increase in phosphodiesterase activity—is also unsettled. Insulin was recently found to stimulate phosphodiesterase in extracts of isolated rat heart,[363] which is consistent with the growing feeling that insulin may act upon phosphodiesterase rather than upon adenyl cyclase. In summary, the evidence presently available indicating that insulin's actions in heart muscle are mediated by the adenyl cyclase system is weak.

## VI. FUNDAMENTAL MECHANISM OF ACTION OF INSULIN

### A. Insulin interaction with the cell

Analogous to the interaction between enzyme and substrate (see appendix), the interaction between insulin and receptor is thought to involve two distinct processes: recognition-binding and activation.

Separation of these features of hormone-receptor interaction is well known for other hormones—glucagon, angiotensin, ACTH, catecholamines—for which hormone inhibitors are known. These inhibitor molecules attach themselves to the receptor adequately but do not effect the anticipated functional change in the receptor tissue. Unfortunately, there is no such inhibitor molecule for insulin which may be used to clearly show the separation in binding and activation processes, since known insulin analogues also bind poorly in proportion to the decrease in activation observed.

The evidence that insulin affects its multivalent actions on the exterior surface of the cell, largely derived from studies of insulin bound to plastic beads and everted "ghost" membranes, will be discussed in a later section.

Some recent studies of the enzymatic digestion of insulin "receptor site" and the effects of receptor-insulin interaction clarify some aspects of the mechanism of action of insulin.[128, 159, 160, 205, 364] According to the mosaic membrane model, the insulin "receptor" would be found in either the membrane protein pool "floating" laterally or be among the amphipathic lipids. When the membrane is treated with phospholipases, the binding capacity for insulin markedly increases rather than decreases. Hence the receptors are not phospholipids, but the data also suggest that a number of "occult" receptor sites may be uncovered, three times as numerous as ordinary sites, which are normally blocked by the polar heads of the phospholipids. This interpretation is further supported by the fact that the same increase in binding capacity may be observed when salts are added to the medium. In the presence of the dissolved ions surrounding the polar heads of the phospholipids, the occult insulin-binding sites become available, and under these circumstances the addition of phospholipases does not further increase the binding sites available.

A portion or all of the insulin receptor may then be assumed to be a polypeptide. Mild trypsin exposure of these sites reduces the receptor affinity for insulin, i.e., greater concentrations are necessary to produce a given effect, without a reduction in the cell's capacity to bind insulin, as measured by labelling experiments. It is thought that such mild trypsin digestion does not destroy insulin receptor sites but alters them sufficiently to "loosen" the binding of insulin by destroying the "fit" of receptor with insulin. Pretreatment of adipose cells with high concentrations of trypsin abolishes the lowering of cyclic AMP levels and increased glucose transport resulting from exposure to insulin regardless of the concentration of insulin used. The cells remain sensitive to other adenyl cyclase and phosphodiesterase stimulants and their glucose transport is responsive to changes in glucose concentration and phloretin. Such cells have reversibly lost the ability to bind insulin.[161] The loss in binding sites may be restored by treatment with phospholipase, which compensates for the trypsin-destroyed binding sites by exposing an even greater number of "occult" binding sites (Fig 22). Treatment with even mild trypsin a second time will result in destruction of the uncovered insulin binding sites. Destruction of both superficial ("physiological") and occult binding sites may be achieved at once by exposure to tetranitromethane, a molecule small enough to gain access to all binding sites.

## B. The insulin receptor is a glycoprotein

The effect of enzymes that cleave sugar residues from membrane structures are also of interest. Neuraminidase detaches the amino sugar sialic acid and abolishes insulin-induced glucose uptake and inhibition of lipolysis (Fig 23). However, the capacity of the cell to bind insulin remains unimpaired. These data are interpreted by Cuatrecasas[205, 364, 365] as showing that the insulin receptor includes one or more sialic acid residues but that these are not part of the receptor *site*. The sialic acid moieties serve to modulate and transfer the information that is imparted by the interaction of insulin and receptor to the remainder of the membrane, which then in turn eventually affects enhanced glucose uptake, inhibition of lipolysis, incorporation of amino acids and other insulin actions. In this case, the two processes of binding and activation are truly different.

Treatment of the insulin-responsive cell with β-galactosidase does not affect the insulin response. However, exposure to neuraminidase first and β-galactosidase second not only results in loss of insulin binding, but also in loss of insulin response. One explanation is that galactose forms a part of the receptor site, and sialic acid is attached to the galactose in a way to cover it from the action of β-galactosidase. These data imply that a chain of sugars forms part of the receptor, with galactose occurring more proximal than sialic acid, which may be the terminal group of the chain, and also defines the insulin receptor as a glycoprotein. Indeed, isolation of the insulin receptor by means of affinity chromatography (Fig 24),[366] has enabled further binding experiments with the pure receptor, and also supports the contention that the insulin receptor site is a glycoprotein with a concentration of 10,000/fat cell with a molecular weight of about 300,000 amu. Although the receptor sites are randomly distributed throughout the membrane, they retain considerable mobility, so that they may quickly

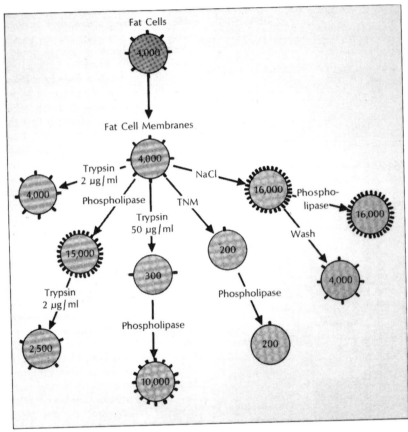

**Figure 22** Changes in cellular binding capacity (numbers indicate counts per minute of labeled insulin) under various manipulations have elucidated the presumed structure of the insulin receptor, depicted in other illustrations. NaCl steps up binding capacity, presumably because its ions neutralize charges on phospholipid heads: TNM a small molecule, can penetrate phospholipid layer to destroy all sites. Reproduced with permission.[365]

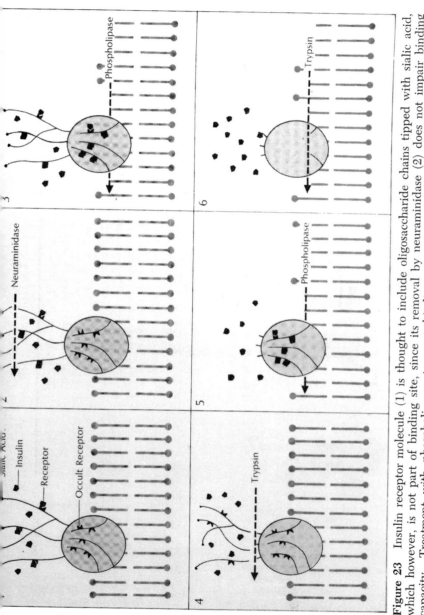

**Figure 23** Insulin receptor molecule (1) is thought to include oligosaccharide chains tipped with sialic acid, which however, is not part of binding site, since its removal by neuraminidase (2) does not impair binding capacity. Treatment with phospholipase steps up binding capacity, exposing "occult" binding sites (3). Trypsin destroys normal binding sites (4), but subsequent phospholipase treatment more than replaces these with occult sites (5). If phospholipase is followed by trypsin, all sites are destroyed (6). Reproduced with permission.[365]

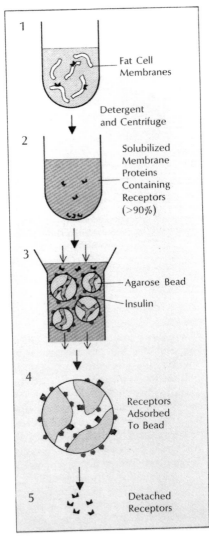

1

Fat Cell
Membranes

Detergent
and Centrifuge

2

Solubilized
Membrane
Proteins
Containing
Receptors
(>90%)

3

Agarose Bead

Insulin

4

Receptors
Adsorbed
To Bead

5

Detached
Receptors

**Figure 24**   Relatively pure preparations of receptor sites are produced by affinity chromatography, in which protein fraction of membranes is passed through column of beads pretreated with insulin. The first step is to obtain isolated membranes from fat cells, from which the protein component can be removed by various detergents; as one would expect, the deproteinized membranes no longer bind insulin. The soluble detergent fraction, separated from the membranes by centrifugation, is a very crude preparation, since it contains a large proportion of the membrane proteins, among which the insulin receptor accounts for less than 1 per cent. After some preliminary purification steps, the mixture is passed through a column of

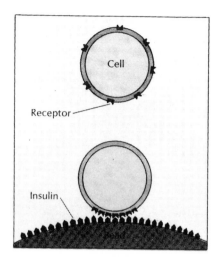

**Figure 25** Probable mobility of receptor sites within plasma membrane is shown by cell's response when it is "treated" with insulin-agarose bead. Cellular response is close to normal, indicating that nearly all its receptor sites must be activated. Reproduced with permission.[365]

concentrate themselves in an area of stimulation on the cell surface to effect maximal intracellular action (Fig 25).

## C. Hypothesis regarding insulin action and cyclic nucleotides

### 1. *Possible mechanisms and cyclic nucleotides*

With these data as background, what are the possible mechanisms which may account for the many intracellular actions of insulin? First, it is possible that the insulin receptor is close to the enzyme adenyl cyclase, which is also thought to be located in the plasma membrane. Perhaps by direct modulation of adenyl cyclase activity and resulting changes in level of cyclic AMP, the many intracellular actions of insulin could be effected, as illustrated in Figure 26, panel 1. The failure of this hypothesis to explain the effects on myocardium have

---

agarose beads—highly porous particles with a correspondingly large surface area. These have been previously prepared by reacting with insulin and certain other substances in such a manner that the insulin is firmly bound to the bead column. The insulin receptors attach themselves to the bead-bound insulin, while most of the rest of the protein passes on through. By delicate chemical manipulation, one can then gently detach the receptor from the bound insulin, thereby obtaining a quite concentrated solution of receptor molecules (a purity of about 50 per cent). Reproduced with permission.[365]

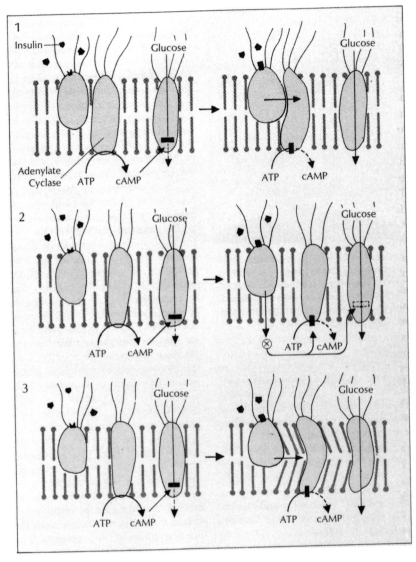

**Figure 26**   Three possible modes of insulin action are shown schematically. Activation of receptor molecule by hormone is known to block cAMP production, which in turn may activate other insulin-dependent processes, typified by glucose transport (1). Or, activation may release "X" substance (perhaps cGMP or a related nucleotide), which both blocks cAMP production and triggers other processes (2). Finally, activation may produce cellular responses by physically deranging membrane structure (3). Reproduced with permission.[365]

already been outlined, for the present evidence does not support a major role for cyclic AMP as mediator of insulin action in the heart. Even in adipose tissue, it is really uncertain whether insulin's primary effect is on adenyl cyclase or phosphodiesterase.

A second, and more likely possibility is that the insulin receptor does not *directly* influence the activity of adenyl cyclase. Rather, insulin interaction with the membrane receptor may cause the liberation of an unknown substance ("X" on Fig 26, panel 2) which independently modifies membrane properties and affects intermediary metabolism. Rasmussen [119, 122, 367] believes ions may function as "second messengers," at least for the cyclic AMP system. Another cyclic nucleotide, 3',5'-guanosine monophosphate (cyclic GMP) has received much attention as a mediator of intracellular events, complementary to cyclic AMP. Although there is no hormone-activated guanyl cyclase as yet identified in the plasma membrane, several hormones which do not influence cyclic AMP activity—insulin, cholinergic (acetylcholine) or other agents (histamine)—now appear to act by way of cyclic GMP, as postulated by Larner [368] even before reliable radioimmunoassay methods were available for measuring cyclic GMP. Illiano and co-workers [369] have recently shown that insulin augments cyclic GMP concentrations in adipose and liver. In addition, there are two distinct protein kinases—one dependent upon cyclic AMP, and the other on cyclic GMP—in other tissues,[370] and it is likely that distinct phosphodiesterases and cyclic nucleotide binding proteins, or phosphokinases exist, which further suggests that the sites of synthesis, degradation and action are different for the two cyclic nucleotides. Of even greater significance is the suggestion that high concentrations of one cyclic nucleotide prevent the formation, metabolism, or action of the other.[371, 372] Goldberg and colleagues [373] hypothesize that a hormone, such as insulin, may exert "monodirectional" control of generating either cyclic AMP or cyclic GMP. Each nucleotide would exert a separate stimulatory effect, and obey the generalization that such a monodirectional control requires the presence of calcium ions. Together, both nucleotides exert "bidirectional" control, in that stimulation or inhibition of a particular process is achieved by a simultaneous drop in concentrations of cyclic AMP as those of cyclic GMP increase (Fig 27). While it is true that cyclic GMP promotes intracellular events that are antagonistic to those stimulated by cyclic AMP, further study is necessary before this "dualism" is accepted. There is firm evidence that the effects of acetylcholine on the heart, "opposite" to those of the catecholamines, is mediated by cyclic GMP and influenced by calcium ions.[379]

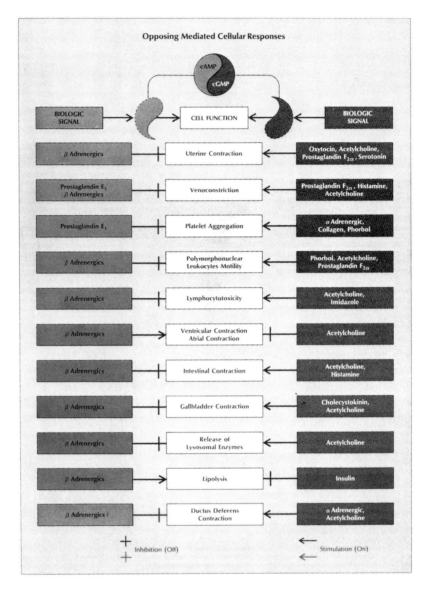

**Figure 27** In a variety of circumstances the actions of cyclic AMP and cyclic GMP "oppose" each other. From the point of view of control theory, this allows finer regulation. Reproduced with permission.[371]

Finally, a third possibility in the mechanism of action of insulin is depicted in Figure 26, panel 3. Activation of the insulin receptor is visualized as changing its shape or charge, inducing some major change in the membrane conformation. According to Changeux,[118] membranes—viewed as lattice protomers—may exist in at least two configurations. If so, a configurational change effected by the interaction of a given protomer with insulin could refold the entire membrane, simultaneously decreasing $P_{Na^+}$ and $P_{K^+}$, increasing $P_{glucose}$ by exposing carriers, and change the rate constants of several enzyme systems. Other actions of insulin—effect on protein synthesis and stimulation of uptake of nucleotides and their incorporation into DNA and RNA, and interaction with mitochondria—remain unexplained even by this unproved and highly controversial hypothesis (Fig 28).

A postulated change in conformation of boundaries of a membrane "channel" and alteration in one or more cyclic nucleotide levels are not mutually exclusive processes. The catecholamines, for instance, in addition to increasing intracellular levels of cyclic AMP in myocardium, also enhance the inward calcium current.[374] Thyroid hormone also shares the ability to increase myocardial cyclic AMP levels by stimulating membrane adenyl cyclase, but appears to have a rather selective influence upon membrane potassium conductance.[384] While the relationship between enhanced cyclic AMP levels and alterations in ion transport effected by these hormones, including insulin, are unknown, it is certainly of interest to note the recent recognition of these dual actions of hormones on the myocyte. Certainly an alteration in membrane conformation might account for the changes in ion transport, while the alterations in cyclic nucleotide levels might provide one explanation for the changes in intermediary metabolism observed.

## 2. *Evidence against cyclic AMP as mediator of insulin actions*

Although there is some evidence that cyclic AMP participates in the many actions of insulin, strict criteria demonstrating such involvement have not been fulfilled. The correlation between the cellular response to insulin and change in cyclic AMP levels is poor.[389-392]

In human adipose-tissue homogenates, the sequence of events leading to lipolysis have recently been delineated.[393-397] Triglyceride lipase is activated by a phosphorylation reaction catalyzed by a protein kinase which itself is activated by cyclic AMP (Fig 29). The binding of cyclic AMP to the regulatory subunits of the kinase (cAMP-R in Fig 29) dissociates the inactive holoenzyme and releases the active subunits (C) which catalyze the phosphorylation and activation of the

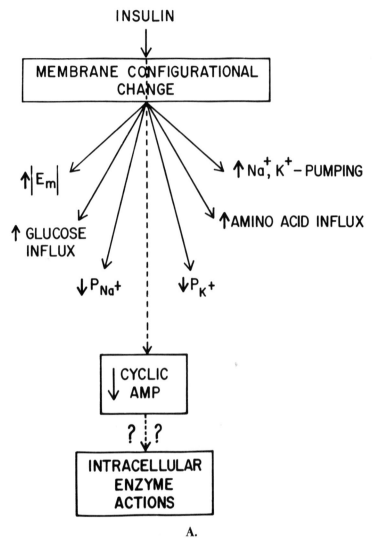

**Figure 28** Highly speculative diagram of possible effects of insulin on ion and molecule movement in heart muscle. (A) depicts an action of insulin mediated by a decrease in cyclic AMP levels, for which there is currently little supporting evidence in heart cells. (B) depicts an action of insulin mediated by an increase in intracellular calcium concentrations, postulated to occur via release from membranes and redistribution between storage depots. cAMP=cyclic AMP; $|E_m|$=absolute value of resting membrane potential; $P_{Na^+}$, $P_{K^+}$=permeability coefficient of respective ion.

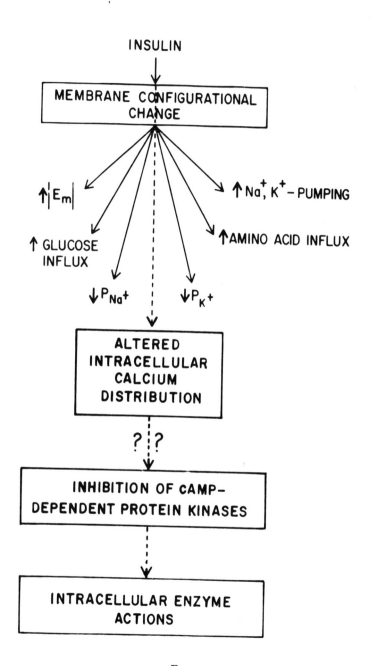

B.

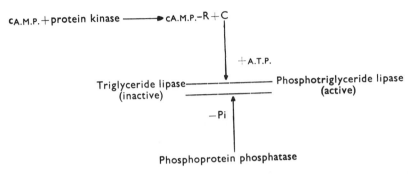

**Figure 29** Current model of activation of triglyceride lipase. This enzyme is activated by a phosphorylation reaction catalyzed by a protein kinase which is itself activated by cyclic AMP. The binding of cyclic AMP to the regulatory subunits of the kinase (cyclic AMP-R) dissociates the inactive holoenzyme and releases the active subunits which catalyze the phosphorylation and activation of the lipase.[394] This sequence is similar to the ones illustrated in Figs 19 and 21 for phosphorylase *b* kinase. Insulin is thought to reduce the activation of the protein kinase involved, and probably also activates phosphoprotein phosphatase.

lipase. This sequence is similar to the protein kinase catalyzed phosphorylation of muscle phosphorylase *b* kinase and glycogen synthetase (Fig 21).[396, 398] In addition, there is a phosphoprotein phosphatase whose activity corresponds to the inactivation of triglyceride lipase, probably providing another means of regulating the reaction.

As expected, epinephrine produces glycerol release and increases in cyclic AMP levels and protein kinase activity, with nearly no change in phosphatase activity. A small dose of insulin at this point sharply reduces glycerol levels while cyclic AMP levels are unaffected. Large doses of insulin produce some fall in cyclic AMP levels, but at a time considerably after lipolysis is decreased.[392] In the presence of insulin, the proportion of activated protein kinase is lowered at a time and to a degree which parallels the decrease in glycerol release. Therefore, at least some of the antilipolytic effect of insulin is due to a decrease in protein kinase activation and subsequent inhibition of triglyceride lipase. There may also be a contribution by activation of phosphoprotein phosphatase by insulin as well. An insulin-induced decrease in protein-kinase activity would lead to inhibition of glycogen phosphorylase and stimulation of glycogen synthetase.

The independence of insulin-induced stimulation of protein synthesis and membrane glucose and amino acid transport has already been discussed. During this process basal tissue cyclic AMP levels are unaltered.[399] The activity of pyruvate dehydrogenase is regulated by a phosphorylation-dephosphorylation cycle involving a kinase which inactivates the enzyme and a phosphatase which reactivates it. The activity of these two regulatory enzymes is not affected by physiologic concentrations of cyclic AMP.[400] Finally, increases in tissue cyclic AMP levels by epinephrine to cause 75% maximal stimulation of lipolysis do not hamper insulin-induced protein synthesis.[389]

## D. Insulin and intracellular calcium

In the search for another "messenger" for some intracellular actions of insulin, there is some evidence to suggest that intracellular calcium may be a candidate in adipose tissue. At the level of the cell membrane, glucose and amino acid permeability are a function of the calcium bound to the membrane.[401] The activity of several enzymes involved in mediating the intracellular actions of insulin is calcium-dependent.[393, 400, 401] In particular, calcium ions may depress cyclic AMP-dependent protein kinase activity, and may also stimulate phosphoprotein phosphatase activity (Figure 29). However, such modulating effects of calcium on various enzymes appears to be tissue-dependent, since $Ca^{++}$ facilitates the conversion of the G-6-P dependent form of glycogen synthetase to the independent form in adipose homogenates,[402] whereas in muscle the activation of glycogenolysis by phosphorylase $b$ kinase is stimulated by $Ca^{++}$ (an effect which is opposite to that produced by insulin).[403] Nonetheless, it is noteworthy that increasing free calcium concentrations from $10^{-8}$ M to $10^{-4}$ M produces a four- to eight-fold rise in pyruvate dehydrogenase phosphatase activity.[400] Finally, the presence of $Ca^{++}$ is required for insulin-induced protein synthesis.[404]

Another interesting relationship recently explored is that between pharmacologic agents which alter intracellular calcium levels and metabolic processes. Procaine hydrochloride inhibits epinephrine-induced calcium efflux from perifused adipocytes,[405] and would be expected to raise intracellular calcium concentrations. Mimicking insulin's actions, the addition of procaine to this preparation decreases the protein kinase activation ratio and increases cyclic AMP levels.[392] Other agents, for instance ouabain, lanthanum, and the $Ca^{++}$ ionophore (A23187) also increase intracellular calcium levels and produce similar metabolic effects in adipose tissue.[406]

In common with other cell types, isolated fat cells contain over 90% of their total calcium content in a complexed form which is non-exchangeable. The remaining exchangeable calcium is distributed among kinetically distinct pools. In adipose tissue three such pools have been identified:[405] one "rapid" located superficially and unaffected by dinitrophenol, and two "slower" pools inhibited by dinitrophenol, one or both of which is postulated to represent calcium "stores" in the plasma membrane and endoplasmic reticulum. In myocardial muscle, kinetic analysis of exchangeable calcium is more complicated, probably because of even greater intracellular compartmentalization, since calcium transfers between pools effect contraction and relaxation (see discussion and references, the work of Langer and associates, Chapter 3, pages 191-198). Insulin decreases the affinity of fat-cell ghosts for calcium, an effect which correlates with glycerol release.[405] Pretreatment with trypsin digests the insulin receptor and renders ghosts made from such cells resistant to the decrease in calcium binding affinity anticipated in the presence of insulin.

Fat cell membranes contain a $Ca^{++}$-sensitive ATPase, as do heart cell membranes, and their cell ghosts are capable of active calcium extrusion against an electrochemical gradient. After steady-state $^{45}Ca^{++}$ efflux is achieved in Krebs' buffer, $^{45}Ca^{++}$-efflux rises sharply after epinephrine is added, followed by glycerol release. This effect is inhibited by dinitrophenol, which suggests that the $^{45}Ca^{++}$ is extruded from an intracellular pool. After perfusion of this preparation with insulin, the subsequent addition of epinephrine is followed by only slight lipolysis and $^{45}Ca^{++}$-efflux. These data suggest that insulin inhibits the release of calcium from intracellular stores, which, in addition to its mobilization of calcium from membrane stores, would tend to increase intracellular calcium.

While these experiments are concerned with adipose tissue, they do provide the framework for a hypothesis of insulin action to account for both the membrane and intracellular actions of insulin. Insulin binding could change membrane configuration and permeabilities of various substrates simultaneously. Calcium would be displaced from high-affinity binding sites together with an inhibition of $Ca^{++}$ release from intracellular pools. The rise in local intracellular $Ca^{++}$ concentrations may then inhibit the cyclic-AMP dependent protein kinase and activate phosphoprotein phosphatase, thereby depressing the activities of triglyceride lipase and glycogen phosphorylase and activating glycogen synthetase. A secondary rise in mitochondrial calcium levels would stimulate pyruvate dehydrogenase as well.

Such a model of hormone action recalls the now classic papers of Rasmussen [122, 407] in which calcium was envisioned as a third messenger in a variety of tissues (Figure 18). Using this general hypothesis (Figure 30), it may well be that calcium is one of the messengers involved in insulin's many actions, or that an unknown cyclic nucleotide or substance is the "second" messenger for insulin.

As mentioned, whether or not some of the actions of insulin are

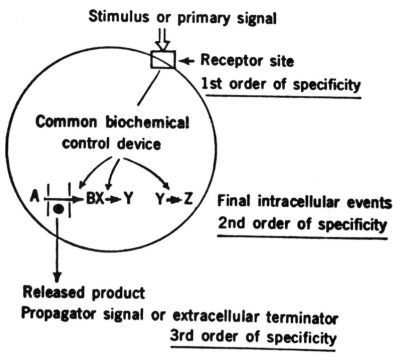

**Stimulus or primary signal**

← **Receptor site**
**1st order of specificity**

**Common biochemical control device**

**Final intracellular events**
**2nd order of specificity**

**Released product**
**Propagator signal or extracellular terminator**
**3rd order of specificity**

**Figure 30** A general schema of intercellular and intracellular control of metabolic, electrical, and secretory processes involved in the production of an end-organ response. Three "orders of specificity" or messenger levels are depicted. Reproduced from Rasmussen [107] with permission. Copyright, 1970, American Association for the Advancement of Science.

mediated by cyclic AMP in the heart is really unknown. Although there is in fact little evidence to indicate it does, there is also no firm data disproving a role for cyclic AMP as mediator of insulin actions. In addition, the molecular mechanisms by which cyclic AMP effects membrane changes is also unclear. One very intriguing association recently described is one between cyclic AMP-mediated reactions and the presence of filamentous proteins, *i.e.*, microtubules, microfilaments, and actin-like proteins in the regulated cell. Acknowledging that the cellular response to hormones mediated by cyclic nucleotides may involve many unidentified and complicated events, Olsen [108] proposes that filamentous proteins are the necessary mediators of many cyclic nucleotide-regulated cell responses. Such a model is depicted in Figure 31, in which the possible effects of filamentous proteins upon membrane activities are summarized. Rapid movement of substances toward, along side of, within, and through membranes could be

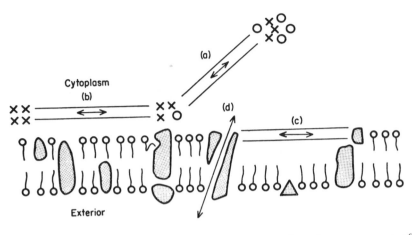

**Figure 31** Function of filamentous proteins in aiding fast movement of molecules through membranes. (a) movement to and away from membrane sites; (b) movement parallel to membrane; (c) movement within one layer of membrane; (d) movement through membrane. Balls and sticks represent lipid molecules; globular structures represent protein molecules; "railroad tracks" represent filamentous proteins; X and O represent cellular molecules and vesicles. Reproduced with permission.[108]

altered by filaments. Figure 31(a) and (b) shows how fast movement of molecules up to and along the membrane could be controlled. There also may be an interaction with globular proteins within the membrane, free to move laterally according to the fluid mosaic membrane theory, thereby affecting molecular movement through the membrane (Figure 31(c)). GTP is required for many microtublar systems to be active. "Contractile activity" of filaments may also open and close membrane pores (Figure 31(d)). This model may also be used to explain how cyclic nucleotides control substrate traffic near intracellular membranes, for instance, mitochondria. In particular, whether this mechanism is operative in the heart cell and whether any effect of insulin is so mediated is unknown, but is certainly of interest.[109]

### E. Conclusion

Plasma membranes in insulin-sensitive tissues contain specific receptors for insulin, in part composed of peptides that face the external surface of the cell. At least in adipose tissue, these receptors have been isolated and are thought to complex with insulin in a simple noncovalent association.

To effect its several actions, insulin generates a "signal" upon complexing with the receptor; each action appears to require a signal of different strength. For the rather immediate and perhaps direct effect on specific ion conductance and membrane transport of amino acids and sugars, insulin need only alter the conformation of its receptor. Amplification of the signal is great and therefore only a small number of insulin receptors must be so changed. In addition, insulin receptors may migrate to cluster near a site of particular stimulation under certain circumstances.

The nature of the signal causing various slower changes in intermediary metabolism is unknown. These anabolic actions include protein synthesis, mediated in part through increased RNA polymerase activity, the initiation of polypeptide chains and enhanced ribosomal aggregation. Also of importance to the ischemic heart, insulin reduces protein catabolism by stabilizing lysosomes.[376]

While insulin may reduce the levels of cyclic AMP in liver and fat cells, there is no evidence that it does so in myocardium. Cyclic GMP has received much attention as a second "second messenger" and it may well be that this or another substance will be identified as a mediator of one or more of insulin's actions.[375, 377, 385]

## VII. INSULIN RESPONSE IN HEART DISEASE

### A. Adrenergic mechanism of insulin release

Epinephrine [162-165] and norepinephrine [166] inhibit the release of insulin in man. While glucagon release appears to be exclusively mediated by a beta-receptor, insulin secretion is regulated by an alpha-,[167-170] and a beta-receptor.[170] For instance, propranolol attenuates the acute insulin response to intravenous glucose.[170a, 170b] Since β-receptor activation is associated with an increase in cyclic AMP levels and α-receptor agonism with a decrease in cyclic AMP levels in other tissues,[171] a similar sequence was suspected in the pancreas.[172] However, recent evidence casts doubt on this hypothesis,[173] and it now appears that epinephrine infusion does in fact cause an initial drop in insulin levels, followed by a recovery phase.[174] Since the early decrease may be blocked by phentolamine and the recovery phase may be delayed by propranolol, recovery of insulin secretion is probably mediated by the β-receptor (Fig. 32).[175] Moreover, the alpha effect is partly a direct suppression of insulin secretion quite independent of the lowering of cyclic AMP levels,[176] possibly mediated by reduced calcium uptake in islet beta cells.[177] These actions may be explained by a two compartment model of insulin secretion in which a small, fast

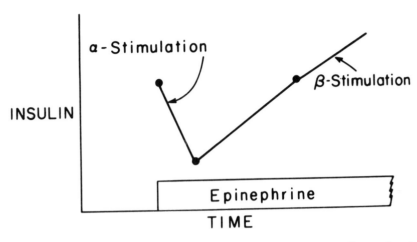

**Figure 32** A schematic explanation for the dual receptor effects of epinephrine on insulin secretion. Reproduced with permission.[175]

storage pool is activated by a sudden change in blood glucose level and a slower, synthesis-dependent pool responds to glucose variation over a longer period of time (Fig. 33).[178, 179] Epinephrine may block insulin output by alpha receptor agonism,[180] while simultaneous activation for both slow and fast pools by the beta receptor account for the catecholamine-effect on insulin secretion.[174, 175, 181, 181a]

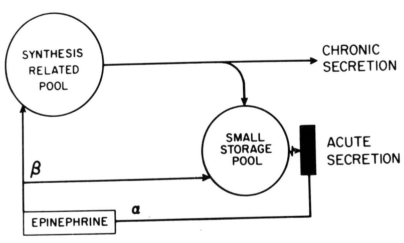

**Figure 33** A proposed two-pool model for insulin secretion, and its interaction with epinephrine. Note dual α-and β-effects on the small storage pool. Reproduced with permission.[175]

Recently the evidence for the presence of a monoaminergic system in the beta cells of the islets was reviewed.[182] Dopamine, serotonin, and norepinephrine are the major monoamines in the islets, which are thought to exert a tonic inhibitory action upon insulin release. An interaction between external insulin secretogogues and an internal beta cell monoaminergic inhibitory system results in insulin secretion.[182]

## B. Nervous regulation of insulin secretion

The autonomic nervous system is critically involved in glucose metabolism,[183] and appears to influence insulin secretion in both the normal and the stressed animal. The suppression and recovery of insulin secretion by administered α and β adrenergic agents was discussed in the above section and is generally accepted.[184, 185] Nonstressed endogenous insulin secretion may be modulated by the sympathetic nervous system, since basal insulin levels change during epinephrine infusion.[182] Since α-blockade raises and β-blockade lowers insulin levels, at least part of basal insulin secretion results from a continuous catecholamine input. This may occur by means of circulating catecholamines or by neurotransmitter release locally in the islets.

Cholinergic drugs and vagal stimulation release insulin, both of which may be blocked by atropine *in vitro* [169, 382] and in laboratory animals.[186, 187] However, no defect in insulin release results from cervical vagotomy in man,[188] and early reports that methacholine stimulated insulin secretion in the dog [189] are unconfirmed in man.[190] On the other hand, the fact that conditioned hypoglycemia could be blocked by atropine or cervical vagotomy suggested a role for the parasympathetic fibers in regulation of insulin secretion.[191] Direct stimulation of the pancreatic nerves was recently shown to increase insulin output.[192] When blocked by atropine, stimulation of the same nerves inhibited glucose-induced insulin release. Thus it appears likely that both the sympathetic and parasympathetic autonomic systems continuously modulate endogenous insulin levels (Fig. 34).[193]

## C. Stress and insulin secretion

An extensive literature confirms that acute stress of different origins activates sympathetic discharge. Under these circumstances, basal insulin levels are lowered but may rebound to normal or above-normal values if the stress is maintained. Teleologically, the associated hyperglycemia, whether from catecholamine-induced hepatic glucose release,[194] direct neural liver stimulation,[195] or mediated by pancreatic glu-

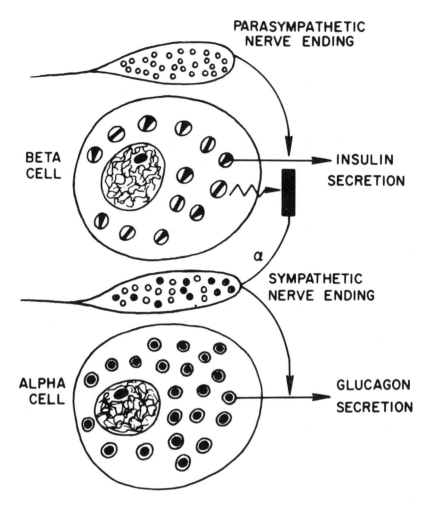

**Figure 34**   Schematic representation of the known neural input to the endocrine pancreas. Reproduced with permission.[175]

cagon[193] as well as by relative insulin deficiency, may have survival value in that glucose is thereby made available to the central nervous system, which is not strongly insulin-responsive. For example, after significant injury [196, 197] with or without shock,[198, 199] carbohydrate intolerance and poor insulin response are related to the extent of tissue damage and shock and are reversible.

In one well-studied experimental model, acute hypoxia in puppies, insulin was lacking in the face of considerable hyperglycemia.[200] Phentolamine reduced the glucose levels in the absence of an insulin response.[201] Other agents, diazoxide and apresoline, which are not alpha blockers but cause vasodilation of similar degree, did not reverse the inhibition of insulin secretion produced by hypothermia.[202] Therefore, diminution in pancreatic blood flow by catecholamines probably was not responsible for the deficient insulin release. When cardiac output is maintained constant, by right heart bypass, insulin secretion is not strongly dependent upon pancreatic blood flow.[203] Hence the predominant influence of the catecholamines is a direct suppression of insulin secretion with the concomitant circulatory changes of secondary importance.[204] This is illustrated on the proposed two-pool model for insulin secretion in Figure 35.

## D. Insulin secretion in heart disease and related systemic metabolic changes

Acute left ventricular power or "pump" failure, as seen after acute myocardial infarction, is accompanied by reflex circulatory changes

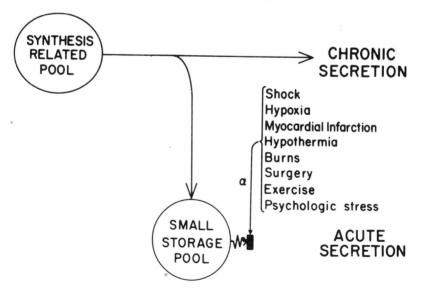

**Figure 35** The effect of stress states on insulin secretion related to a proposed two-pool model for insulin secretion. Reproduced with permission.[175]

that are "compensatory" in the sense that they maintain central aortic pressure.[206] These are mediated by increased sympathetic drive, resulting in vasoconstriction in the "noncritical" cutaneous, splanchnic and renal vascular beds.[207-210] Both the adrenal medulla and the peripheral sympathetic nerve endings release supportive catecholamines, resulting in elevated plasma and urinary levels of catecholamines and their metabolic products.[211-220]

Elevations in the levels of plasma cortisol,[221-225] glucagon, and growth hormone[226] accompany the stress response to decreased cardiac output (Fig. 36). The more severe the hemodynamic insult, the greater the alpha-sympathetic output, and the poorer the prognosis.[227] In fact, the elevations of plasma cortisol and catecholamine levels and the associated free fatty acidemia may all be used to predict the severity of myocardial infarction.[228] The relationship among these reactants is illustrated in Figure 37.

Hyperglycemia is frequently noted in association with low cardiac outputs, especially following acute myocardial infarction.[229-231] While

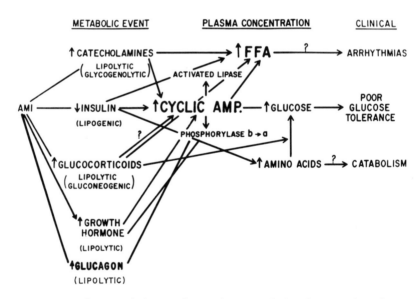

Figure 36   The metabolic markers of myocardial infarction (AMI) are shown. The physiological property of each substance in the first column appears beneath it. For instance, insulin, normally lipogenic, is reduced in amount, thus leading to an increase in free-fatty acid (FFA) content in the blood. Catecholamine levels are increased and their effects—lipolysis and glycogenolysis—are correspondingly enhanced. FFA levels are elevated, which may predispose to the development of arrhythmias.

several hormones with glycogenolytic properties are secreted (Fig. 36), the alpha-adrenergic catecholamine output chiefly accounts for the early hyperglycemia observed. Hepatic glycogen stores are limited, and glucocorticoid-induced gluconeogenesis may also raise plasma glucose levels.[222, 232] However, the persistence of this hyperglycemia led to the suspicion that failure of peripheral glucose uptake was largely responsible. Failure of an insulin response to hyperglycemia or to intravenous tolbutamide was subsequently demonstrated [231, 233] and the suppression of insulin secretion correlated with the severity of left ventricular power failure. Severe hyperglycemia and low insulin levels were also observed in infants undergoing hypothermic cardiovascular surgery.[234] In general, cardiovascular surgery may be associated with early complete suppression of the insulin response to glucose.[235-238] Since glucose was regularly infused during these procedures, severe hyperglycemia and osmotically-induced hyponatremia were reported, especially in association with hypothermia.[239-241] These changes spontaneously reversed after surgery and the resultant insulin rebound raised cellular glucose and potassium uptake to the extent that arrhythmias were precipitated.[235, 242] Thus, whether the low cardiac output syndrome results from open-heart surgery,[243] acute myocardial infarction,[231] or chronic heart failure due to rheumatic heart disease,[244] insulin

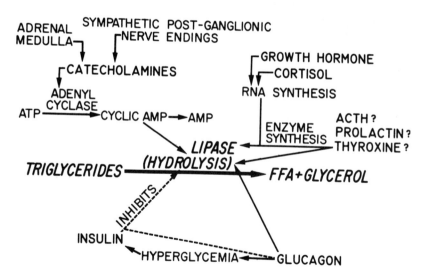

**Figure 37**  The interrelationship between cortisol, FFA, and catecholamines is diagrammatically shown. Reproduced with permission from Prakash et al.[228] Copyright 1972, American Heart Association, Inc.

secretion is depressed and is quantitatively related to the extent of hemodynamic abnormality.[245, 246]

The observed recovery of insulin secretion, as the patient with a low cardiac output improves, has been explained by invoking the inhibition of epinephrine actions by digitalis.[247] However, this has not been confirmed in man to date.[248]

Two mechanisms for insulin suppression have been suggested: reduced pancreatic blood flow and increased sympathetic activity, including elevations in levels of circulating catecholamines. While pancreatic blood flow may be compromised when cardiac output is reduced, the data presently available indicate that pancreatic blood flow *in vivo* is not an important determinant of insulin secretion.[203, 204] However, the experimental and clinical evidence that the catecholamine response to low cardiac output may account for suppressed insulin release is considerable. Therefore, considering the data cited above, it appears reasonable to attribute the hyperglycemia of low cardiac output states to augmented adrenergic drive and reduced insulin release. Presumably the catecholamines affect the islet alpha cells directly (Fig. 35).

### E. Significance of reduced insulin secretion in heart disease

The ischemic myocyte is dependent upon anaerobic pathways to provide ATP, and its survival is a direct function of glucose utilization.[249-251, 260] This anaerobic alternative method of energy production is activated in the ischemic heart,[45, 252, 253] although submaximally,[259] but even when optimal cannot meet the ATP needs of the normally contracting mammalian heart. However, the extent of glycolytic glucose metabolism depends upon adequate glucose transport into the cell and an increased rate of phosphorylation.[254] Adenosine di- and monophosphate and inorganic phosphate accumulate intracellularly and may increase the rate of glucose phosphorylation.[255-257] However, the transport of glucose into the myocyte is critically insulin-dependent.[254, 258] Under these conditions, insulin-lack may deprive the heart of intracellular glucose concentrations, even more important during anaerobic metabolism, and reduce energy available in the form of ATP.

## VIII. CONCLUSION

Insulin has many actions on cell metabolism and may independently and directly influence ion transport while effecting additional changes in intermediary metabolism. Insulin accelerates the "carrier-mediated" transport of glucose passively and hence only hastens equilibration of intracellular and extracellular glucose concentrations. Facilitated glucose transport is a rate-limiting step in glucose utilization. Amino acid transport is active, is coupled in some instances to sodium transport, and leads to amino acid accumulation against an electrochemical gradient. The importance of augmented transmembrane amino acid transport as mediator of insulin's stimulatory affect on polypeptide synthesis is unknown. At present, there is no convincing evidence that such a role is of major consequence.

Insulin alters the rates of many reactions in its target cells. Binding of insulin to cell membranes is specific, of high affinity, stereospecific, selective, and reversible. Few insulin molecules are able to exert significant actions over a considerable tissue area, *i.e.*, the amplification of the system is high. Some intracellular actions of insulin may be mediated by lowered levels of cyclic adenylate in adipose tissue, either a result of stimulated membrane-bound phosphodiesterase and/or inhibition of adenyl cyclase, but this is not true in the heart.

Insulin hyperpolarizes membranes and the changes in ionic permeability caused by insulin are probably due to a direct membrane interaction, involving the formation of a simple noncovalent association between insulin and its receptor.

The importance of insulin in heart disease has been recently underscored by the realization that the failing heart is highly dependent on glucose for its energy needs and the finding that insulin release is compromised as the cardiac index is reduced. Increased alpha adrenergic drive associated with left ventricular "power" failure and elevated levels of circulating catecholamines directly reduces insulin secretion in the alpha cells of the pancreas, only partially mediated through lowered pancreatic cyclic AMP levels. Inhibition of insulin release and lack of its effect in the myocardium may preclude maximal energy production and further reduce heart performance.

## References

1. Goulston, A.: West Indian cane sugar in the treatment of certain forms of heart diseases. *Brit Med J* **2**:693-695, 1912.
2. Budingen, T.: Ueber die Moeglichkeit einer Ernaehrungs behandlung des Herzmuskels durch Einbringen von Tranbenzuckerlasungen in den grossen Kreislaug. *Dt Arch Klin Med* **114**:534-579, 1914.
3. Pick, E. P.: Ueber das primum und ultimum morieus rin Herzen. *Klin Wochenschrift* **3**:662-667, 1924.
4. Loeper, M., Lemaine, A., Degos, R.: L'insulin dans la nutrition du coeur des cardiaques. *Presse Medicale* **38**:1361-1363, 1930.
5. Osato, S.: Ueber die Wirkung von insulin-glucose auf nicht diabetische Schwere Krankheitszustande. *Z Exp Med* **51**:488-496, 1926.

6. Rimbaud, L., Balmes, A., Anselne-Martin, G.: L'association sucre-insuline en therapeutique cardiaque. *Presse Med* **39**:1647-1650, 1931.

7. Wiener, J.: L'insulinotherapie dans les affections cardiaques. *Bruxelles-Medical* **8**:188-191, 1932.

8. Shirley-Smith, K.: Insulin and glucose in the treatment of heart disease. *Brit Med J* **1**:1-8, 1933.

9. Kones, R. J., Phillips, J. H.: Glucagon-present status in cardiovascular disease. *Clin Pharm Ther* **12**:427-444, 1971.

10. Vance, J. E., Buchanan, K. D., Challoner, D. R., et al.: Effect of glucose concentration on insulin and glucagon release from isolated islets of Langerhans of the rat. *Diabetes* **17**:187-193, 1968.

11. Williams, R. H., Ensick, J. W.: Secretion rates and actions of insulin and related products. *Diabetes* **15**:623-654, 1966.

12. Aschcroft, S. J. H., Randle, P. J.: Glucose metabolism and insulin release by pancreatic islets. *Lancet* **1**:278-279, 1968.

13. Seltzer, H. S.: Quantitative effects of glucose, sulfonylureas, salicylate and indole-3-acetic acid on the secretion of insulin activity into pancreatic venous blood. *J Clin Invest* **41**:289-300, 1962.

14. Montagne, W., Howell, S. L., Taylor, K. W.: Pentitols and the mechanism of insulin release. *Nature* **215**:1088-1089, 1967.

15. Greenberger, N. J., Tzagournis, N., Graves, T. N.: Stimulation of insulin secretion in man by medium chain triglycerides. *Metabolism* **17**:796-801, 1968.

16. Fajans, S. S., Floyd, J. C., Knopf, R. F., et al.: A difference in mechanism by which leucine and other amino acids induce insulin release. *J Clin Endocrinol* **27**:1600-1606, 1967.

17. Floyd, J. C., Fajans, S. S., Conn, J. W., et al.: Insulin secretion in response to protein ingestion. *J Clin Invest* **45**:1479-1486, 1966.

18. Lefebre, P., Unger, R. M.: *Glucagon.* Pergamon Press, New York, 1972.

19. Unger, R. H., Ohneda, A., Valverde, I., et al.: Characterization of the responses of circulating glucagon-like immuno-reactivity to intraduodenal and intravenous administration of glucose. *J Clin Invest* **47**:48-55, 1968.

20. Jarrett, R. J., Cohen, N. M.: Intestinal hormones and plasma-insulin—Some observations on glucagon, secretion and gastrin. *Lancet* **2**:861-863, 1967.

21. Deckert, T.: Stimulation of insulin secretion by glucagon and secretin. *Acta Endocrinol* **57**:578-584, 1968.

22. Kones, R. J., Phillips, J. H.: Glucagon in congestive heart failure. *Chest* **59**:392-397, 1971.

23. Kones, R. J., Dombeck, D. H., Phillips, J. H.: Glucagon in cardiogenic shock. *Angiology* **23**:525-535, 1972.

24. Kones, R. J.: Glucagon: a new agent for the treatment of low cardiac output syndromes. *Jap Heart J* **13**:266-271, 1972.

25. Arnould, Y., Cantraine, F., Ooms, H. A., et al.: Kinetics of plasma disappearance of labelled iodoinsulins following intravenous injections. *Arch Int Pharmacodyn* **166**:225-237, 1967.

25a. Sherwin, R. S., Kramer, K. J., Tobin, J. D., et al.: A model of the kinetics of insulin in man. *J Clin Invest* **53**:1741-1792, 1974.

26. Stimmler, L.: Disappearance of immunoreactive insulin in normal and adult-onset diabetic subjects. *Diabetes* **16**:652-655, 1967.

27. Rubenstein, A. H., Lowry, C., Welborn, T. A., et al.: Urine insulin in normal subjects. *Metabolism* **16**:234-244, 1967.

28. Spitz, I. M., Rubenstein, A. H., Bersohn, L., et al.: Urine insulin in renal disease. *J Lab Clin Med* **75**:998-1005, 1970.

29. Kones, R. J.: Topics in biological transport. I. Ionic and particular diffusion. *J Mol Cell Cardiol* **3**:179-192, 1971.

30. Danielli, J. F.: The present position in the field of facilitated diffusion and selective active transport. *Proc Symp Colston Res Soc* **7**:1-4, 1954.
31. Morgan, H. E., Regen, D. M., Park, C. R.: Identification of a mobile carrier-mediated sugar transport in muscle. *J Biol Chem* **239**:369-374, 1964.
32. Park, C. R., Morgan, H. E., Henderson, M. J., et al.: Hormones and organic metabolism. V. The regulation of glucose uptake in muscle as studied in the perfused rat heart. *Recent Progr Hormone Res* **17**:493-538, 1961.
33. Henderson, M. J.: Uptake of glucose into cells and the role of insulin in glucose transport. *Can J Biochem* **42**:933-944, 1964.
34. Wilbrandt, W., Rosenberg, T.: The concept of carrier transport and its corollaries in pharmacology. *Pharm Rev* **13**:109-183, 1961.
35. LeFevre, P. G.: Evidence of active transfer of certain nonelectrolytes across the human red cell membrane. *J Gen Physiol* **31**:505-527, 1948.
36. Rosenberg, T., Wilbrandt, W.: Uphill transport induced by counterflow. *J Gen Physiol* **41**:289-296, 1957.
37. Kones, R. J.: Topics in biological transport. III. Active and coupled transport, facilitated diffusion, bulk transport (pinocytosis) and the Law of the Capillary. In preparation.
37a. Singer, S. J.: Architecture and topography of biologic membranes. *Hosp Practice* **8**:81-90 (May), 1973.
37b. Singer, S. J.: The molecular organization of biological membranes, in *Structure and Function of Biological Membranes,* edited by Rothfield, L. I., Academic Press, New York, 1971, pp. 145-222.
37c. Singer, S. J., Nicolson, G. L.: The fluid mosaic model of the structure of cell membranes. *Science* **175**:720-731, 1972.
38. Britton, H. G.: Induced uphill and downhill transport: relationship to the Ossing criterion. *Nature* **198**:190-191, 1966.
39. Mitchell, P.: Reversible coupling between transport and chemical reactions, in *Membranes and Ion Transport,* edited by Bittar, E. E., John Wiley & Sons, New York, Vol. 1, 1970, pp. 192-256.
40. Davis, R. P.: Biochemical and metabolic aspects of transport, in *Biological Membranes,* edited by Dowben, R. M., Little Brown & Co., Boston, 1969, pp. 109-156.
41. Park, C. R., Reinwein, D., Henderson, M. J., et al.: The action of insulin in the transport of glucose through the cell membrane. *Amer J Med* **26**: 674-684, 1959.
42. Battaglia, F. C., Randle, P. J.: Regulation of glucose uptake by muscle. The specificity of monosaccharide-transport systems in rat-diaphragm muscle. *Biochem J* **75**:408-416, 1960.
43. LeFevre, P. G.: Sugar transport in the red blood cell: Structure-activity relationships in substrates and antagonists. *Pharmacol Rev* **13**:39-70, 1961.
44. Lundsgaard, E.: On the mode of action of insulin. *Uppsala Lokareforen Forh* **45**:143-152, 1939.
45. Morgan, H. E., Henderson, M. J., Regen, D. M., et al.: Regulation of glucose uptake in muscle. I. The effects of insulin and anoxia on glucose transport and phosphorylation in the isolated perfused heart of normal rats. *J Biol Chem* **236**:253-261, 1961.
46. Kones, R. J.: Metabolism of the acutely ischemic and hypoxic heart. *Crit Care Med* **1**:321-330, 1973.
47. Park, C. R., Johnson, L. H.: Effect of insulin on transport of glucose and galactose into cells of rat muscle and brain. *Amer J Physiol* **182**:17-23, 1955.
48. Park, C. R., Post, R. L., Kalman, C. F., et al.: The transport of glucose and other sugars across cell membranes and the effect of insulin, in *Ciba Foundation Colloquia on Endocrinology, Internal Secretions of the Pancreas,* edited

by Wolstenholme, G. E. W., O'Connor, C. M., Little Brown, Boston, 1956, Vol. 9, pp. 240-260.

49. Morgan, H. E., Cadenas, E., Regen, D. M., et al.: Regulation of glucose uptake in muscle. II. Rate-limiting steps and effects of insulin and anoxia in heart muscle from diabetic rats. *J Biol Chem* **236**:262-272, 1961.

50. Post, R. L., Morgan, H. E., Park, C. R.: Regulation of glucose uptake in muscle. III. The interaction of membrane transport and phosphorylation in the control of glucose uptake. *J Biol Chem* **236**:269-272, 1961.

51. Narahara, H. T., Ozand, P.: Studies of tissue permeability. IX. The effect of insulin on the penetration of 3-methylglucose-H[3] in frog muscle. *J Biol Chem* **238**:40-49, 1963.

52. Henderson, M. J., Morgan, H. E., Park, C. R.: Regulation of glucose uptake in muscle. V. The effect of growth hormone on glucose transport in the isolated perfused rat heart. *J Biol Chem* **236**:2157-2161, 1961.

53. Manchester, K. L., Randle, P. J., Young, F. B.: The effect of growth hormone and of cortisol on the response of isolated rat diaphragm to the stimulating effect of insulin on glucose uptake and on incorporation of amino acids into protein. *J Endocrinol* **18**:395-408, 1959.

54. Hjalmarson, A.: Influence of growth hormone on the sensitivity of rat diaphragm to insulin. *Acta Endocrinol* **57** (suppl) **126**:49-60, 1968.

55. Morgan, H. E., Neely, J. R., Wood, R. E., et al.: Factors affecting glucose transport in heart muscle and erythrocytes. *Fed Proc* **24**:1040-1045, 1965.

56. Henderson, M. J., Morgan, H. E., Park, C. R.: Regulation of glucose uptake in muscle. IV. The effect of hypophysectomy on glucose transport, phosphorylation, and insulin sensitivity in the isolated, perfused heart. *J Biol Chem* **236**:273-277, 1961.

57. Helmreich, E., Cori, C. F.: Studies of tissue permeability. II. The distribution of pentoses between plasma and muscle. *J Biol Chem* **224**:663-679, 1957.

58. Morgan, H. E., Randle, P. J., Regen, D. M.: Regulation of glucose uptake by muscle. 3. The effect of insulin anoxia, salicylate, and 2:4 dinitrophenol on membrane transport and intracellular phosphorylation of glucose in the isolated rat heart. *Biochem J* **73**:573-579, 1959.

59. Neely, J. R., Liebermeister, H., Morgan, H. E.: Effect of pressure development on membrane transport of glucose in isolated rat heart. *Amer J Physiol* **212**:815-822, 1967.

60. Neely, J. R., Bowman, R. H., Morgan, H. E.: Effects of ventricular pressure development and palmitate on glucose transport. *Amer J Physiol* **216**:804-811, 1969.

61. Christensen, H. N.: Free amino acids and peptides in tissues, in *Mammalian Protein Metabolism*, edited by Munro, H. N., Academic Press, New York, 1964, Vol. 1, pp. 105-124.

62. Oxender, D. L., Christensen, H. N.: Transcellular concentration as a consequence of intracellular accumulation. *J Biol Chem* **234**:2321-2324, 1959.

63. Begin, N., Scholefield, P. G.: The uptake of amino acids by mouse pancreas in vitro. II. The specificity of the carrier systems. *J Biol Chem* **240**:332-337, 1965.

64. Vidaver, G. A., Romain, L. F., Haurowitz, F.: Some studies on the specificity of amino acid entry routes in pigeon erythrocytes. *Arch Biochem Biophys* **107**:82-87, 1964.

65. Riggs, T. R., Walker, L. M., Christensen, H. N.: Potassium migration and amino acid transport. *J Biol Chem* **233**:1479-1484, 1958.

66. Kipnis, D. M., Parrish, J. E.: Role of Na$^+$ and K$^+$ on sugar (2-deoxglucose) and amino acid ($\alpha$-aminoisobutyric acid) transport in striated muscle. *Fed Proc* **24**:1051-1059, 1965.

67. Christensen, H. N.: Linked ion and amino acid transport, in *Membranes and Ion Transport* edited by Bittar, E. E., Wiley-Interscience, New York, 1970, Vol. 1, pp. 365-394.
68. Christensen, H. N.: Amino acid transport and nutrition. *Fed Proc* **22**:1110-1114, 1963.
69. Christensen, H. N.: Concept of the reactive site in biological transport, in *Physical Principles of Biological Membrane* edited by Snell, F., Walken, J., Iverson, G., et al., Gordan and Breach, New York, 1970, pp. 397-416.
70. Christensen, H. N.: Introduction. *FEBS Symposium*, Academic Press, London, **20**:81-85, 1970.
71. Sinex, F. M., MacMullen, J., Hastings, A. B.: The effect of insulin on the incorporation of C¹⁴ into protein of rat diaphragm. *J Biol Chem* **198**:615-619, 1952.
72. Manchester, K. L., Wool, I. G.: Insulin and incorporation of amino acids into protein of muscle. 2. Accumulation and incorporation studies with the perfused rat heart. *Biochem J* **89**:202-209, 1963.
73. Manchester, K. L.: The control by insulin of amino acid accumulation in muscle. *Biochem J* **117**:457-465, 1970.
74. Scharff, R., Wool, I. G.: Accumulation of amino acids in muscle of perfused rat heart. Effects of insulin in the presence of puromycin. *Biochem J* **97**:272-276, 1965.
75. Morgan, H. E., Earl, D. C. N., Broadus, A., et al.: Regulation of protein synthesis in heart muscle. I. Effect of amino acids on protein synthesis. *J Biol Chem* **246**:2152-2162, 1971.
76. Rennels, D. E., Jefferson, L. S., Hjalmarson, A. C., et al.: Maintenence of protein synthesis in hearts of diabetic animals. *Biochem Biophys Res Commun* **40**:1110-1116, 1970.
77. Morgan, H. E., Jefferson, L. S., Wolpert, E. B., et al.: Regulation of protein synthesis in muscle. II. Effects of amino acid levels and insulin on ribosomal aggregation. *J Biol Chem* **246**:2163-2170, 1971.
78. Wool, I. G., Castles, J. J., Leader, D. P., et al.: Insulin and the function of muscle ribosomes, in *Handbook of Physiology, Endocrinology*, edited by Greep, R. D., Astwood, E. B., Steiner, D. F., et al., American Physiological Society, Washington, D.C., 1972, Section 7, Vol. 1, pp. 385-394.
79. Gross, N. J., Getz, G. S., Rabinowitz, M.: Apparent turnover of mitochondrial deoxyribonucleic acid and mitochondrial phospholipids in the tissues of the rat. *J Biol Chem* **244**:1552-1562, 1969.
80. Rabinowitz, M., Aschenbrenner, V., Albin, R., et al.: Synthesis and turnover of heart mitochondria in normal, hypertrophied, and hypoxic heart, in *Cardiac Hypertrophy*, edited by Alpert, N. R., Academic Press, New York, 1971, pp. 283-299.
80a. Gibson, K., Harris, P.: Aminoacyl-t RNA synthetase activities specific to twenty amino acids in rat, rabbit and human myocardium. *J Mol Cell Cardiol* **5**:419-425, 1973.
80b. Rothschild, M. A., Schreiber, S. S., Oraty, M.: Hepatic and cardiac protein synthesis. *N Y State J Med* **73**:2887-2890, 1973.
81. Zak, R., Rabinowitz, M.: Metabolism of the ischemic heart. *Med Clin NA* **57**:93-103, 1973.
82. Morkin, E., Kimata, S., Skillman, J. J.: Myosin synthesis and degradation during development of cardiac hypertrophy. *Circ Res* **30**:690-702, 1972.
83. Rabinowitz, M.: Protein synthesis and turnover in normal and hypertrophied heart. *Amer J Cardiol* **31**:202-210, 1972.
83a. Rabinowitz, M.: Control of metabolism and synthesis of macromolecules in the normal and ischemic heart. *J Mol Cell Cardiol* **2**:277-292, 1971.
84. Aschenbrenner, V., Druyan, R., Albin, R., et al.: Heme *a*, cytochrome *c*

and total protein turnover in mitochondria from rat heart and liver. *Biochem J* **119**:157-160, 1970.

85. Nair, K. G., Cutilletta, A. F., Zak, R., et al.: Biochemical correlates of cardiac hypertrophy. I. Experimental model: changes in heart weight, RNA content, and nuclear RNA polymerase activity. *Circ Res* **23**:451-462, 1968.

86. Fanburg, B. L.: Experimental cardiac hypertrophy. *New Eng J Med* **282**: 723-732, 1970.

87. Rabinowitz, M., Zak, R.: Biochemical and cellular changes in cardiac hypertrophy. *Ann Rev Med* **23**:245-262, 1972.

88. Gudbjarnason, S., DeSchryver, C., Chiba, C., et al.: Protein and nucleic acid synthesis during the reparative processes following myocardial infarction. *Circ Res* **15**:320-326, 1964.

89. Lochner, A., Brunk, A. J., Brink, A., et al.: Protein synthesis in myocardial ischemia and infarction. *J Mol Cell Cardiol* **3**:1-14, 1971.

89a. Lochner, A., Brink, A., Bestler, A. J.: Nucleic acid synthesis in myocardial ischemia and infarction. *J Mol Cell Cardiol* **5**:301-309, 1973.

90. Albin, R., Aschenbrenner, V., Rabinowitz, M.: Increased turnover of mitochondrial constituents in cardiac hypertrophy and acute hypoxia in the rat. *J Clin Invest* **49**:2A, 1970.

91. Aschenbrenner, V., Zak, R., Rabinowitz, M.: Effect of hypoxia on the turnover of mitochondrial components in rat cardiac muscle. *Amer J Physiol* **221**:1418-1425, 1971.

92. Regan, T. J., Frank, M. J., Lehan, P. H., et al.: Relationship of insulin and strophanthidin to myocardial metabolism and function. *Amer J Physiol* **205**: 790-794, 1963.

93. Hazlewood, C. F., Zierler, K. L.: Insulin-induced hyperpolarization of skeletal muscle from normal and from hypophesectomized rats. *Johns Hopkins Med J* **121**:188-193, 1967.

94. Zierler, K. L.: Effect of insulin on membrane potential and potassium content of rat muscle. *Amer J Physiol* **197**:515-523, 1959.

95. Zierler, K. L.: Increase in resting membrane potential of skeletal muscle produced by insulin. *Science* **126**:1067-1068, 1957.

96. Zierler, K. L.: Hyperpolarization of muscle by insulin in a glucose free environment. *Amer J Physiol* **197**:524-526, 1959.

97. Zierler, K. L., Rogus, E., Hazlewood, C. F.: Effect of insulin on potassium flux and water and electrolyte content of muscles from normal and from hypophysectomized rats. *J Gen Physiol* **49**:433-456, 1966.

98. Ussing, H. H.: The distinction by means of tracers between active transport and diffusion. *Acta Physiol Scand* **19**:43-56, 1950.

99. Hoshiko, T., Lindley, B. D.: Macroscopic definition of ideal behavior of tracers. *J Theoret Biol* **26**:315-320, 1970.

100. Kedem, O., Essio, A.: Isotope flows and flux ratios in biological membranes. *J Gen Physiol* **48**:1047-1070, 1965.

101. Keynes, R. D.: The ionic movements during nervous activity. *J Physiol* **114**:119-150, 1951.

102. Zierler, K. L.: Effect of insulin on potassium efflux from rat muscle in the presence and absence of glucose. *Amer J Physiol* **198**:1066-1070, 1960.

103. Gourley, D. R. H.: Effect of insulin on potassium exchange in normal and ouabain-treated skeletal muscle. *J Pharmacol Exp Ther* **148**:339-347, 1965.

104. Creese, R.: Sodium exchange in rat muscle. *Nature* **201**:505-506, 1964.

105. Creese, R.: Sodium fluxes in diaphragm muscle and the effects of insulin and serum proteins. *J Physiol* **197**:255-278, 1968.

106. Kernan, R. P.: The role of lactate in the active excretion of sodium by frog muscle. *J Physiol* **162**:129-137, 1962.

107. Moore, R. D.: The ionic effects of insulin. *Abstr, 9th Biophys Soc Ann Meeting,* San Francisco, 1965, p. 122.

108. Bittar, E. E.: Insulin and the sodium pump of the Maia muscle fiber. *Nature* 214:726-727, 1967.

109. Ussing, H. H., Zeralin, K.: Active transport of sodium as the source of electric current in the short-circuited isolated frog skin. *Acta Physiol Scand* 23:110-127, 1951.

110. Herrera, F. C.: Effect of insulin on short-circuit current and sodium transport across toad urinary bladder. *Amer J Physiol* 209:819-824, 1965.

111. Herrera, F. C., Whittenbury, G., Planchart, A.: Effect of insulin on short-circuit current across isolated frog skin in the presence of calcium and magnesium. *Biochem Biophys Acta* 66:170-172, 1963.

112. Andre, R., Crabbe, J.: Stimulation by insulin of active sodium transport by toad skin: influence of aldosterone and vasopressin. *Arch Intern Physiol Biochem* 74:538-540, 1966.

113. Bittar, E. E.: Regulation of ion transport by hormones, in *Membranes and Ion Transport,* edited by Bittar, E. E., Wiley-Interscience, New York, 1971, Vol. 3, pp. 297-316.

114. Bittar, E. E., Dick, D. A. T., Fry, D. J.: Action of insulin on sodium efflux from the toad oocyte. *Nature* 217:1280-1281, 1968.

115. Rogus, E., Price, T., Zierler, K. L.: Sodium plus potassium-activated, ouabain-inhibited adenosine trophosphatase from a fraction of rat skeletal muscle, and lack of insulin effect on it. *J Gen Physiol* 54:188-202, 1969.

115a. Hadden, J. W., Hadden, E. M., Wilson, E. E., et al.: Direct action of insulin on plasma membrane ATPase activity in human lymphocytes. *Nature New Biol* 235:174-177, 1972.

115b. Brodal, B. P., Jebens, E., Oy, V., et al.: Effect of insulin on (Na+, K+)-activated adenosine triphosphatase activity in rat muscle sarcolemma. *Nature* 249:41-43, 1974.

116. Skou, J. C.: Enzymatic basis for active transport of Na+ and K+ across cell membrane. *Physiol Rev* 45:596-617, 1965.

117. Zierler, K. L.: Insulin, ions, and membrane potentials, in *Handbook of Physiology, Endocrinology,* edited by Greep, R. O., Astwood, E. B., Steiner, D. F., et al., American Physiological Society, Washington, D.C., 1972, Section 7, Vol. 1, pp. 347-368.

118. Changeux, J.-P., Thiery, J., Tuno, Y., et al.: On the cooperativity of biological membranes. *Proc Natl Acad Sci USA* 57:335-341, 1967.

119. Kones, R. J.: The ionic and molecular basis of altered myocardial contractility. *Res Commun Chem Path Pharmacol* 5 (suppl 1): 1-84, 1973.

120. Butcher, R. W., Robinson, G. A., Sutherland, E. W.: Cyclic AMP and hormone action, in *Biochemical Actions of Hormones,* edited by Litwack, G., Academic Press, New York, 1972, Vol. 2, pp. 21-54.

120a. Cuatrecasas, P.: Membrane receptors. *Ann Rev Biochem* 43:169-214, 1974.

121. Epstein, S. E., Skelton, C. L., Levey, G. S., et al.: Adenyl cyclase and myocardial contractility. *Ann Int Med* 72:561-578, 1970.

122. Rasmussen, H., Tenenhouse, A.: Parathyroid hormone and calcitouin, in *Biochemical Actions of Hormones,* edited by Litwack, G., Academic Press, New York, 1970, Vol. 1, pp. 365-413.

123. Grahame-Smith, D. G., Butcher, R. W., Ney, R. L., et al.: Adenosine 3',5'-monophosphate as the intracellular mediator of the action of adrenocorticotropic hormone on the adrenal cortex. *J Biol Chem* 242:5535-5538, 1967.

124. Beck, N. P., Field, J. B., Davis, B.: Effect of prostaglandin E, (PGE$_1$), chlorpropamide (CPM) and vasopressin (VP) on cyclic 3',5' adenosine monophosphate (CAMP) in renal medulla of rats. *Clin Res* 18:494, 1970.

125. Bourne, H., Melmon, K.: Beta-adrenergic receptors control synthesis of cyclic AMP in human leukocytes. *Clin Res* **19**:178, 1971.

126. Singer, J. J., Goldberg, A. L.: Cyclic AMP and transmission at the neuromuscular junction, in *Role of Cyclic AMP in Cell Function*, edited by Greengard, P., Costa, E., New York, Raven Press, 1970, pp. 335-348.

127. Goldstein, R. E., Skelton, C. L., Levey, G. S., et al.: Effects of glucagon on contractility and adenyl cyclase activity of human papillary muscles. *Circulation* **42**:III-158, 1970.

128. Kono, T.: Destruction and restoration of the insulin effector of isolated fat cells. *J Biol Chem* **244**:5777-5784, 1969.

129. Rodbell, M., Birnbaumer, L., Pohl, S. L.: Adenyl cyclase in fat cells. III. Stimulation by secretion and the effects of trypsin on the receptors for lipolytic hormones. *J Biol Chem* **245**:718-722, 1970.

130. Birnbaumer, L., Rodbell, M.: Adenyl cyclase in fat cells. II. Hormone receptors. *J Biol Chem* **244**:3477-3482, 1969.

131. Bitensky, M. W., Russell, V., Blanco, M.: Independent variation of glucagon and epinephrine responsive components of hepatic adenyl cyclase as a function of age, sex, and steroid hormones. *Endocrinol* **86**:154-159, 1970.

132. Bitensky, M. W., Russell, V., Robertson, W.: Evidence for separate epinephrine and glucagon responsive adenyl cyclase systems in rat liver. *Biochem Biophys Res Comm* **31**:706-712, 1968.

133. Krebs, E. G., DeLange, R. J., Kemp, R. G., et al.: Activation of skeletal muscle phosphorylase. *Pharmacol Rev* **18**:163-171, 1966.

134. Walsh, D. A., Parkins, J. P., Krebs, E. G.: An adenosine 3',5'-monophosphate-dependent protein kinase from rabbit skeletal muscle. *J Biol Chem* **243**:3763-3774, 1968.

135. Larner, J., Villar-Palasi, C., Goldberg, N., et al.: Hormonal and nonhormonal control of glycogen synthesis control of transferase I kinase. *Adv Enzyme Reg* **6**:409-423, 1968.

136. Sobel, B. E., Mayer, S. E.: Cyclic adenosine monophosphate and cardiac contractility. *Circ Res* **32**:407-414, 1973.

137. Erlichman, J., Hirsch, A. H., Rosen, O. M.: Interconversion of cyclic nucleotide-activated and cyclic nucleotide-independent forms of a protein kinase from beef heart. *Proc Nat Acad Sci USA* **68**:731-735, 1971.

138. Katz, A. M., Repke, D. I.: Calcium-membrane interactions in the myocardium: effects of ouabain, epinephrine, and 3',5'-cyclic adenosine monophosphate. *Amer J Cardiol* **31**:193-201, 1973.

139. Pastan, I.: Cyclic AMP. *Scientific Amer* **227**:97-104 (Aug), 1972.

140. Cheung, W. Y.: Adenosine 3',5'-monophosphate: on its mechanism of action. *Persp Biol Med* **15**:221-235, 1972.

141. Rizack, M. A.: Activation of an epinephrine-sensitive lipolytic activity from adipose tissue by adenosine 3',5'-phosphate. *J Biol Chem* **239**:392-395, 1964.

142. Butcher, R. W., Baird, C. E., Sutherland, E. W.: Effects of lipolytic and antilipolytic substances on adenosine 3',5'-monophosphate levels in isolated fat cells. *J Biol Chem* **243**:1705-1712, 1968.

143. Butcher, R. W., Sneyd, J. G. T., Park, C. R., et al.: Effect of insulin on adenosine 3',5'-monophosphate in the rat epididymal fat pad. *J Biol Chem* **24**:1651-1653, 1966.

144. Robison, G. A., Park, C. R.: Cyclic adenylate in mammalian tissues, in *Diabetes Mellitus: Theory and Practice*, edited by Ellenberg, M., Rifkin, H., McGraw-Hill Book Co., New York, 1970, pp. 132-149.

144a. Robison, G. A., Butcher, R. W., Sutherland, E. W.: *Cyclic AMP*, Academic Press, New York, 1971, pp. 171, 174, 183.

145. Jringas, R. L.: Role of cyclic 3',5'-AMP in the response of adipose tissue to insulin. *Proc Natl Acad Sci USA* **56**:757-763, 1966.
146. Blecher, M., Merlino, N. S., Ro'Ane, J. T.: Control of the metabolism and lipolytic effects of cyclic 3',5'-adenosine monophosphate in adipose tissue by insulin, methyl xanthines, and nicotinic acid. *J Biol Chem* **243**:3973-3977, 1968.
147. Muller-Oerlinghausen, B., Schwab, U., Hasselblatt, A., et al.: Activity of cyclic 3',5'-AMP phosphodiesterase in liver and adipose tissue of normal and diabetic rats. *Life Sci* **7**:593-598, 1968.
148. Jefferson, L. S., Exton, J. H., Butcher, R. W., et al.: Role of adenosine 3',5'-monophosphate in the effects of insulin and anti-insulin serum on liver metabolism. *J Biol Chem* **243**:1031-1038, 1968.
149. Exton, J. M., Jefferson, L. S., Butcher, R. W.: Gluconeogenesis in the perfused liver: the effects of fasting, alloxan diabetes, glucagon, epinephrine, adenosine 3',5'-monophosphate and insulin. *Am J Med* **40**:709-715, 1966.
150. Exton, J. H., and Park, C. R.: The role of cyclic AMP in the control of liver metabolism. *Advan Enzyme Regulation* **6**:391-407, 1968.
151. Bishop, J. S., and Larner, J.: Rapid activation inactivation of liver uridine diphosphate glucose-glycogen transferase and phosphorylase by insulin and glucagon in vivo. *J Biol Chem* **242**:1354-1356, 1967.
152. DeWulf, H., and Hers, H. G.: The stimulation of glycogen synthesis and of glycogen synthetase in the liver by glucocorticoids. *European J Biochem* **6**:552-557, 1968.
153. Exton, J. H., Lewis, S. B., Ho, R. J., et al.: The role of cyclic AMP in the interaction of glucagon and insulin in the control of liver metabolism. *Ann NY Acad Sci* **185**:85-100, 1971.
154. Villar-Palasi, C., and Wenger, J. I.: In vivo effect of insulin on muscle glycogen synthetase: identification of the action pathway. *Federation Proc* **26**:563, 1967.
155. Villar-Palasi, C., Larner, J., Shen, L. C.: Glycogen metabolism and the mechanism of action of cyclic AMP. *Ann NY Acad Sci* **185**:74-84, 1971.
156. Goldberg, N. D., Villar-Palasi, C., Sasko, H., et al.: Effects of insulin treatment on muscle 3',5'-cyclic adenylate levels in vivo and in vitro. *Biochem Biophys Acta* **148**:665-671, 1967.
157. Robison, G. A., Butcher, R. W., Sutherland, E. W.: *Cyclic AMP*, Academic Press, New York, 1971, pp. 271-278.
158. Morgan, H. E., Whitfield, C. F., Neely, J. R.: Regulation of glucose transport in heart muscle and erythrocytes, in *The Role of Membranes in Metabolic Regulation*, edited by Mehlman, M. A., Hanson, R. W., Academic Press, New York, 1972, pp. 133-148.
159. Park, C. R., Crofford, O. B., Kono, T.: Mediated (nonactive) transport of glucose in mammalian cells and its regulation. *J Gen Physiol* **52**:296-305, 1968.
160. Kono, T.: Restoration of response of fat cells to insulin after abolition by trypsin. *Fed Proc* **28**:508, 1969.
161. Crofford, O. B.: The uptake and inactivation of native insulin by isolated fat cells. *J Biol Chem* **243**:362-369, 1968.
162. Porte, D., Jr., Grober, A. L., Kuzuya, T., et al.: The effect of epinephrine on immunoreactive insulin levels in man. *J Clin Invest* **45**:228-236, 1966.
163. Porte, D., Jr., Graber, A., Kuzuya, T., et al.: Epinephrine inhibition of insulin release. *J Clin Invest* **44**:1087, 1965.
164. Loubatieres, A., Mariani, M. M., Chapal, J., et al.: Actions nocive de l'adrenaline pour la structure histologique ilots de Langherhans du pancreas. *Diabetologia* **1**:13-20, 1965.

165. Coore, H. G., Roudle, P. J.: Regulation of insulin secretion with pieces of rabbit pancreas incubated in vitro. *Biochem J* **93**:66-78, 1964.

166. Porte, P. Jr., Williams, R. H.: Inhibition of insulin release by norepinephrine in man. *Science* **152**:1248-1250, 1966.

167. Iverson, J.: Adrenergic receptors and the secretion of glucagon and insulin from the isolated, perfused canine pancreas. *J Clin Invest* **52**:2102-2116, 1973.

168. Porte, P., Jr.: A receptor mechanism for the inhibition of insulin release by epinephrine in man. *J Clin Invest* **46**:86-94, 1967.

169. Malaisse, W., Malaisse-Lagae, F., Wright, P. H., et al.: Effects of adrenergic and cholinergic agents upon insulin secretion *in vitro*. *Endocrinology* **80**: 975-978, 1967.

170. Malaisse, W. J., Malaisse-Lagae, F., Mayhew, D.: A possible role for adenylcyclase system in insulin secretion. *J Clin Invest* **46**:1724-1734, 1967.

170a. Cerasi, E., Luft, R., Effendic, S.: Effect of adrenergic blocking agents in insulin response to glucose infusion in man. *Acta Endocrinol (Kbh)* **69**:335-346, 1972.

170b. Raptis, S., Dollinger, H., Chrissiku, M., et al.: The effect of the beta-receptor blockade (Propranolol) on the endocrine and exocrine pancreatic function in man after the administration of intestinal hormones (secretin and cholecystokinin-pancreaoymin). *Eur J Clin Invest* **3**:163-168, 1973.

171. Kones, R. J.: The molecular and ionic basis for altered myocardial contractility. *Res Commun Chem Path Pharmacol* **5** (suppl 1): 1-84, 1973.

172. Turtle, J. R., Kipnis, D. M.: An adrenergic receptor mechanism for the control of cyclic 3′,5′-adenosine monophosphate synthesis in tissues. *Biochem Biophys Res Commun* **28**:797-802, 1967.

173. Feldman, J. M., Lebovitz, H. E.: Mechanism of epinephrine and serotonin inhibition of insulin release in the golden hamster in vitro. *Diabetes* **19**:480-486, 1970.

174. Robertson, R. P., Porte, D., Jr.: Adrenergic modulation of basel insulin secretion in man. *Diabetes* **22**:1-8, 1973.

175. Porte, D., Jr., Robertson, R. P.: Control of insulin secretion by catecholamines, stress and the sympathetic nervous system. *Fed Proc* **32**:1792-1996, 1973.

176. Montagne, W., Cook, J. R.: The role of adenosine 3′,5′-cyclic monophosphate in the regulation of insulin release by isolated rat islets of Langerhans. *Biochem J* **122**:115-120, 1971.

177. Malaisse, W. J., Brisson, G., Malaisse-Lagae, F.: The stimulus-secretion coupling of glucose induced insulin release. I. Interaction of epinephrine and alkaline earth cations. *J Lab Clin Med* **76**:895-902, 1970.

178. Porte, D., Jr., Bagdade, J. D.: Human insulin secretion: an integrated approach. *Ann Rev Med* **21**:219-240, 1970.

179. Porte, D., Jr., Pupo, A. A.: Insulin responses to glucose: evidence for a two pool system in man. *J Clin Invest* **48**:2309-2319, 1969.

180. Lerner, R. L., Porte, D., Jr.: Epinephrine: selective inhibition of the acute insulin response to glucose. *J Clin Invest* **50**:2453-2457, 1971.

181. Robertson, R. P., Porte, D., Jr.: The glucose receptor. A defective mechanism in diabetes mellitus distinct from the beta adrenergic receptor. *J Clin Invest* **52**:870-876, 1973.

181a. Hedstrand, H., Aberg, H.: Insulin response to intravenous glucose during beta-adrenergic blockade. *N Eng J Med* **290**:910, 1974.

182. Lebovitz, H. E., Feldman, J. M.: Pancreatic biogenic amines and insulin secretion in health and disease. *Fed Proc* **32**:1797-1802, 1973.

183. Brodows, R. G., Pi-Sunyer, F. X., Campbell, R. G.: Neural control of

counter-regulatory events during glucopenia in man. *J Clin Invest* **52**:1841-1844, 1973.

184. Porte, D., Jr.: Beta adrenergic stimulation of insulin release in man. *Diabetes* **16**:150-155, 1967.

185. Porte, D., Jr.: Sympathetic regulation of insulin secretion. *Arch Int Med* **123**:252-260, 1969.

186. Kaneto, A., Kosaka, K., Nakao, K.: Effects of stimulation of the vagus nerve on insulin secretion. *Endocrinology* **80**:530-536, 1967.

187. Daniel, P. M., Henderson, J. R.: The effect of vagal stimulation on plasma insulin and glucose levels in the baboon. *J Physiol* **192**:317-327, 1967.

188. Frohman, L. A., Ezdinkli, E. Z., Javid, R.: Effect of vagal stimulation on insulin secretion. *Diabetes* **15**:522, 1966.

189. Kaneto, A., Kajinuma, H., Kosaka, K., et al.: Stimulation of insulin secretion by parasympathomimetic agents. *Endocrinology* **83**:651-658, 1968.

190. Majid, P. A., Saxton, C., Dykes, J. R. W., et al.: Autonomic control of insulin secretion and the treatment of heart failure. *Brit Med J* **4**:328-334, 1970.

191. Woods, S. C.: Conditioned hypoglycemia: effect of vagotomy and pharmacological blockade. *Amer J Physiol* **223**:1424-1427, 1972.

192. Porte, D., Jr., Girardier, L., Seydoux, J., et al.: Neural regulation of insulin secretion in the dog. *J Clin Invest* **52**:210-214, 1973.

193. Porte, D., Jr., Marliss, E. B., Girardier, L., et al.: Neural regulation of pancreatic glucagon secretion. *J Clin Invest* **51**:75a, 1972.

194. Himms-Hagen, J.: Sympathetic regulation of metabolism. *Pharmacol Rev* **19**:367-461, 1967.

195. Shimazu, T., Fukuda, A.: Increased activities of glycogenolytic enzymes in liver after splanchnic-nerve stimulation. *Science* **150**:1607-1608, 1965.

196. Cryer, P. E., Herman, C. M., Sode, J.: Carbohydrate metabolism in the baboon subjected to gram-negative (E. coli) septicemia. I. Hyperglycemia with repressed plasma insulin concentrations. *Ann Surg* **174**:91-100, 1971.

197. King, L. R., Knowles, K. C., Jr., McLaurin, R. L., et al.: Glucose tolerance and plasma insulin in cranial trauma. *Ann Surg* **173**:337-343, 1971.

198. Carey, L. C., Lowery, B. D., Cloutier, C. T.: Blood sugar and insulin response of humans in shock. *Ann Surg* **172**:342-350, 1970.

199. Cerchio, G. M., Moss, G. S., Popovich, P. A., et al.: Serum insulin and growth hormone response to hemorrhagic shock. *Endocrinology* **88**:138-143, 1971.

200. Baum, D., Porte, D., Jr.: A mechanism for regulation of insulin release in hypoxia. *Amer J Physiol* **222**:695-699, 1972.

201. Baum, D., Porte, D., Jr.: Alpha-adrenergic inhibition of immunoreactive insulin release during deep hypothermia. *Amer J Physiol* **221**:303-311, 1971.

202. Baum, D., Dillard, D. H., Porte, D., Jr.: Inhibition of insulin release in infants undergoing deep hypothermic cardiovascular surgery. *New Eng J Med* **279**:1309-1314, 1968.

203. Mandelbaum, I., Morgan, C. R.: Relationship between pancreatic blood flow and insulin secretion. *Diabetes* **17**:333-334, 1968.

204. Rappaport, A. M., Kawamura, T., Davidson, J. K., et al.: Effects of hormones and of blood flow on insulin output of isolated pancreas in situ. *Amer J Physiol* **221**:343-348, 1971.

205. Cuatrecasas, P.: Insulin receptor of liver and fat cell membranes. *Fed Proc* **32**:1838-1846, 1973.

206. Kones, R. J.: *Cardiogenic Shock: Mechanisms and Management*, Futura Publishing Co., Mt. Kisco, N.Y., 1975.

207. Gregg, D. E.: Haemodynamic factors in shock. In *Shock, Pathogenesis and*

*Therapy, Ciba Foundation International Symposium on Shock*, edited by Bock, K. D., Springer-Verlag, Berlin, 1962.

208. Selkurt, E. E., Alexander, R. S., Patterson, M. S.: The role of mesenteric circulation in the irreversibility of haemorrhagic shock. *Amer J Physiol* **149**: 732-743, 1947.

209. Selkurt, E. E., Brecher, G. A.: Solanchnic hemodynamics and $O_2$ utilization during hemorrhagic shock in the dog. *Circ Res* **4**:693-704, 1956.

210. Levy, M. M.: Influence of levarterenol on portal venous flow in acute hemorrhage. *Circ Res* **6**:587, 1958.

211. Jewitt, D. E., Mercer, C. J., Reid, D., et al.: Free noradrenaline and adrenaline excretion in relation to the development of cardiac arrhythmias and heart failure in patients with acute myocardial infarction. *Lancet* **1**: 635-641, 1969.

212. Tomomatsu, T., Ueba, Y., Matsomoto, T., et al.: Catecholamines in congestive heart failure. *Jap Heart J* **4**:13-24, 1963.

213. Valori, C., Thomas, M., Shillingford, J. P.: Urinary excretion of free noradrenaline and adrenalin following acute myocardial infarction. *Lancet* **1**:127-130, 1967.

214. Chidsey, C. A., Braunwald, E., Morow, A. G.: Catecholamine excretion and cardiac stores of norepinephrine in congestive heart failure. *Amer J of Med* **39**:442-445, 1965.

215. Gazes, P. C., Richardson, J. A., Woods, E. F.: Plasma catecholamine concentrations in myocardial infarction and angina pectoris. *Circulation* **19**: 657-661, 1959.

216. Klein, R. F., Troyer, W. G., Thompson, H. K., et al.: Catecholamine excretion in myocardial infarction. *Arch Intern Med* **122**:476-482, 1968.

217. Januszewica, W., Sznajderman, M., Wocial, B., et al.: Urinary excretion of free norepinephrine and free epinephrine in patients with acute myocardial infarction in relation to its clinical course. *Amer Heart J* **76**:345-352, 1968.

218. Valori, C., Thomas, M., Shillingford, J.: Free noradrenaline and adrenaline excretion in relation to clinical syndromes following myocardial infarction. *Amer J Cardiol* **20**:605-617, 1967.

219. McDonald, L., Baker, C., Bray, C., et al.: Plasma-catecholamines after cardiac infarction. *Lancet* **2**:1021-1023, 1969.

220. Hayashi, K. D., Moss, A. J., Yu, P. N.: Urinary catecholamine excretion in myocardial infarction. *Circulation* **40**:473-481, 1969.

221. Connolly, C. K., Wills, M. R.: Plasma cortisol levels in heart failure. *Brit Med J* **2**:25-27, 1967.

222. Logen, R. W., Murdock, W. R.: Blood-levels of hydrocortisone, transminases, and cholesterol after myocardial infarction. *Lancet* **2**:521-524, 1966.

223. Bailey, R. R., Abernethy, M. H., Beaven, D. W.: Adrenocortical response to the stress of an acute myocardial infarction. *Lancet* **1**:970-973, 1967.

224. Klein, A. J., Palmer, L. A.: Plasma cortisol in myocardial infarction. *Amer J Cardiol* **11**:332-337, 1963.

225. Hansen, B., Beck-Nielsen, J., Juul, J., et al.: Plasma-hydrocortisone values in heart disease. *Acta Med Scand* **186**:411-416, 1969.

226. Goetz, R. H., Bregman, D., Esrig, B., et al.: Unidirectional intraaortic balloon pumping in cardiogenic shock and intractible lift ventricular failure. *Amer J Cardiol* **29**:213-222, 1972.

227. Ratshin, R. A., Rackley, C. E., Russel, R. O., Jr.: Hemodynamic evaluation of left ventricular function in shock complicating myocardial infarction. *Circulation* **45**:127-139, 1972.

228. Prakash, R., Parmley, W. W., Howat, M. H., et al.: Serum cortisol, plasma free fatty acids, and urinary catecholamines as indicators of complications in acute myocardial infarction. *Circulation* **45**:736-745, 1972.

229. Mackenzie, G. J., Taylor, S. H., Flenley, D. C., et al.: Circulatory and respiratory studies in myocardial infarction and cardiogenic shock. *Lancet* **2**:825-832, 1964.

230. Ellenberg, M., Oserman, K. E., Pollack, H.: Hyperglycemia in coronary thrombosis. *Diabetes* **1**:16-21, 1952.

231. Taylor, S. H., Saxton, C., Majid, P. A., et al.: Insulin secretion following myocardial infarction with particular respect to the pathogenesis of cardiogenic shock. *Lancet* **2**:1373-1378, 1969.

232. Connolly, D. K., Wills, M. R.: Plasma cortisol levels in heart failure. *Brit Med J* **2**:25-27, 1967.

233. Allison, S. P., Chamberlain, M. J., Hinton, P.: Intravenous glucose tolerance, insulin, glucose and free fatty acid levels after myocardial infarction. *Brit Med J* **4**:776-778, 1969.

234. Baum, D., Dillard, D. H., Porte, D.: Inhibition of insulin release in infants undergoing deep hypothermic cardiovascular surgery. *New Eng J Med* **279**: 1309-1314, 1968.

235. Allison, S. P.: Changes in insulin secretion during open heart surgery. *Brit J Anaesthesia* **43**:138-143, 1971.

236. Mandelbaum, I., Morgan, L. R.: Effect of extracorporeal circulation upon insulin. *J Thorac Cardiovasc Surg* **55**:526-534, 1968.

237. Allison, S. P., Prowse, K., Chamberlain, M. J.: Failure of insulin response to glucose load during operation and after myocardial infarction. *Lancet* **1**:478-481, 1967.

238. Allison, S. P., Tomlin, P. J., Chamberlain, M. J.: Some effects of anaesthesia and surgery on carbohydrate and fat metabolism. *Brit J Anaesthesia* **41**:588-593, 1969.

239. Wright, H. K., Gaun, D.: Hyperglycemic hyponatremia in nondiabetic patients. *Arch Int Med* **112**:344-346, 1963.

240. Wynn, V.: Electrolyte disturbances associated with failure to metabolize glucose during hypothermia. *Lancet* **2**:575-578, 1954.

241. Moffitt, E. A., Rosevear, J. M., Molnar, G. D., et al.: Myocardial metabolism in open heart surgery. Correlation with insulin response. *J Thorac Cardiovasc Surg* **59**:691-706, 1970.

242. Moffitt, E. A., Rosevear, J. W., Molnar, G. D., et al.: The effect of glucose-insulin-potassium solution on ketosis following cardiac surgery. *Anesthesis Analgesia Current Res* **50**:291-297, 1971.

243. Majid, P. A., Ghosh, P., Pakrashi, B. C., et al.: Insulin secretion after open heart surgery with particular respect to the pathogenesis of low cardiac output state. *Brit Heart J* **33**:6-11, 1971.

244. Sharma, B., Majid, P. A., Pakrashi, B. C., et al.: Insulin secretion in heart failure. *Brit Med J* **2**:396-398, 1970.

245. Ettinger, P. O., Oldewurtel, H. O., Dzindzio, B., et al.: Glucose intolerance in nonischemic cardiac disease. Role of cardiac output and adrenergic function. *Circulation* **43**:809-823, 1971.

246. Ettinger, P. O., Oldewurtel, H. O., Weisse, A. B., et al.: Diminished glucose tolerance and immunoreactive insulin response in patients with nonischemic cardiac disease. *Circulation* **38**:559-567, 1968.

247. Triner, L., Papayoanou, J., Killian, P., et al.: Effects of ouabain on insulin secretion in the dog. *Circ Res* **25**:119-127, 1969.

248. Saxton, C., Majid, P. A., Taylor, S. H.: Effect of ouabain on insulin secretion in man. *Clin Sci*, in press, 1971.

249. Scheuer, J.: Myocardial metabolism in cardiac hypoxia. *Amer J Cardiol* **19**:385-392, 1967.

250. Cascarano, J., Chick, W. L., Siedman, L.: Anaerobic rat heart: Effect of

glucose and Krebs cycle metabolites on rate of breathing. *Proc Soc Exper Biol Med* **127**:25-30, 1968.

251. Weissler, A., Kruger, F. A., Baba, N., et al.: Role of anaerobic metabolism in preservation of functional capacity and structure of anoxic myocardium. *J Clin Invest* **47**:403-416, 1968.

252. Owen, P., Thomas, M., Opie, L.: Relative changes in free fatty acid and glucose utilization by ischemic myocardium after coronary artery occlusion. *Lancet* **1**:1187-1190, 1969.

253. Klarwein, M., Kako, K., Chrysohou, A., et al.: Effect of atrial and ventricular tachycardia on carbohydrate metabolism of the heart. *Circ Res* **9**:819, 1961.

254. Neely, J. R., Whitfield, C. F., Morgan, H. E.: Regulation of glycogenolysis in hearts: effects of pressure development, glucose, and FFA. *Amer J Physiol* **219**:1083-1088, 1970.

255. Michal, G., Naegle, S., Darforth, W., et al.: Metabolic changes in heart muscle during anoxia. *Amer J Physiol* **197**:1147-1151, 1959.

256. Lemley, J. M., Meneely, G.: Effects of anoxia on metabolism of myocardial tissue. *Amer J Physiol* **169**:66-73, 1952.

257. Regan, D. M., Davis, W. W., Morgan, H. E., et al.: The regulation of hexokinase and phosphofructokinase activity in heart muscle. *J Biol Chem* **239**:43-49, 1964.

258. Darforth, W. H., McKinsey, J. J., Stewart, J. T.: Transport and phosphorylation of glucose of the dog heart. *J Physiol, London* **162**:367-384, 1962.

259. Kubler, W., Spieckermann, P. G.: Regulation of glycolysis in the ischemic and the anoxic myocardium. *J Mol Cell Cardiol* **1**:351-377, 1970.

260. Neely, J. R., Rovetto, M. J., Whitner, J. T., et al.: Effects of ischemia on function and metabolism of the isolated working rat heart. *Amer J Physiol* **225**:651-658, 1973.

261. Posner, B. I., Mierzwinski, L., Fallen, E. L.: Studies on amino acid levels and transport in the mechanically stressed heart. *J Mol Cell Cardiol* **5**:221-223, 1973.

262. Morbein, E.: Activation of synthetic processes in cardiac hypertrophy. *Circ Res* **34-35** (suppl II): 37-48, 1974.

263. Badeer, H. S.: Development of cardiomegaly. A unifying hypothesis explaining the growth of muscle fibers, blood vessels and collagen of heart. *Cardiology* **57**:247-261, 1972.

264. Cohen, J.: Role of endocrine factors in the pathogenesis of cardiac hypertrophy. *Circ Res* **34-35** (suppl II): 49-57, 1974.

265. Lesch, M., Gorlin, M., Sonnenblick, E. H.: Myocardial amino acid transport in the isolated rabbit right ventricular papillary muscle: General characteristics and effect of passive stretch. *Circ Res* **27**:445-461, 1970.

266. Meerson, F. Z. : The myocardium in hyperfunction, hypertrophy, and heart failure. *Circ Res* **24-25** (suppl II): 1-163, 1969.

267. Meerson, F. Z.: Development of modern components of the mechanism of cardiac hypertrophy. *Circ Res* **34-35** (suppl II): 58-63, 1974.

268. Christensen, H. N.: *Biological Transport*, WA Benjamin, New York, 1962, p. 114.

269. Arvill, A.: Relationship between the effects of contraction and insulin on the metabolism of the isolated levator ani muscle of the rat. *Acta Endocr* (Kobenhavn) **56** (suppl 122): 27-41, 1967.

270. Lesch, M., Gorlin, R., Sonnenblick, E. H.: Myocardial amino acid transport in the isolated rabbit right ventricular papillary muscle. General characteristics and effects of passive stretch. *Circ Res* **27**:445-460, 1970.

271. Peterson, M. B., Lesch, M.: Protein synthesis and amino acid transport in the isolated rabbit right ventricular papillary muscle. *Circ Res* **31**:317-327, 1972.

272. Ahren, K., Hjalmarson, A., Isaksson, O.: In vitro work load and rat heart metabolism: II. Effect on amino acid transport. *Acta Physiol Scan* **86**:257-270, 1972.
273. Schreiber, S. S., Oratz, M., Rothschild, M. A.: Initiation of protein synthesis in the acutely overloaded perfused heart, in *Cardiac Hypertrophy*, edited by Alpert, N. A., Academic Press, New York, 1971, pp. 215-245.
274. Peterson, D. T., Alford, F. P., Reaven, E. P., et al.: Characteristics of membrane-bound and free hepatic ribosomes from insulin-deficient rats. I. Acute experimental diabetes mellitus. *J Clin Invest* **52**:3201-3211, 1973.
275. Wiener, R., Spitzer, J. J.: Substrate utilization by myocardium and skeletal muscle in alloxan-diabetic dogs. *Amer J Physiology* **225**:1288-1294, 1973.
276. Koide, T., Ozeki, K.: Increased amino acid transport in experimentally hypertrophied rat heart. *Jap Heart J* **12**:177-184, 1971.
277. Morkin, E., Kimata, S., Skillman, J. J.: Myosin synthesis and degradation during development of cardiac hypertrophy in the rabbit. *Circ Res* **30**:690-702, 1972.
278. Skosey, J. L., Zak, R., Martin, A. F., et al.: Biochemical correlates of cardiac hypertrophy: V. Labeling of collagen, myosin, and nuclear DNA during experimental myocardial hypertrophy in the rat. *Circ Res* **31**:145-157, 1972.
279. Hider, R. C., Fern, E. B., London, D. R.: Relationship between intracellular amino acids and protein synthesis in the extensor digitorum longus muscle of rats. *Biochem J* **114**:171-178, 1969.
280. Righetti, P., Little, E. P., Wolf, G.: Reutilization of amino acids in protein synthesis in hela cells. *J Biol Chem* **246**:5724-5732, 1971.
281. Rabinowitz, M.: Overview on pathogenesis of cardiac hypertrophy. *Circ Res* **34-35** (suppl II): 3-11, 1974.
282. Bleehen, N. M., Fisher, R. B.: The action of insulin in the isolated rat heart. *J Physiol* **123**:260-276, 1954.
283. Crass, M. F., McCaskill, J. C., Shipp, J. C., et al.: Metabolism of endogenous lipids in cardiac muscle: effect of pressure development. *Am J Physiol* **220**:428-435, 1971.
284. Rannels, D. E., Hjalmarson, A. C., Morgan, H. E.: Effects of noncarbohydrate substances on protein synthesis in muscle. *Amer J Physiol* **226**:528-539, 1974.
285. Wool, I. G., Stirewalt, W. S., Moyer, A. N.: Effect of diabetes and insulin on nucleic acid metabolism of heart muscle. *Amer J Physiol* **214**:825-831, 1968.
286. Atkinson, D. E.: The energy charge of the adenylate pool as a regulatory parameter. Interaction with feedback modifiers. *Biochemistry* **7**:4030-4034, 1968.
287. Bergmann, F. H., Berg, P., Dieckmann, M.: The enzymatic synthesis of amino acyl derivatives of ribonucleic acid. *J Biol Chem* **236**:1735-1740, 1961.
288. Ibuki, F., Moldave, K.: Evidence for the enzymatic binding of aminoacyl transfer ribonucleic acid to rat liver ribosomes. *J Biol Chem* **243**:791-798, 1968.
289. Lin, S. Y., McKeehan, L., Culp, W., et al.: Partial characterization of the enzymatic properties of the aminoacyl transfer ribonucleic acid binding enzyme. *J Biol Chem* **244**:4340-4350, 1969.
290. Siler, J., Moldave, K.: Studies on the kinetics of peptidyl transfer RNA translocase from rat liver. *Biochem Biophys Acta* **195**:138-144, 1969.
291. Buse, M., Willingham, M. C., Biggers, J. F.: Inhibition of protein synthesis by fatty acids in the perfused rat heart. *Diabetes* **18** (suppl 1): 338, 1969.
292. Takahashi, A.: Myocardial protein metabolism following coronary occlusion. *Jap Heart J* **31**:581-599, 1967.

293. Bajusz, E.: *Conditioning Factors for Cardiac Necroses,* Intercontinental Medical Book Co., Basel:Karger, New York, 1963, pp. 250-271.
294. Wicken, D. E. L., Shorey, C. D., Eikens, E.: Repair of muscle cells after myocardial infarction: Ultrastructural evidence. *Cardiovascular Research,* p. 324, Abstracts of papers, VI World Congress of Cardiology, 1970.
295. Cohen, J., Aroesty, J. M., Rosenfeld, M. G.: Determinants of thyroxine-induced cardiac hypertrophy in mice. *Circ Res* **18**:388-397, 1966.
296. Lochner, A., Brink, A. J.: Oxidative phosphorylation and glycolysis in the muscular dystrophy of the Syrian hamster. *Clin Sci* **33**:409-423, 1967.
297. Wannenmacher, R. W., Jr., McCoy, J. R.: Regulation of protein synthesis in the ventricular myocardium of hypertrophied hearts. *Amer J Physiol* **216**:781-787, 1969.
298. Bester, A. J., Brink, A. J., Lochner, A., et al.: Effects of ischaemia and infarction on metabolism and function of isolated, perfused rat heart. *Cardiovasc Res* **6**:284-294, 1972.
299. Gudbjarnason, S., DeSchryver, C.: Nuclear ribosomes, an early factor in tissue reparation. *Biochem Biophy Res Commun* **14**:12-16, 1964.
300. Grove, D., Zak, R., Nair, K. G., et al.: Biochemical correlates of cardiac hypertrophy. IV. Observations on the cellular organization of growth during myocardial hypertrophy in the rat. *Circ Res* **25**:483, 1964.
301. Cohen, J., Feldman, R. E., Whitbeck, A. A.: Effects of energy availability in protein synthesis in isolated rat atria. *Amer J Physiol* **216**:76-81, 1969.
302. Hollenberg, M.: Effect of oxygen on growth of cultured myocardial cells. *Circ Res* **28**:148-157, 1971.
303. Peterson, M., Sonnenblick, E. H., Lesch, M.: Preservation of cellular viability during anoxia with high levels of glucose. *Circ* **45-46**:II-121, 1972.
304. Peterson, M., Lesch, M.: Studies on the reversibility of anoxic damage to the myocardial protein synthetic mechanism: effects of glucose. *J Mol Cell Cardiol* **7**:175-190, 1975.
305. Gudbjarnason, S., Fenton, J. C., Wolf, P. L., et al.: Stimulation of reparative processes following experimental myocardial infarction. *Arch Int Med* **118**:33-40, 1966.
306. Pozefsky, T., Felig, P., Tobin, J. D., et al.: Amino acid balance across tissues of the forearm in postabsorptive man. Effects of insulin at two dose levels. *J Clin Invest* **48**:2273-2282, 1969.
307. Crofford, O. B.: The uptake and inactivation of native insulin by isolated fat cells. *J Biol Chem* **243**:362-369, 1968.
308. Kono, T., Barham, F. W.: Insulin like effects of tryspin on fat cells. Localization of the metabolic steps and the cellular site affected by the enzyme. *J Biol Chem* **246**:6204-6209, 1971.
309. House, P. D. R.: Kinetics of $^{125}$I-insulin binding to rat liver plasma membranes. *FEBS Lett* **16**:339-342, 1971.
310. El Allawy, R. M., Gliemann, J.: Trypsin treatment of adipocytes: effect on sensitivity to insulin. *Biochem Biophys Acta* **273**:97-109, 1972.
311. Hammond, J. M., Jarett, L., Mariz, I. K., et al.: Heterogeneity of insulin receptors on fat cell membranes. *Biochem Biophys Acta* **49**:1122-1128, 1972.
312. Kono, T., Barham, F. W.: The relationship between the insulin-binding capacity of fat cells and the cellular response to insulin. Studies with intact and tryspin-treated fat cells. *J Biol Chem* **246**:6210-6216, 1971.
313. Wohltmann, H. J., Narahara, H. T.: Binding of insulin-131I by isolated frog partorius muscles. Relationship to changes in permeability to sugar caused by insulin. *J Biol Chem* **241**:4931-4939, 1966.
314. Cuatrecasas, P.: The nature of insulin-receptor interactions, in *Insulin Action,* edited by Fritz, I. B., Academic Press, New York, 1972, pp. 137-166.
315. Garratt, C. J., Cameron, J. S., Menzinger, G.: The association of (131-I)

iodo-insulin with rat diaphragm muscle and its effect on glucose uptake. *Biochem Biophys Acta* **115**:179-186, 1966.

316. Cuatrecasas, P.: Properties of the insulin receptor isolated from liver and fat cell membranes. *J Biol Chem* **247**:1980-1991, 1972.

317. Cuatrecasas, P.: Isolation of the insulin receptor of liver and fat-cell membranes (detergent-solubilized, 125-I) insulin-polyethylene glycol precipitation-sephadex. *Proc Nat Acad Sci USA* **69**:318-322, 1972.

318. Crofford, O. B., Okayama, T.: Insulin-receptor interaction in isolated fat cells. *Diabetes* **19**:369, 1970.

319. Crofford, O. B., Rogers, N. L., Russell, W. G.: The effect of insulin on fat cells: an insulin degrading system extracted from plasma membranes of insulin responsive cells. *Diabetes* **21**: Suppl 2, 403-413, 1972.

320. Freychet, P., Kahn, R., Roth, J., et al.: Insulin interactions with liver plasma membranes. Independence of binding of the hormone and its degradation. *J Biol Chem* **247**:3953-3961, 1972.

321. Cadenas, E., Kaji, H., Park, C. R., et al.: Inhibition of the insulin effect on sugar transport by N-ethylmaleimide. *J Biol Chem* **236**:PC63-PC64, 1961.

322. Fong, C. T., Silver, L., Popenoe, E. A., et al.: Some observations on insulin-receptor interaction. *Biochim Biophys Acta* **56**:190-192, 1962.

323. Whitney, J. E., Cutler, O. E., Wright, F. E.: Inhibition of insulin-finding to tissues by P-hydroxymercuribenzoate and N-ethylmaleimide. *Metabolism* **12**:352-358, 1963.

324. Freychet, P., Roth, J., Neville, D. M., Jr.: Insulin receptors in the liver: specific binding of (125 I) insulin to the plasma membrane and its relation to insulin bioactivity. *Proc Nat Acad Sci USA* **68**:1833-1837, 1971.

325. Pilkis, S. J., Johnson, R. A., Park, C. R.: Characterization of the insulin receptor of rat liver plasma membranes. *Diabetes* **21**: Suppl 1, p. 335, 1972.

326. Weis, L. S., Narahara, H. T.: Regulation of cell membrane permeability in skeletal muscle. I. Action of insulin and trypsin on the transport system for sugar. *J Biol Chem* **244**:3084-3091, 1969.

327. Kuo, J. F., Dill, I. K., Holmland, E. C.: Comparison of the effects of Bacillus subtilis protease, type 8 (subtilopeptidase A), and insulin on isolated adipose cells. *J Biol Chem* **242**:3659-3664, 1967.

328. Kono, T.: Destruction and restoration of the insulin effector system of isolated fat cells. *J Biol Chem* **244**:5777-5784, 1969.

329. Minemura, T., Crofford, O. B.: Insulin-receptor interaction in isolated fat cells. I. The insulin-like properties of p-chloromercuribenzene sulfonic acid. *J Biol Chem* **244**:5181-5188, 1969.

330. Cuatrecasas, P.: Perturbation of the insulin receptor of isolated fat cells with proteolytic enzymes. Direct measurement of insulin-receptor interactions. *J Biol Chem* **246**:6522-6531, 1971.

331. Cuatrecasas, P., Desbuquois, B., Krug, F.: Insulin-receptor interactions in liver cell membranes. *Biochem Biophys Res Commun* **44**:333-339, 1971.

332. Crofford, O. B., Minemura, T., Kono, T.: Insulin-receptor interaction in isolated fat cells. *Adv Enzyme Regul* **8**:219-238, 1970.

333. Crofford, O.: Unpublished.

334. Cuatrecasas, P.: Interaction of insulin with the cell membrane: the primary action of insulin. *Nat Acad Sci USA* **63**:450-457, 1969.

335. Kones, R. J., Dombeck, D. H., Phillips, J. H.: Glucagon in cardiogenic shock. *Angiology* **23**:525-535, 1972.

336. Kones, R. J.: Glucagon and the heart. *Medikon (Belgium)* **3**:2-12, 1974.

337. Kahn, C. R., Neville, D. M., Jr., Gorden, P., et al.: Insulin receptor defect in insulin resistance: studies in the obese-hyperglycemic mouse. *Biochem Biophys Res Commun* **48**:135-142, 1972.

338. Wool, I. G., Stirewalt, W. S., Kurihara, K., et al.: Mode of action of

insulin in the regulation of protein biosynthesis in muscle. *Recent Progr Horm Res* **24**:139-213, 1968.

339.  Morgan, H. E., Jefferson, L. S., Wolpert, E. B., et al.: Regulation of protein synthesis in heart muscle. II. Effect of amino acid levels and insulin on ribosomal aggregation. *J Biol Chem* **246**:2163-2170, 1971.

340.  Manchester, K. L., Krahl, M. E.: Effect of insulin on the incorporation of C14 from C14 labeled carbosylic acids and bicarbonate into the protein of isolated rat diaphragm. *J Biol Chem* **234**:2938-2942, 1959.

341.  Manchester, K. L.: Effect of insulin on protein synthesis. *Diabetes* **21**: Suppl 2:447-452, 1972.

342.  Wool, I. G., Cavicchi, P.: Protein synthesis by skeletal muscle ribosomes. Effect of diabetes and insulin. *Biochemistry* **6**:1231-1242, 1967.

343.  Wool, I. G., Cavicchi, P.: Insulin regulation of protein synthesis by muscle ribosomes: effect of the hormone on translation of messenger RNA for a regulatory protein. *Proc Nat Acad Sci USA* **56**:991-998, 1966.

344.  Martin, T. E., Wool, I. G.: Formation of active hybrids from subunits of muscle ribosomes from normal and diabetic rats. *Proc Nat Acad Sci USA* **60**:569-574, 1968.

345.  Stirewalt, W. S., Castles, J. J., Wool, I. G.: Skeletal muscle ribosomes subunits and peptidyl transfer ribonucleic acid. *Biochemistry* **10**:1594-1598, 1971.

346.  Wool, I. G., Wettenhall, R. E. H., Klein-Bremhaar, H., et al.: Insulin and the control of protein synthesis in muscle, in *Insulin Action*, edited by Fritz, I. B., Academic Press, New York, 1972, pp. 415-429.

347.  Jefferson, L. S., Koehler, J. O., Morgan, H. E.: Effect of insulin on protein synthesis in skeletal muscle of an isolated perfused preparation of rat hemicorpus. *Proc Nat Acad Sci USA* **69**:16-820, 1972.

348.  Rannels, D. E., Jefferson, L. S., Hjalmarson, A. C., et al.: Maintenance of protein synthesis in hearts of diabetic animals. *Biochem Biophys Res Commun* **40**:1110-1116, 1970.

349.  Chain, E. B., Sender, P. M.: Protein synthesis by perfused hearts from normal and insulin-deficient rats. Effect of insulin in the presence of glucose and after depletion of glucose, glucose 6-phosphate and glycogen. *Biochem J* **132**:593-601, 1973.

350.  Gould, M. K., Chaudry, I. H.: The action of insulin on glucose uptake by isolated rat soleus muscle. I. Effects of cations. *Biochem Biophys Acta* **215**:249-257, 1970.

351.  Gould, M. K., Chaudry, I. H.: The action of insulin on glucose uptake by isolated rat soleus muscle. II. Dissociation of a priming effect of insulin from its stimulatory effect. *Biochem Biophys Acta* **215**:258-263, 1970.

352.  Tarui, S., Saito, Y., Suzuki, F., et al.: Parallel stimulation of sugar transport and glycogen formation by a synthetic insulin-dextron complex in diaphragms. *Endocrinology* **91**:1442-1446, 1972.

353.  Larner, J., Villar-Palasi, C.: in Current Topics in Cellular Regulation, edited by Horecker, B., Stadtman, E. W., **3**:195-236, 1972.

354.  Chain, E. B., Mansford, K. R., Opie, L. H.: Effects of insulin on the pattern of glucose metabolism in the perfused working and Langendorff heart of normal and insulin-deficient rats. *Biochem J* **115**:537-546, 1969.

355.  Beitner, R., Kalant, N.: Stimulation of glycolysis by insulin. *J Biol Chem* **246**:500-503, 1971.

356.  Ozand, P., Narahara, H. T.: Regulation of glycolysis in muscle. 3. Influence of insulin, epinephrine, and contraction of phosphofructokinase activity in frog skeletal muscle. *J Biol Chem* **239**:3246-3252, 1964.

357.  Schonhofer, P. S., Skidmore, I. F., Krishna, G.: Effects of insulin on the

lipolytic system of rat fat cells. *Hormone and Metabolic Res* **4**:447-454, 1972.
358. Goldberg, N. D., Villar-Palasi, C., Sasko, H., et al.: Effects of insulin treatment on muscle 3′,5′-cyclic adenylate levels in vivo and in vitro. *Biochim Biophys Acta* **148**:665-672, 1967.
359. Walaas, O., Walaas, E., Wick, A. N.: The stimulatory effect by insulin on the incorporation of 32 P radioactive inorganic phosphate into intracellular inorganic phosphate, adenine nucleotides and guanine nucleotides of the intact isolated rat diaphragm. *Diabetologia* **5**:79-87, 1969.
360. Cryer, P. E., Jarett, L., Kipnis, D. M.: Nucleotide inhibition of adenyl cyclase activity in fat cell membranes. *Biochim Biophys Acta* **177**:586-590, 1969.
361. Keely, S. L., Corbin, J. D., Park, C. R.: Regulation of heart AMP-dependent protein kinase. *Fed Proc* **32**:643, 1974.
362. Morgan, H. E.: Unpublished data.
363. Das, I., Chain, E. B.: An effect of insulin on the adenosine 3′,5′-cyclic monophosphate phosphodiesterase and guanosine 3′,5′-cyclic monophosphate phosphodiesterase activities in the perfused Langendorff and working hearts of normal and diabetic rats. *Biochem J* **128**:95P-96P, 1972.
364. Cuatrecasas, P.: Membrane receptors. *Ann Rev Biochem* **43**:169-214, 1974.
365. Cuatrecasas, P.: Hormone-receptor interactions and the plasma membrane. *Hosp Practice* **9** (July): 73-80, 1974.
366. Cuatrecasas, P.: Affinity chromatography of macromolecules, in *Advances in Enzymology*, edited by Meister, A., John Wiley and Sons, New York, Vol. 36, 1972, pp. 29-89.
367. Rasmussen, H.: Ions as "second messengers." *Hosp Practice* **9** (June): 99-107, 1974.
368. Larner, J.: Insulin and glycogen synthase. *Diabetes* **21**: Suppl 2:428-438, 1972.
369. Illiano, G., Tell, G. P. E., Siegel, M., et al.: Guanosine 3′:5′-cyclic monophosphate and the action of insulin and acetylcholine. *Proc Natl Acad Sci USA* **70**:2443-2447, 1973.
370. Kuo, J. F., Greengard, P.: Cyclic nucleotide-dependent protein kinases. VI. Isolation and partial purification of a protein kinase activated by guanosine 3′,5′-monophosphate. *J Biol Chem* **245**:2493-2498, 1970.
371. Goldberg, N. D.: Cyclic nucleotides and cell function. *Hosp Practice* **9** (May): 127-142, 1974.
372. Goldberg, N. D., Estensen, R. D., Hill, H. R., et al.: Cyclic GMP and cell movement. *Nature* **245**:458-460, 1973.
373. Goldberg, N. D., O'Dea, R. F., Haddox, M. K.: Cyclic GMP, in *Advances in Cyclic Nucleotide Research* edited by Greengard, P., Robison, G. A., Ravin Press, New York, 1974, Vol. 3.
374. Vassort, G., Rougier, O., Garnier, D., et al.: Effects of adrenaline on membrane inward currents during the cardiac action potential. *Arch Physiol Menschen Tiere* **309**:70-81, 1969.
375. Kolata, G. B.: Cyclic GMP: cellular regulatory agent. *Science* **182**:149-151, 1973.
376. Rannels, D. E., Kao, R., Morgan, H. E.: Effect of insulin on lysosomal enzyme activity in perfused rat heart. *Circulation* **47-48** (suppl IV): 25, 1973.
377. Editorial: From Cyclic AMP to cyclic GMP. *Nature* **246**:186-187, 1973.
378. Kao, R., Rannels, D. E., Morgan, H. E.: Effects of insulin on the inhibition of protein synthesis in hypoxic, anoxic, and ischemic myocardium. *Fed Proc* **33**:386, 1974.
379. Ignarro, L. J., White, L. E., Wilkerson, R. D., et al.: Cardiac guanyl

cyclase: stimulation by acetylcholine and calcium. *Circulation* **47-48** (suppl IV): 12, 1973.
380. Barasio, P. G., Vassalle, M.: Dibutyryl cyclic AMP and potassium transport in cardiac Purkinje fibers. *Amer J Physiol* **226**:1232-1237, 1974.
381. Jordan, F.: The electronic structure of and conformational energy barrier to rotation around the C-N glycosidic linkage in adenosine 3',5'-cyclicmonophosphate (cyclic AMP) and its phosphonate analog. *J Theoret Biol* **41**: 23-40, 1973.
382. Sharp, R., Culbert, S., Cook, J., et al.: Cholinergic modification of glucose-induced biphasic insulin release in vitro. *J Clin Invest* **53**:710-716, 1974.
383. Morgan, H. E., Rannels, D. E., Kao, R. L.: Factors controlling protein turnover in heart muscle. *Circ Res* **34-35** (suppl III): 22-29, 1974.
384. Johnson, P. N., Freedberg, A. S., Marshall, J. M.: Action of thyroid hormone on the transmembrane potentials from sinoatrial node cells and atrial muscle cells in isolated atria of rabbits. *Cardiology* **58**:272-289, 1973.
385. Fritz, I. B.: Insulin actions on carbohydrate and lipid metabolism, in *Biochemical Actions of Hormones*, edited by Litwack, G., Academic Press, New York, 1972, Vol. 2, pp. 165-214.
386. Ookhtens, M., Marsh, D. J., Smith, S. W., et al.: Fluctuations of plasma glucose and insulin in conscious dogs receiving glucose infusions. *Amer J Physiol* **226**:910-919, 1974.
387. Hladky, S. B., Gordon, L. G. M., Haydon, D. A.: Molecular mechanisms of ion transport in lipid membrane. *Ann Rev Phys Chem* **25**:11-38, 1974.
388. Gitler, C.: Plasticity of biological membranes. *Am Rev Biophys Bioeng* **1**:51-92, 1972.
389. Fain, J. N., Rosenberg, L.: Antilipolytic action of insulin on fat cells. *Diabetes* **21** (suppl II): 414-425, 1971.
390. Khoo, J. C., Steinberg, D., Thompson, B., et al.: Hormonal regulation of adipocyte enzymes. The effects of epinephrine and insulin on the control of lipase, phosphorylase kinase, phosphorylase, and glycogen synthetase. *J Biol Chem* **248**:3823-3830, 1973.
391. Siddle K., Hales, C. N.: The relationship between the concentration of adenosine 3',5'-cyclic monophosphate and the anti-lipolytic action of insulin in isolated rat fat cells. *Biochem J* **142**:97-103, 1974.
392. Kissebah, A. H., Tulloch, B. R., Vydelingum, N., et al.: The role of calcium in insulin action. II. Effects of insulin and procaine hydrochloride on lipolysis. *Horm Metab Res* **6**:357-364, 1974.
393. Kissebah, A. H., Vydelingum, N., Tulloch, B. R., et al.: The role of calcium in insulin action. I. Purification and properties of enzymes regulating lipolysis in human adipose tissue: effects of cyclic AMP and calcium ions. *Horm Metab Res* **6**:247-255, 1974.
394. Soderling T. R., Corbin J. D., Park, C. R.: Regulation of adenosine 3',5'-monophosphate-dependent protein kinase. II. Hormonal regulation of the adipose tissue enzyme. *J Biol Chem* **248**:1822-1829, 1973.
395. Huttunen, J. K., Steinberg, D.: Activation and phosphorylation of purified adipose tissue hormone-sensitive lipase by cyclic AMP-dependent protein kinase. *Biochim Biophys Acta* **239**:411-427, 1971.
396. Walsh, D. A., Ashby, D., Gonzales, C., et al.: Purification and characterization of a protein inhibitor of adenosine 3',5'-monophosphate-dependent protein kinases. *J Biol Chem* **246**:1977-1985, 1971.
397. Coors, H. G., Denton, R. M., Martin, B. R., et al.: Regulation of adipose tissue pyruvate dehydrogenase by insulin and other hormones. *J Biochem* **125**:115-127, 1971.
398. Soderling, T. R., Hickenbottom, J. P., Reimann, E. H., et al.: Inactivation of glycogen synthetase and activation of phosphorylase kinase by muscle

adenosine 3′,5′-monophosphate-dependent protein kinases. *J Biol Chem* **245**: 6317-6328, 1970.

399. Mangeniello, V. C., Murad, F., Vaughan, M.: Effects of lipolytic and anti-polytic agents on cyclic 3′,5′-adenosine monophosphate in fat cells. *J Biol Chem* **246**:2195-2202, 1971.
400. Randle, P. J., Denton, R. M., Pask, H. T.: in *Calcium and Cell Regulation* (edited by R. M. S. Smellie), p. 75, London, 1974.
401. Krahl, M. E.: Insulin like and anti-insulin effects of chelating agents on adipose tissue. *Fedn Proc* **25**:832-834, 1966.
402. Hope-Gill, H. F., Kissebah, A. H., Tulloch B. R., et al.: VII Cong Int Diabetes Fedn. *Excerpta Med Abst* **54**:123, 1971.
403. Bronstrom, C. O., Hunkeler, F. L., Krebs, E. G.: The regulation of skeletal muscle phosphorylase kinase by Ca²⁺. *J Biol Chem* **246**:1961-1967, 1971.
404. Cameron, L. E., Lejohn, H. B.: On the involvement of calcium in amino acid transport and growth of the fungus *Achyla*. *J Biol Chem* **247**:4729-4739, 1972.
405. Kissebah, A. H., Clarke, P., Vydelingum, N., et al.: *Eur J Clin Invest* (in the press).
406. Clarke, P., Kissebah, A. H., Vydelingum, N., et al.: Regulation of glycogenesis through changes in intracellular calcium. *Horm Metab Res* **6**:525, 1974.
407. Rasmussen, H.: Cell communication calcium ion, and cyclic adenosine monophosphate. *Science* **170**:404-412, 1970.
408. Olsen, R. W.: Filamentous protein model for cyclic AMP-mediated cell regulatory mechanisms. *J Theor Biol* **49**:263-287, 1975.
409. Bryan, J.: Microtubules. *Bioscience* **24**:701-711, 1974.

# CHAPTER 3

# POTASSIUM AND CALCIUM

The relationship between potassium $[K^+]$ and the heart has fascinated investigators for over a century. Although there have been recent advances in the understanding of the influence of altered potassium levels—intracellular and extracellular—there is still much to be learned about potassium and the heart. In this chapter intracellular $K^+$ metabolism in the normal and ischemic heart will be considered.

## I. TRANSMEMBRANE POTENTIAL: "PASSIVE" PROPERTIES

### A. Generation of electrical potentials by ions

Electrical potential differences exist at the boundaries between two solutions of electrolytes which are composed of ions with different mobility or concentrations on either side. For instance, under certain experimental circumstances two different concentrations of the same electrolyte in contact with each other through a porous filter may generate a potential, $\mathcal{E}$, given by:

$$\mathcal{E} = \frac{RT}{F} \frac{u^+ - v^-}{u^+ + v^-} \ln \frac{a_1}{a_2}$$ (Equation 1)

where R is the gas constant, T the absolute temperature, F is the Faraday, $u^+$ and $v^-$ the mobilities of the positive and negative ions respectively, and $a_1$, $a_2$, the geometric mean activity of the two ions on each side, approximated by their concentrations. The interposition of a membrane impermeable to the cation reduces $u^+$ to 0 and thus

$$\mathcal{E} = \frac{RT}{F} \ln \frac{a_2}{a_1}.$$ (Equation 2)

In the instance where two solutions of dissimilar cations are in contact, for example, NaCl and KCl:

$$\mathcal{E} = \frac{RT}{F} \ln \frac{u_{Na^+} + v_{Cl^-}}{u_{K^+} + v_{Cl^-}}$$ (Equation 3)

The sarcolemma separates an interstitium rich in sodium from intracellular fluid rich in potassium (Fig. 1). For the purposes of this discussion, the cell membrane has finite measurable values of basic constants such as specific membrane resistance (on the order of 20,000 $\Omega cm^{-2}$ for Purkinje fibers), conductance (on the order of 1 mho $cm^{-2}$), susceptance (measured as capacitance, about 1 $\mu Fcm^{-2}$), and internal specific resistance (223 $\Omega cm$ for "synthetic strands").[266] The passive rate of ion penetration through the membrane is in large part a function of the concentration gradient, the voltage gradient, and the permeability of the membrane to the ion under consideration.

## B. The Goldman-Hodgkin-Katz equation

An ion is at *equilibrium* across a membrane if no net ion movement occurs.[1] If a membrane were permeable to only potassium, the side of lowest concentration would be positively charged because of diffusion of $K^+$ down the concentration gradient. The membrane potential at which no net $K^+$ current would flow is given by the equation:

$$\mathcal{E}_{K^+} = \frac{RT}{F} \ln \frac{[K^+]_i}{[K^+]_o} \qquad \text{(Equation 4)}$$

where $\mathcal{E}_{K^+}$ is *the equilibrium potential of $K^+$*. For heart muscle, $\mathcal{E}_{K^+}$

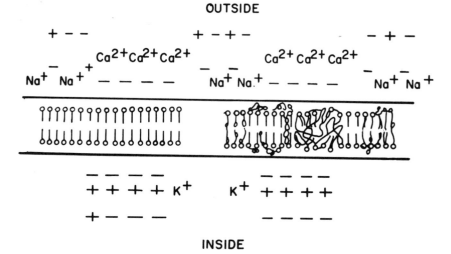

**Figure 1**  The myocardial membrane according to the Davson-Danielli model. Left, lipid bilayer, right, intermixed with protein.

$= -92.6$ mV and $\mathcal{E}_{Na^+} = +84$ mV.[*] Since $\mathcal{E}_{K^+}$ is close to the actual membrane potential, $K^+$ is the most permeable ion and hence the most important one in maintaining the resting membrane potential (RMP or $\mathcal{E}_m$). $\mathcal{E}_m$ is not exactly $\mathcal{E}_{K^+}$ because other ions influence the resting potential according to the Goldman-Hodgkin-Katz relation:

$$\mathcal{E}_m = \frac{RT}{F} \ln \frac{P_{Na^+}[Na^+]_i + P_{K^+}[K^+]_i + P_{Cl^-}[Cl^-]_o}{P_{Na^+}[Na^+]_o + P_{K^+}[K^+]_o + P_{Cl^-}[Cl^-]_i} \qquad \text{(Equation 5)}$$

where $_{o, i}$ refer to ions extracellularly and intracellularly respectively, and P is permeability.

## C. The Na⁺, K⁺-pump

It is now well established that cardiac muscle and other excitable cells utilize an energy-dependent ionic pump to expel $Na^+$, which may accumulate intracellularly, and restore $K^+$ to the intracellular space.[2, 3] By this means, a high intracellular $[K^+]_i$ (approximately 140 mM compared with approximately 5 mM $= [K^+]_o$) and high $[Na^+]_o$ (approximately 150 mM compared with approximately 30 mM $= [Na^+]_i$) is supported. The maintenance of the ionic concentration gradients by active $Na^+$—for—$K^+$ exchange results in the separation of charge and hence generates at least part of the transmembrane potential. The extent of the contribution of the pump to the membrane potential is a function of the net difference between pumping and leakage rates, and for this reason the process is called "electrogenic." From intact membrane preparations in which the semipermeable characteristics permit study of pump direction and stoichiometry (red blood cell ghosts and squid axon), the Na⁺, K⁺-pump relations are:

$$\left\{ \begin{array}{c} 3[Na^+]_i \rightarrow 3[Na^+]_o \\ 2[K^+]_i \leftarrow 2[K^+]_o \\ ATP^{-4} + H_2O \rightarrow ADP^{-3} + P_i^{-2} + H^+ \end{array} \right\}$$

Since three sodium ions leave for every two potassium ions entering the cell, the pump should be electrogenic. The extent to which this effect is neutralized by proton uptake and movements of other ions is uncertain.

The ATPase system supplying energy for ionic pumping is located within the sarcolemma and is asymmetrical with respect to pumping

---

[*] The substitution of concentration values for chemical activities in the Nernst equation may result in significant errors, especially when calculating $\mathcal{E}_{Na^+}$. Therefore, these values are approximate ones.

of $Na^+$ and $K^+$.[1] The $Na^+$-pump is sensitive to changes in $[Na^+]_i$ within the cell, and therefore has been considered to be under negative feedback control (Fig. 2A).[5] Consistent with this view is the observation that the substitution of extracellular $Na^+$ by choline$^+$ reduces net $K^+$ uptake.[267] However, $Na^+$ extrusion is almost insensitive to a change in $[K^+]_o$. The $Na^+$, $K^+$-pump also regulates cell volume, since any reduction in its activity results in a greater concentration of osmotically-active particles intracellularly.

Activation of the $Na^+$, $K^+$-ATPase by $Na^+$ and $K^+$ may be explained by considering that separate sites exist on the enzyme with high affinities for $Na^+$ and $K^+$, and some cross competition exists between the ions for the two species of loci. The $Na^+$-activation site would have high affinity for $Na^+$ and low affinity for $K^+$; $Na^+$ at the site would activate ATP hydrolysis and be inhibited by $K^+$. The $K^+$-activation site would have high affinity for $K^+$ and low affinity for $Na^+$. The sodium activation sites are located on the internal side of the membrane and the potassium-activation sites are located on the exterior surface. ATP acts with an internal site, after which ADP and $P_i$ return to the intracellular pool (Fig 2B). This arrangement is consistent with the fluid mosaic model for membrane structure since surfaces are exposed to both sides of the membrane.

The unanswered questions regarding the spatial and temporal aspects of $Na^+$, $K^+$-pump action are underscored by comparing two models (Fig 2C). In one, $Na^+$ and $K^+$ are exchanged simultaneously,

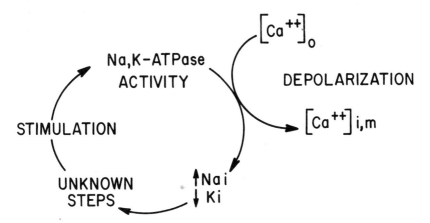

**Figure 2A**   Net sodium influx and potassium efflux attends each depolarization cycle. These changes are reversed by $Na^+$, $K^+$-pumping, energized by $Na^+$, $K^+$-ATPase. Calcium influx also occurs during the action potential.

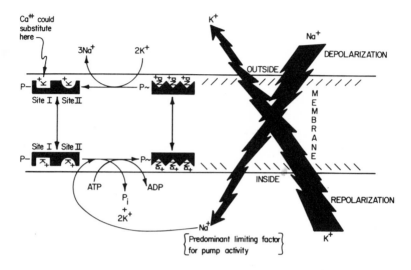

**Figure 2B**  Diagrammatic details of the role of the sodium pump in maintaining sodium and potassium concentration gradients across the cell membrane. The possibility that calcium substitutes for potassium is hypothesis (see text). P∼ and P− represent different forms of a phosphomembrane complex. Reproduced with permission.[318]

whereas in the sequential model, a single site is involved which first accepts one ion, "flips" to release the ion and, presumably due to a change in configuration, accepts the complementary ion.[331]

When $Na^+$ is present in high concentrations, $Na^+$, $K^+$-ATPase activity increases in sigmoidal fashion upon presentation of increasing $K^+$ concentrations. This property of the enzyme may be explained either by cooperativity between activation sites or by the existence of multiple independent sites.

The energy changes occurring during the operation of the sodium pump are: [319]

| Reactions of Energy Changes | G(calories) |
|---|---|
| 1. Energy released from the hydrolysis of one ATP molecule | − 13,017 |
| 2. Osmotic work required to extrude three sodium ions | + 4,927 |
| 3. Osmotic work required to take up two potassium ions | + 4,177 |
| 4. Electrical work required to move one net positive charge out of the cell | + 207 |
| Net free energy change | − 3,706 |

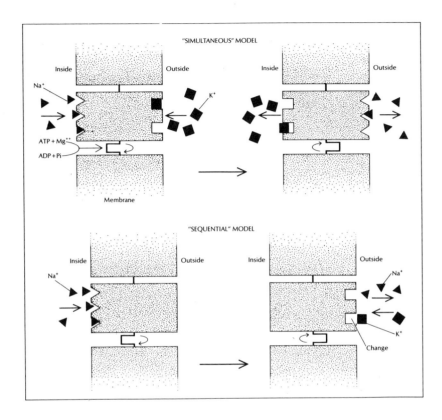

**Figure 2C** Both "simultaneous" and "sequential" models of action have been proposed for the $Na^+$-$K^+$ pump, as schematics suggest. In simultaneous model, $Na^+$ binds to inside of cell membrane while $K^+$ binds to exterior. ATP breakdown changes configuration of pump protein in such a way that the protein shifts the ions across the membrane, somewhat like a revolving door, with the $K^+$ presumably dephosphorylating the protein as the ions pass through. In the sequential model, only one type of site is involved. This first accepts $Na^+$ from interior of cell, then, perhaps by becoming phosphorylated, moves $Na^+$ to the outside. Since its shape has been changed by phosphorylation, the site now accepts $K^+$. Additional clues to the pump's action have been obtained by studying the effect of inhibitory substances, such as calcium, that block pump action by preventing dephosphorylation of the phosphoproteins. Cardiotonic glycosides inhibit the pump only from the cell's outside; it is thought that by binding to $K^+$-sensitive sites they impede the "cooperative" action of $Na^+$ and $K^+$ needed for the pump to operate. Reproduced with permission.[331]

The mechanism by which this $Na^+$, $K^+$-exchange occurs may be (i) penetration through channels lined with carbonyl groups or fixed negative charges, (ii) complex with carrier, and (iii) penetration by tight initial binding to membrane with subsequent distortion in membrane structure such that bound ions are exposed to the opposite surface, and affinities decrease to allow dissociation of the cation.

Transduction of the energy by $Na^+$, $K^+$-ATPase from ATP for ion exchange occurs in the following sequence. In the absence of $Mg^{++}$ and $Na^+$:

$$ATP + E \rightleftharpoons ATP \cdot E.$$

In the presence of $Mg^{++}$ and $Na^+$, the terminal $\sim P$ of ATP is transferred:

$$ATP \cdot E \xrightleftharpoons{Mg^{++}, Na^+} ADP + (E \sim P)_1,$$

where $\sim P$ may be a covalent bond between orthophosphate and an acyl group on the enzyme. In another step, with $Mg^{++}$ present, another change of the enzyme occurs:

$$(E \sim P)_1 \xrightleftharpoons{Mg^{++}} (E \sim P)_2.$$

Finally, a $K^+$-activated dephosphorylation step completes the enzyme turnover cycle:

$$(E - P)_2 \xrightarrow{K^+} E + P_i.$$

### D. Ion conductances and membrane potential

Ohm's law states

$$R_i = \frac{\mathcal{E}_m}{I_i} \qquad \text{(Equation 6)}$$

Where $R_i$ is resistance to $i^{th}$ ion, $I_i$ is the current carried by ion $i$ and $\mathcal{E}_m$ is the membrane potential. Ion conductance, $g_i$, is defined by

$$g_i = \frac{1}{R_i} \qquad \text{(Equation 7)}$$

and therefore

$$g_{K^+} = I_{K^+}/\mathcal{E}_m - \mathcal{E}_{K^+},$$

$$g_{Na^+} = I_{Na^+}/\mathcal{E}_m - \mathcal{E}_{Na^+}$$

$$g_{Cl^-}/\mathcal{E}_m - \mathcal{E}_{Cl^-}$$

and

where $(\mathcal{E}_m - \mathcal{E}_i)$ is the driving force "behind" each ion.

Using a very simple circuit with three "DC sources" for sodium, potassium and negatively charged ions ("leakage"), *e.g.*,

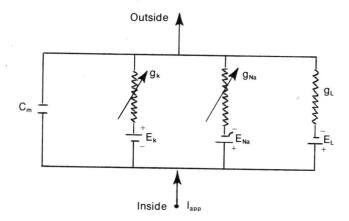

for purposes of illustration, by elementary circuit analysis we may calculate

$$\mathcal{E}_m = \left(\frac{g_{K^+}}{g_{K^+}+g_{Na^+}+g_{L^-}}\right)\mathcal{E}_{K^+} + \left(\frac{g_{Na^+}}{g_{K^+}+g_{Na^+}+g_{L^-}}\right)$$
$$\mathcal{E}_{Na^+} + \left(\frac{g_{L^-}}{g_{K^+}+g_{Na^+}+g_{L^-}}\right)\mathcal{E}_{L^-} \qquad \text{(Equation 8)}$$

or, setting $g_{K^+}+g_{Na^+}+g_{L^-}=g$, from

$$\mathcal{E}_m = \frac{1}{g}(g_{K^+}\cdot\mathcal{E}_{K^+}+g_{Na^+}\cdot\mathcal{E}_{Na^+}+g_{L^-}\cdot\mathcal{E}_{L^-}). \qquad \text{(Equation 9)}$$

At rest $g_{K^+}$ is high, and $I_{K^+}$, $g_{Na^+}$, and $I_{Na^+}$ are low, so $\mathcal{E}_m$ is close to $\mathcal{E}_{K^+}$. Variations in external $[K^+]_o$ alter $\mathcal{E}_m$ roughly logarithmically over a wide range if $g_{K^+}$ is unchanged.

After adrenalectomy the resting membrane potential of rat hearts falls from $-86$ mV to $-68$ mV.[268] There is a rise in $[K^+]_o$ from 4.3 to approximately 7.0 mM, and a drop of $[K^+]_i$ from 132 to 126 mM, which cannot totally explain the change in resting potential. Perfusion of the coronary vessels with Tyrode's solution preparation does not restore the low resting potential. Replacement therapy with adrenocortical hormones does result in an increase in membrane potential toward normal values. Difficult to understand, in the context of the "classical" view of the generation of resting transmembrane potential, is why $[K^+]_o$ does not fall below 6 mM when resting membrane potential is restored.

## E. The association-induction hypothesis

All of the preceding discussion is based upon conventional membrane theory. Although much data has been interpreted with this model, a recent alternative deserves consideration. In question is the assumption that the cellular ions and water are in free solution and maintained in their characteristic patterns of distribution by energy-consuming pumps, and that the cellular potentials reflect charge separations caused by diffusion of ions through membranes of controlled, selective permeability. Ling and others [224-228] postulate that the concept of membrane-situated pumps is thermodynamically untenable because of their excessive energy requirements. In addition, other recent data suggest that cellular water exists in an ordered state which greatly diminishes its solvent capacity for ions, and that the bulk of intracellular ions are adsorbed.[229-231] Ling [225] proposes the "Association-Induction Hypothesis" as an alternative model to explain ion accumulation and the electrophysiology of the cell.

According to the association-induction hypothesis, most of the intracellular ions are adsorbed to cellular proteins. Because of the electron densities of the adsorption sites and the association energies of $K^+$ and $Na^+$, $K^+$ is adsorbed preferentially and cooperatively. Ordering of the cellular water by the proteins greatly reduces the solutility of $Na^+$ and largely excludes that ion from the cell. The concentration of $K^+$ in the intracellular water is approximately the same as that in the extracellular water. In this model, $K^+$ tends to dissociate from the fixed anionic sites on the surface, and when the equilibrium between adsorbed $K^+$ and dissolved $K^+$ is reached, some anionic sites are unoccupied, producing the negative cellular potential. The action potential occurs when the electron densities of the adsorption sites are altered by a propagated inductive effect, and temporarily, $Na^+$ is adsorbed preferentially. Repolarization is established by restoration of the preference for $K^+$, with desorption of $Na^+$. According to this model,[232]

$$\mathcal{E}_m = A - \frac{RT}{F} \ln \left( K_{K^+}[K^+]_o + K_{Na^+}[Na^+]_o \right) \qquad \text{(Equation 10)}$$

where A, a constant includes partition functions and a parameter for the fixed anionic sites at the cell surface, RT and F have their usual meanings, and $K_{K^+}$ and $K_{Na^+}$ are the association energy constants for $K^+$ and $Na^+$, respectively. At rest (diastole), $K_{K^+} \gg K_{Na^+}$, and during the action potential, $K_{Na^+} \gg K_{K^+}$. Hence, the resting and action potentials are related closely to the external concentrations of $K^+$ and $Na^+$, respectively.

In the normal range of $[K^+]_o$, the ratio $K_{K^+}/K_{Na^+}$ is such that some $Na^+$ associates with the fixed surface charges during diastole, reducing $\mathcal{E}_m$ to less than the value predicted by consideration only of $[K^+]_o$ and $K_{K^+}$. In addition, at $[K^+]_o$ less than the physiological range, $Na^+$ association may increase cooperatively,[233] causing an absolute decrease of potential.

A comparison of the association-induction equation relating $\mathcal{E}_m$ to ionic activities and the Hodgkin-Goldman-Katz equation immediately shows that the former contains no expression for the dependence of $\mathcal{E}_m$ on $[Cl^-]_o$, $[Cl^-]_i$, $[K^+]_i$, $[Na^+]_i$.

For a further discussion of electrochemical information transfer, the reader is referred to a recent fascinating presentation by Pilla.[330]

## II. DEPOLARIZATION AND REPOLARIZATION: "ACTIVE PROPERTIES"

The propagation of the depolarization wave or action potential throughout adjacent cells is easier to describe quantitatively than the local membrane changes because the membrane relies upon both positive and negative feedback to produce pulses, but the peak values for action potentials are controlled by many local processes within the cell.

### A. Some relations between membrane potential and conductance

The action potential is described by the forms of $g_{K^+} = f_1 (\mathcal{E}_m, t)$, $g_{Na^+} = f_2 (\mathcal{E}_m, t)$ and the circuit properties of the network representing the sarcolemma. Implicit in these functions and in the remarks to follow are the following general assumptions:

(a) the total ionic current is composed of three independent parts, sodium, potassium, and "leakage,"
(b) the sodium and potassium pathways are infinitely selective,

(c) the flow of any ion down its electrochemical gradient is independent of the flow of any other ion of the same or different species (independence principle),
(d) equilibrium potentials do not change with time or current flow,
(e) the ionic current through each channel can be represented by the product of a chord conductance, which at short times is independent of potential (linear instantaneous current voltage relation), and an electrical potential difference,
(f) the transient sodium permeability change following changes in membrane potential can be represented by two independent processes (activation and inactivation).

When a stimulus is applied to responsive heart muscle in the form of an electric pulse or propagating action potential, $\mathcal{E}_m$ becomes less negative. If $I_{app}$ is the stimulating current in the membrane, and for the moment restricting the discussion to a simple equivalent electric circuit composed of Na$^+$, K$^+$ and L$^-$ cells, from Kirchoff's Law we have:

$$I_{app} = I_{K^+} + I_{Na^+} + I_{L^-} + I_C. \qquad \text{(Equation 11)}$$

Assuming that the capacitance, $C_m$, is constant, we may write

$$I_c = C_m \frac{d\mathcal{E}_m}{dt}. \qquad \text{(Equation 12)}$$

Since the ionic currents are assumed to reflect specific driving forces and conductances (e.g., $I_{K^+} = g_{K^+} (\mathcal{E}_m - \mathcal{E}_{K^+})$), substituting in equation 11:

$$\frac{d\mathcal{E}_m}{dt} = \frac{1}{C_m} [g_{K^+}(\mathcal{E}_m - \mathcal{E}_{K^+}) + g_{Na^+}(\mathcal{E}_m - \mathcal{E}_{Na^+}) + g_{L^-}(\mathcal{E}_m - \mathcal{E}_{L^-})].$$
$$\text{(Equation 13)}$$

This equation explicitly describes the dependence of $\mathcal{E}_m$ on the values of $g$. The term $g_{L^-}$ is assumed to be constant throughout. The dependence of the $g_{K^+}$ and $g_{Na^+}$ on membrane potential takes the following form, derived directly from experimental results. Let $n$, $m$, and $h$ be three parameters varying from 0 to 1, such that

$$g_{K^+} = n^4 \cdot \overline{g}_{K^+}, \quad g_{Na^+} = m^3 h \cdot g_{Na^+}$$

where $\overline{g}_{K^+}$ and $\overline{g}_{Na^+}$ are constants corresponding to the maximum respective conductances. $m$ is the dimensionless, voltage-dependent, Na$^+$-

system activation variable, and $h$ is the voltage-dependent, $Na^+$-system inactivation variable.

The quantities $n$, $m$, and $h$ are defined by the following differential equations:

$$dn/dt = \alpha_n(1-n) - \beta_n n,$$
$$dm/dt = \alpha_m(1-m) - \beta_m m,$$
$$dh/dt = \alpha_h(1-h) - \beta_h h. \qquad \text{(Equation 14)}$$

The $\alpha$'s and $\beta$'s are functions of membrane potential and temperature only. For convenience, the membrane potential scale may be translated to zero at the normal resting value $\mathcal{E}_r$ by defining

$$V = \mathcal{E}_m - \mathcal{E}_r. \qquad \text{(Equation 15)}$$

On this scale, the $\alpha$'s and $\beta$'s are defined by the formulas

$$\alpha_n = \frac{0.01(V+10)}{\exp[(V+10)/10]-1}, \quad \beta_n = 0.125 \exp\left(\frac{V}{80}\right),$$

$$\alpha_m = \frac{0.1(V+25)}{\exp[(V+25)/10]-1}, \quad \beta_m = 4 \exp\left(\frac{V}{18}\right) \qquad \text{(Equations 16)}$$

$$\alpha_h = 0.07 \exp\left(\frac{V}{20}\right), \qquad \beta_h = \frac{1}{\exp[(V+30)/10]+1}.$$

Equation (13) can be rewritten as

$$\frac{dV}{dt} = \frac{1}{C_m}[g_{K^+}(V-V_{K^+}) + g_{Na^+}(V-V_{Na^+}) + g_L(V-V_L)]. \qquad \text{(Equation 17)}$$

Equations (14), (16), and (17) then constitute the quantitative model. This is clearly a nonlinear system, which can only be integrated numerically. The study of current carriers is made possible by the voltage-clamp technique, the purpose of which is to measure the current required to hold the potential across a given area of membrane at a known value. The goal is to define the instantaneous current-voltage relationship for each charged carrier. These relations vary, depending upon the excitable tissue involved. For instance, for the squid giant axon in normal seawater, the current carried by $Na^+$ and $K^+$ is linear, *i.e.*, obeys Ohm's Law. On other tissues, the relationship is nonlinear and may be approximated by the Goldman-Hodgkin-Katz constant field equation (equation 5), which upon rearrangement and substitution for the $Na^+$-current becomes:

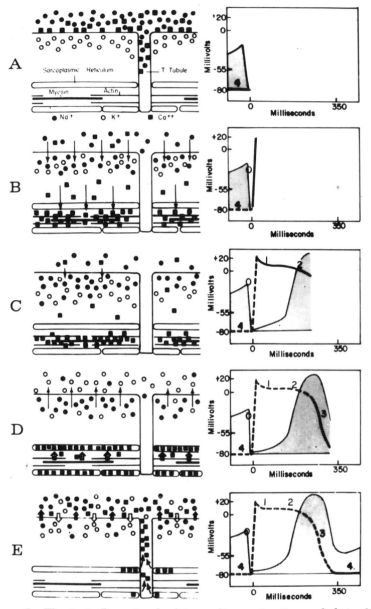

**Figure 3**   The ionic fluxes involved in cardiac contraction and their electrical consequences. After repolarization (A), the extracellular environment
is rich in sodium and the intracellular environment is rich in potassium,
with calcium probably concentrated in the region of the sarcolemma and
its specialized invaginations, the T system. The sarcoplasm has a charge of

$$I_{Na^+} = \left(\frac{P_{Na^+} + F^2 \mathcal{C}_m}{RT}\right)\left(\frac{[Na^+]_o - [Na^+]_i \exp[F\mathcal{C}_m/RT]}{1 - \exp[F\mathcal{C}_m/RT]}\right).$$ (Equation 18)

For cardiac tissue, the instantaneous current-voltage functions for each carrier are quite complex and have not yet been precisely written.

## B. Phases of the action potential

At a critical value of $\mathcal{C}_m$, the "threshold potential" at which regenerative depolarization is initiated, perhaps $-70$ mV,[279] $g_{Na^+}$ increases more than 100-fold, and $Na^+$ enters the cell in response to this primary increase in $P_{Na^+}$ (Fig 3, Panel B).

Entry of Na into the cell during early depolarization, the "fast-inward" current, describes *phase 0* of the action potential, as $\mathcal{C}_m$ approaches $\mathcal{C}_{Na^+}$ (Fig 4, phase 0, rapid upstroke.)[6] Although phase 0 only lasts approximately 1 msec, an influx of 50 $\mu$moles $Na^+$/Kg tissue/depolarization occurs.[9] The rate of rise of the action potential, dV/dt, closely reflects the magnitude of the inward $Na^+$ current,[8] which is in turn a function of the level of the resting potential, $\mathcal{C}_m$, and $[Na^+]_o$. Availability of $m$ "opens" $Na^+$-gates or channels, while availability of $h$ "closes" $Na^+$-gates (Fig 4).[9] At the rate of influx mentioned, if the $Na^+$ were not pumped out of the myocyte by the $Na^+$, $K^+$-pump, intracellular $Na^+$ would nearly double every five minutes and result in cell rupture.

The maximum rate of rise in action potential, $\mathcal{C}_{max}$ (or $V_{max}$) is a function of $\mathcal{C}_m$ (Fig 5). In general, a reduction in $\mathcal{C}_m$ depresses dV/dt and conduction velocity. Membrane *responsiveness*, the rate of depolarization with respect to the resting membrane potential, is reduced when dV/dt is depressed. The chance of decremental conduction,

---

about $-80$ millivolts in relationship to the interstitium. With the influx of sodium (B) the cell is depolarized to $+20$ mv, firing as the threshold (about $-55$ mv) is crossed. Calcium moves into the region of the sarcomere, producing actomyosin linking and contraction. During plateau of the action potential (C) $Na^+$ influx slows and $K^+$ efflux is delayed, and $Ca^{+2}$ probably sustains the inward current. Although not illustrated, while $g_{K^+}$ is decreased at this time, $K^+$-efflux is increased because of the outward electrochemical gradient with respect to $K^+$ during the depolarized state. Subsequently, $K^+$ efflux increases rapidly to repolarize the cell as $Ca^{+2}$ influx ceases and the $Ca^{+2}$ is pumped into the sarcoplasmic reticulum, allowing relaxation to occur (D). The $Na^+$-$K^+$ pump returns sodium to the outside and potassium to the intracellular space. At the same time, the stored $Ca^{+2}$ diffuses from the sarcoplasmic reticulum to the extracellular space (E). Grey shaded area is total membrane resistance.

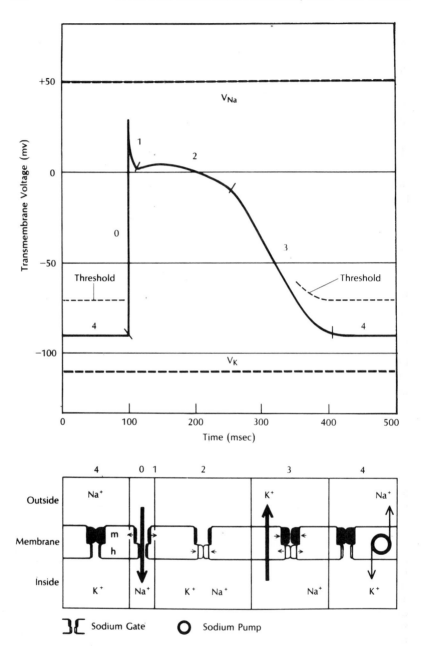

**Figure 4**  A schematic diagram of a cardiac action potential is shown at top, and the events that determine the time voltage course of the action potential are shown in the lower diagram. When the cell is quiescent (phase

blockage, and also reentrant rhythms increases with poor membrane responsiveness.

Phase 1 of the action potential, or rapid repolarization, is marked by decreasing $g_{Na^+}$ and by an inward chloride current [280] (not shown in Figs 3 and 4). Phase 2 of repolarization—the plateau—was thought to be present in cardiac muscle because of the delay in outward potassium flow. However, considerable evidence now supports the contention that inward calcium current occurs during this period (Fig 3, panel C, Fig 6).[10, 12, 15-17, 269-271] In ventricular muscle, decreasing $I_{Na^+}$ is important in the generation of the plateau of the action potential, and in Purkinje fibers the contribution of $I_{K^+}$ to the plateau is also significant. When $[Ca^{++}]_o$ is reduced, the calcium equilibrium potential is shifted to much lower values. The fact that electrical activity is possible in $Ca^{++}$-free solutions is explained by assuming that $Na^+$ and/or other ions can replace $Ca^{++}$ within the "slow system".[272] A number of pharmacologic agents are known which depress the slow inward current, for instance $Mn^{++}$,[272, 273] $La^{++}$ [273] and verapamil.[270, 271] For further discussion of divalent cations as charge carriers the reader is referred to two recent reviews on the subject.[274, 275]

Phase 3, final repolarization, is mediated through a marked increase in potassium conductance, for which there are four potassium channels presently known (Figs 4 and 6),[281] and the cell returns to the resting membrane potential. To account for phase 3, a time-dependent decrease in inward current ($Na^+ \pm Ca^{++}$) has also been proposed.[282] Ex-

---

4), its membrane is much more permeable to potassium than any other ion, so that its resting transmembrane voltage is near the potassium equilibrium potential ($V_{K^+}$). At excitation (0), the cell membrane suddenly becomes permeable to sodium; the intense inward sodium current carries sufficient positive charge into the cell to carry the transmembrane voltage to a value near the sodium equilibrium potential ($V_{Na^+}$). In the several phases of repolarization (1 through 3), changes in transmembrane action potential initially reflect the decreasing sodium conductance and subsequently the marked increase in potassium conductance, which returns the membrane potential to its resting value. Movement of sodium across the cell membrane from outside to inside is controlled by two component sodium channels, $m$ and $h$, which appear to work in opposition to each other. With sufficient depolarization, activation of the $m$ site permits rapid influx of sodium. In succeeding phases of the depolarization-repolarization cycle, sodium conductance is decreased by closure of the $h$ site; in phase 4 the sodium-carrying system is again available and awaiting activation. In this figure the supernormal period is ignored. Reproduced with permission from Bigger: *Hospital Practice* **7**:70, 1972.

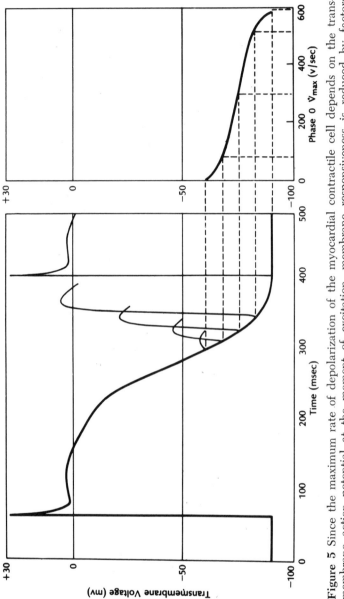

**Figure 5** Since the maximum rate of depolarization of the myocardial contractile cell depends on the transmembrane action potential at the moment of excitation, membrane responsiveness is reduced by factors causing depolarization, *e.g.*, excitation before the repolarization phase is complete and the cell returns to its resting state. As shown diagrammatically at left, response to excitation is minimal at an action potential in the range of $-60$ mv but increases as the potential moves toward the resting value ($-90$ mv). Maximum rates of depolarization ($V_{max}$) at various transmembrane voltage levels are shown at right. Reproduced with permission from Bigger: *Hospital Practice* **7**:70, 1972.

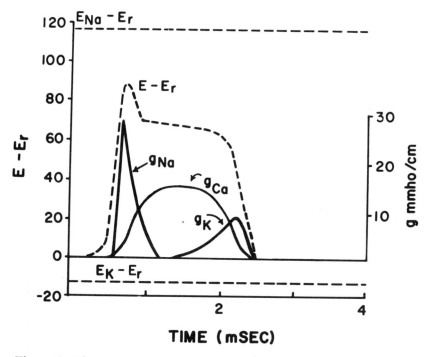

**Figure 6** The components of the cardiac action potential (anomalous rectification is not shown here).

actly which process appears to be manifest is a function of the tissue and experimental design employed.

The time- and voltage-dependence of ion conductances are explained by the opening of ion channels, controlled by gates. One possibility is that charged flexible polar end groups of membrane phospholipids alter their position, thus allowing changes in ion conductance. This hypothesis has led to the search for "gating currents," caused by the opening and closing of the gates. In the axon, such currents have been identified.[11] An equivalent circuit based upon the above sequence appears in Fig 7A.

## C. Inward-going rectification

The Goldman-Hodgkin-Katz equation predicts only a flattening of the $[K^+]_o$-potential curve and does not account for the reduction of potential which occurs in cardiac Purkinje fibers in $[K^+]_o$ less than

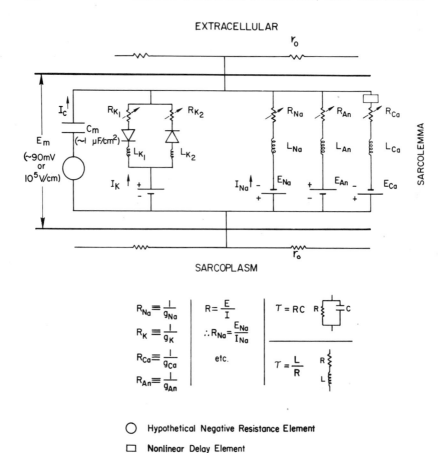

○ Hypothetical Negative Resistance Element

□ Nonlinear Delay Element

**Figure 7A** An equivalent electric circuit for the events depicted in Figure 6. In a uniform membrane, current density (amp/cm²) may be composed of ionic current and capacity current, given by $I_m = I_i + C_m(dV/dt)$.

$$g_{K^+} = \frac{1}{R_{K_1^+}} + \frac{2}{R_{K_2^+}}$$

about 2 mM. Cardiac Purkinje cells have been shown to pass current inward more easily than outward, and the difference of resistance has been related to difference of $K^+$ conductance, $g_{K^+}$.[219] It has been shown further that the permeability of the cell to $^{42}K^+$ increases or decreases as $[K^+]_o$ is increased or decreased.[220] Using "conventional" theory, this effect is a function of the electrochemical gradient of $K^+$ and $\mathcal{E}_m - \mathcal{E}_{K^+}$.[221] Hence, as $[K^+]_o$ is decreased $\mathcal{E}_m - \mathcal{E}_{K^+}$ increases, and $g_{K^+}$ decreases (Fig 7B).[278]

The relative contribution of $C_{Na^+}$ to $C_m$ should be increased by a decrease of $g_{K^+}$, providing an explanation for the deviation of $C_m$ from $C_{K^+}$ at normal to low levels of $[K^+]_o$. Supporting this notion is the observation that the decrease in $C_m$ of cardiac Purkinje cells in $[K^+]_o$ less than 2 mM can be prevented by removing $Na^+$ from the bathing solution.[222, 223]

## III. POTASSIUM LEVELS AND MEMBRANE POTENTIAL

### A. Potassium and the Nernst equation

The Goldman-Hodgkin-Katz relation (equation 5) may be reduced to the following approximation, assuming $Cl^-$ to be passively distributed and $[Na^+]_i$ to be very small in comparison with $[Na^+]_o$:

$$[K^+]_i \approx \left[ [K^+]_o + \frac{P_{Na^+}}{P_{K^+}}[Na^+]_o \right] \exp \frac{C_m F}{RT} \quad \text{(Equation 19)}$$

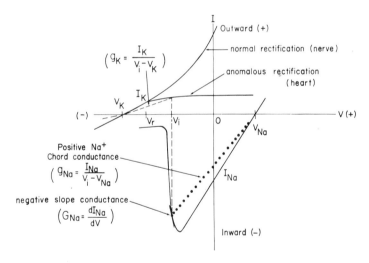

**Figure 7B** Schematic illustration of $Na^+$ and $K^+$ current-voltage relations that might exist early in the depolarization phase of an action potential showing anomalous rectification in heart muscle. Solid lines in upper quadrants contrast normal and anomalous rectification relations for $I_K$. Solid line in lower quadrants shows $I_{Na}$ relation. The dotted line shows $Na^+$ chord conductance at arbitrary potential $V_i$ contrasted with $Na^+$ slope conductance (negative slope) at $V_i$. Dashed line in upper left quadrant shows positive $K^+$ chord conductance at $V_i$. $V_{Na}$, $V_K$, and $V_r$ are $Na^+$ equilibrium potential, $K^+$ equilibrium potential, and membrane resting potentials, respectively.

Equation nineteen explicitly states that the potassium concentration within the cell is a function of extracellular potassium concentration, the ratio of permeabilities of sodium and potassium, extracellular sodium concentration, and the resting membrane potential. Since other terms appear in the right side of equation nineteen, serum potassium need not reflect intracellular potassium nor total body $K^+$.

Concentrating only upon $K^+$ as the primary determinant of passive resting membrane potential, we have

$$\mathcal{E}_m = 6.15 \log_{10} \frac{[K^+]_i}{[K^+]_o} \qquad \text{(Equation 20)}$$

This Nernst equation states that raising $[K^+]_o$ will reduce $\mathcal{E}_m$ (less negative) and the membrane will be depolarized. The extent of $g_{Na^+}$ increase during depolarization will lessen, the upstroke velocity of the action potential $(dV/dt)$ and its amplitude will decrease [60] (Table I). Permeability to $K^+$ is also increased.[61] Decreased membrane potential would be expected to reduce conduction velocity.[62] * However, reduction in the resting membrane potential simultaneously brings the membrane potential closer to the threshold potential, thus lowering the strength of the stimulus necessary to bring $\mathcal{E}_m$ to threshold. For this reason, conduction velocity may first increase due to the proximity of the reduced $\mathcal{E}_m$ to threshold (Fig 8). An increase in $P_{K^+}$ tends to accelerate repolarization and shorten the action potential duration.[63]

### B. Further effects of altering potassium on other electrophysiologic properties

In automatic fibers increasing $[K^+]_o$ lowers the slope of diastolic depolarization (phase 4) as well as reduces the resting membrane potential, both of which would depress automaticity. Closeness of the resting membrane potential to the threshold potential facilitates automaticity. Hence if increasing $[K^+]_o$ reduces membrane potential more than it does threshold potential, the rate of spontaneous discharge may remain unaffected while the slope of phase 4 is less steep.[64]

Lowered $[K^+]_o$ concentrations hyperpolarizes ventricular muscle,[65]

---

* Conduction velocity, $\theta$, is given by

$$\theta = \frac{\text{(a) } d^2 \mathcal{E}_m / dt^2}{2R_i[(C_m)d\mathcal{E}_m/dt + I_m]} \qquad \text{(equation 21)}$$

where a = fibre radius, $\mathcal{E}_m$ = membrane voltage, $C_m$ = specific membrane capacitance, $I_m$ = membrane current density, $R_i$ = resistance.

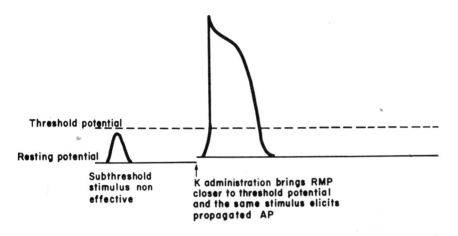

**Threshold potential**

**Resting potential**

**Subthreshold stimulus non effective**

**K administration brings RMP closer to threshold potential and the same stimulus elicits propagated AP**

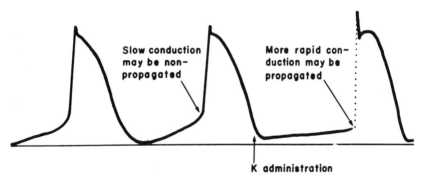

**Slow conduction may be non-propagated**

**More rapid conduction may be propagated**

**K administration**

**Figure 8** Diagrammatic presentation of two mechanisms which may explain increased conduction velocity produced by slight increase in extracellular $K^+$ concentration. Reproduced with permission.[70]

but hypopolarizes Purkinje fibers in most species. Action potential duration is prolonged by decreasing $[K^+]_o$,[64, 65] and the slope of the diastolic depolarization curve is elevated and may induce automatic activity in a fiber with latent pacemaker properties.

Considerable variation exists in specialized fiber sensitivity to the ratio $[K^+]_i/[K^+]_o$. Atrial fibers are most sensitive, ventricular cells less so, and specialized sinoatrial node, internodal atrial tracts and bundle of His fibers are least sensitive. Some fibers exist from the sinoatrial node to the ventricle which are capable of sinoventricular conduction when electrical activity of the atria are suppressed by high $[K^+]_o$.[65a]

Table I  Effects of electrolyte alterations on electrophysiologic properties of the heart.  Reproduced with permission from Zipes.[74]

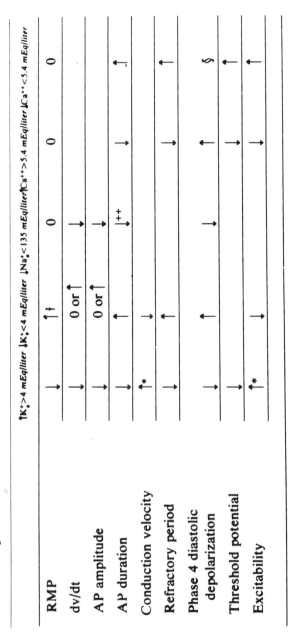

| | $\uparrow K^+_o > 4$ mEq/liter | $\downarrow K^+_o < 4$ mEq/liter | $\downarrow Na^+_i < 135$ mEq/liter | $\uparrow Ca^{++} > 5.4$ mEq/liter | $\downarrow Ca^{++} < 5.4$ mEq/liter |
|---|---|---|---|---|---|
| RMP | ↓ | ↑† | 0 | 0 | 0 |
| dv/dt | ↓ | 0 or ↑ | ↓ | 0 | 0 |
| AP amplitude | ↓ | 0 or ↑ | ↓ | 0 | 0 |
| AP duration | ↓ | ↓ | ↓†† | ↓ | ↑-¶ |
| Conduction velocity | ↑* | ↓ | ↓ | ↓ | ← |
| Refractory period | ↓ | ↑ | | ↓ | ↑ |
| Phase 4 diastolic depolarization | ↓ | ↑ | ↓ | | § |
| Threshold potential | ↓ | | | ↑ | ↑ |
| Excitability | ↑* | ↑ | | ↓ | ↑ |

↑ = increase; ↓ = decrease; 0 = no change (in absolute values).
*When plasma K exceeds about 6 mEq/liter, opposite changes occur.
†For ventricular muscle; opposite for Purkinje fibers when K < 2.7 mEq/liter.
††Species variation, degree of $Na^+$ depletion and substance substituted for $Na^+$ all affect this variable.[1]
§Reduction to less than 0.54 mEq/liter increases the slope of diastolic depolarization, reduces resting membrane potential and abolishes the overshoot.[1]
RMP = resting membrane potential; AP = action potential.

In addition to the final level of $[K^+]_i/[K^+]_o$, the rate at which this ratio changes is an important determinant of the effect on impulse formation and conduction. Rapid correction of $[K^+]_o$ in a $K^+$-depleted preparation shortens action potential duration and slows diastolic depolarization. Thus selective inhibition in pacemaker activity—the Zwaardemaker-Libbrecht phenomenon—may result in bradycardia, cardiac arrest, or depressed conduction,[66] probably due to an increase in $\mathcal{E}_m$ mediated by increased $g_{K^+}$. Finally, other modifiers of the response of cardiac fibers to variations in $[K^+]_i/[K^+]_o$ include pH, $pO_2$, and concentrations of other electrolytes. These may become important in seriously-ill patients, for instance, with the cardiogenic shock syndrome.

Intracellular kaliopenia reduces $\mathcal{E}_m$ and action potential duration (Fig 9). Since it is the ratio $[K^+]_i/[K^+]_o$ which alters membrane properties, the response to reduction in the numerator may be similar to a rise in the denominator.

The electrophysiologic actions of $[K^+]_i/[K^+]_o$ changes are reflected clinically in disorders of impulse formation and conduction.[62, 67-78] Because changes in $[K^+]_i/[K^+]_o$ are responsible for the generation and maintenance of the transmembrane potential, the disturbances in impulse formation and conductance, leading to serious arrhythmias, are seen within clinically common ranges of $[K^+]_o$. Of all ions present physiologically, potassium is the most important and the only one with clinically significant antiarrhythmic properties.[1, 70-78]

## IV. EXCITATION-CONCENTRATION COUPLING

A complex relation exists between potassium and calcium metabolism within the normal and ischemic heart cell. For this reason, excitation-contraction coupling and the effect of ischemia on calcium kinetics in the myocardium will be discussed in the following sections.

### A. Role of calcium in initiation of contraction

Electrical depolarization initiated by the pacemaker is propagated down the sarcolemma and into its continuation, the T-tubules, or invaginations of the membrane into the sarcomeres (Fig 10). A separate system of channels—the sarcoplasmic reticulum—have dilated lateral cisternae which abut on the canals of the T-system. Coincident with and shortly after rapid depolarization, there is a direct and possibly indirect influx of calcium from the T-tubular fluid, the latter via a regenerative release of calcium from the sarcoplasmic reticulum (Table II). In cardiac muscle the bulk of the calcium for contraction is derived from the extracellular fluid, in contrast with skeletal muscle. The magnitude of $Ca^{+2}$ influx is insufficient to effect contraction, and it

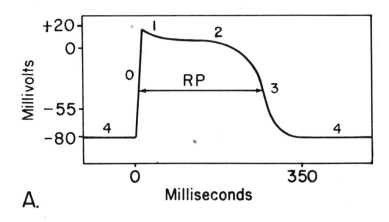

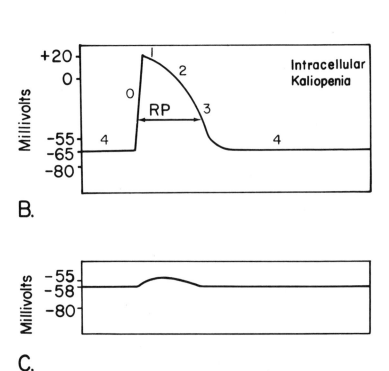

**Figure 9**   A reduction in $[K^+]_i/[K^+]_o$ abbreviates the refractory period, and lowers resting membrane potential. The electrophysiologic changes effected by ischemia and hypoxia may be similar.

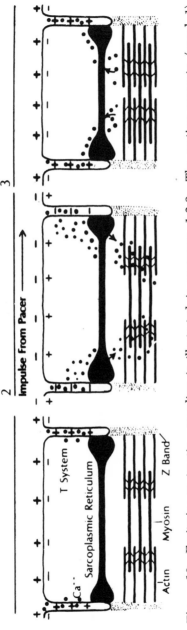

**Figure 10** Excitation-contraction coupling is illustrated in sequence 1-2-3. The resting myocyte (panel 1) depolarized (panel 2) with simultaneous consequent calcium influx (panel 2) to produce contraction (panel 3). Calcium is actively bound to sarcoplasmic reticulum to initiate relaxation (panel 3).

**Table II**    The events connecting action potential transmission of the cardiac impulse and contraction.

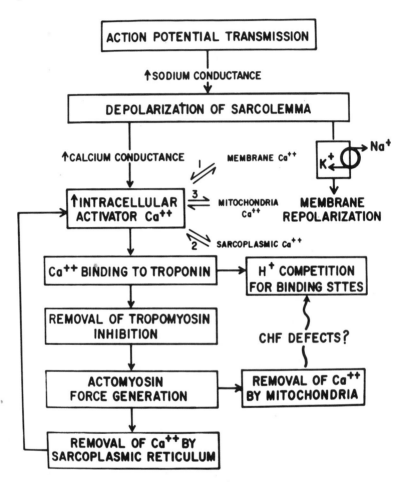

therefore is probable that the $Ca^{++}$ derived from the extracellular fluid "triggers" the release of additional $Ca^{++}$ from internal sites, the binding sites within the sarcoplasmic reticulum. In the relaxed muscle $[Ca^{++}]_i$ is approximately $10^{-7}$ M, which increases by a multiple of 2-3 during excitation. After diffusion to the myofilaments, calcium is thought to interact with its protein receptor on the myofibrillar protein troponin. Further interaction with a second regulatory protein, tropomyosin, results in exposure of postulated sites on myosin. Thus calcium ion causes a decrease in the inhibitory actions of the troponin-tropomyosin complex rather than directly stimulating actin or myosin. Actin and myosin filaments slide, in close association with cleavage of ATP by heavy meromyosin ATPase. Contractile strength is directly related to the quantity of calcium available to actomyosin. Calcium ions appear to control the number of sites at which cross-bridges between actin and myosin are formed, but have no significant effect on the kinetics of a single bridge. Therefore, the number of cross-bridges formed may explain variations in contractility. ADP is rephosphorylated to ATP within the same contraction cycle (Fig 11). Relaxation is attended by dissociation of calcium and rapid active calcium sequestration by the sarcoplasmic reticulum, also called the "relaxing" system (Fig 12). Some calcium also finds its way into mitochondria. The time course of fall of force after contraction is essentially that of calcium removal from the filaments. Sarcotubular calcium is then eventually exchanged with sodium at the sarcolemma via a $Na^+$, $Ca^{++}$-pump (to be further discussed in a later section) and returned to the extracellular fluid within the T-system.

## B. Source of activator calcium

Considerable evidence now supports the contention that significant amounts of calcium from the interstitium enter the cell during the plateau of the action potential.[12, 335-338] The intensity of such a calcium current is a function of the availability of calcium in the extracellular fluid, within the sarcolemma and the intracellular calcium pools, and the duration of the active state. The ratio of $[Ca^{++}]_o/[Ca^{++}]_i$ at rest is of the order of magnitude of $10^5$:1 (from the Nernst equation, $\mathcal{E}_{Ca^{++}} = RT/2F \ln ([Ca^{++}]_o/[Ca^{++}]_i)$ and $P_{Ca^{++}}$ increases significantly during excitation. Myocardial contractility directly depends upon the calcium influx during depolarization.[13-18, 339] These data fit with a large body of related information: $Na^+$-$Ca^{++}$ antagonism in nonmammalian membrane systems; augmented contractility resulting from lengthened phase 2 of the action potential; [16, 18] positive inotropic action of elevated extracellular calcium concentrations [15-21] and reduced extracellular sodium or potassium concentrations; [5, 7, 13, 22, 23] and influence of pharmacologic agents: the digitalis glycosides,[24] the catecholamines,[25] glucagon,[26] the beta-adrenergic blocking agents, verapamil,[27] and some local anesthetics.[28]

The actual source of activator calcium and the details of excitation-contraction coupling remain speculative. Hence the control that membrane electrical activity exerts on myofilament contractility is also unclear. Recently Nayler [11] wrote: "the sites at which the $Ca^{2+}$ exert their effect, therefore, must be in close proximity to the extracellular

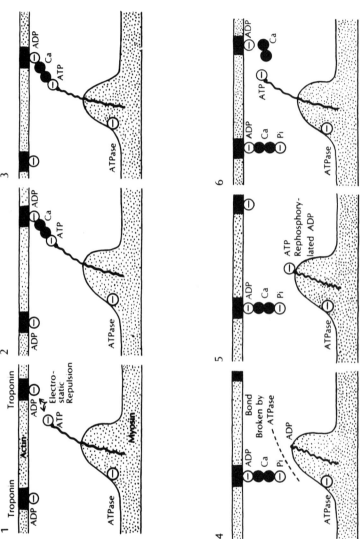

**Figure 11**   The sliding filament model may operate as illustrated above: ATP-heavy meromyosin and ADP-troponin electrostatically repel each other at rest (panel 1). Divalent calcium binds these sites (panel 2), causing a conformational change in the globular myosin head (panel 3). Actin then actively slides along the myosin filament, whence ATP is hydrolyzed by myosin ATPase (panel 4). ADP is rephosphorylated (panel 5), leaving the contractile apparatus ready for the following contraction (panel 6).

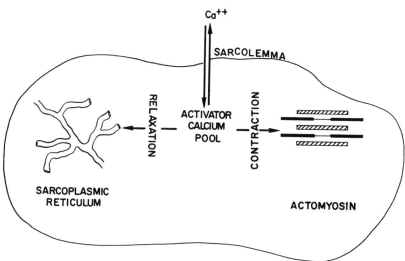

**Figure 12**  The distribution of intracellular calcium. Mitochondria may also significantly sequester calcium.

space, *i.e.*, they must be superficially-located sites. Possibly, there is rapid, direct exchange of $Ca^{2+}$ between intra- and extracellular phases. Alternatively, the $Ca^{2+}$ exchange involved may not reflect a direct exchange of $Ca^{2+}$ between intra- and extracellular phases but instead the displacement of $Ca^{2+}$ from superficially-located binding sites in the immediate vicinity, or within, the cell membrane itself."

Recent information from laboratories using three different techniques bear on the problem: $^{45}Ca^{++}$ washout from ventricular muscle, kinetic analysis of $Ca^{++}$-binding and $Ca^{++}$-uptake by myocardial microsomes, and voltage clamp data. The rate of decline in peak-developed tension upon exposure to 0 concentration of extracellular $^{45}Ca^{++}$ ($t_{1/2} \leq 1$ min) in rabbit ventricular muscle indicates that a source of $Ca^{++}$ in rapid equilibrium with the interstitium must provide the activator $Ca^{++}$.[29] Displacement of $Ca^{++}$ by lanthanum produces an abrupt initial decline in tension and subsequent depression in contractility until lanthanum is removed.[30]

Lanthanum uncouples excitation-contraction coupling such that membrane depolarization is not followed by tension development. Also cited is the fact that the volume of the sarcoplasmic reticulum in heart muscle is less than in skeletal muscle, but the volume of the transverse tubule is greater. These data support the hypothesis that the interstitial space is the primary source of coupling calcium on a beat-to-beat basis and that intermediate sites at or near the cell surface exist to supply the myofilaments. Bailey and co-workers [31] have recently provided additional washout data also suggesting the working sequence of events as follows: activator $Ca^{++}$ enters the cell from the interstitium, is temporarily stored in superficial binding sites, is released during depolarization to effect actomyosin sliding, accumulates in the sarcoplasmic reticulum to initiate relaxation, and is ultimately removed from the cell by an active process (Fig 10).

In summary, although the $Ca^{++}$ derived from the extracellular space is physiologically important, it is quantitatively insufficient to account for the activation of contraction. As mentioned, the calcium comprising the initial influx is presently regarded as a trigger pool, promoting the release of further $Ca^{++}$ from the sarcoplasmic reticulum.

## C. An alternate hypothesis

A provocative alternate theory was proposed by Schwartz.[318] Suppose $Na^+$, $K^+$-ATPase is activated by $K^+$ in a two non-equivalent site model:

$$\frac{v}{Vm} = \left\{ \left[ 1 + \frac{0.213}{[K^+]}\left( 1 + \frac{[Na^+]}{13.7} \right) \right] \left[ 1 + \frac{0.091}{[K^+]}\left( 1 + \frac{[Na^+]}{74.1} \right) \right] \right\}^{-1}$$

$$\qquad\qquad\quad \text{Site I} \qquad\qquad\qquad\quad \text{Site II}$$

(Concentrations are in mM)

Calcium decreases the amount of potassium necessary to activate the enzyme half-maximally, possibly by interaction around site I (Fig 2B). Under normal conditions $Ca^{++}$ partially substitutes for $K^+$ at site I, but $K^+$ binds to site II such that the pump couples $Na^+$ efflux with $K^+$ and $Ca^{++}$ influx. At site I, interactions with $Ca^{++}$ are a function of the dissociation constants for $Na^+$, $K^+$ and $Ca^{++}$ of site I and the extracellular activities of these ions:

$$\% \text{ of site I bound to calcium} = \left\{ \left[ 1 + \frac{K_c}{[Ca^{2+}]}\left( 1 + \frac{[Na^+]}{13.7} + \frac{[K^+]}{0.213} \right) \right] \right\}^{-1}$$

where $K_c$ is a dissociation constant for calcium.

Such a hypothesis may be used to explain the actions of the digitalis glycosides as an $Na^+$, $K^+$-ATPase inhibitor, and the Bowditch effect. A scheme outlining how $Ca^{++}$ influx may be coupled to net $K^+$ loss appears in Figure 14A (page 209). Site I is the $K^+$-activation site at which $Ca^{++}$ may replace $K^+$. $Ca^{++}$ influx and $K^+$ efflux could be coupled in such a way that calcium moves "down" its electrochemical gradient, as potassium moves "down" its concentration gradient, both on a carrier "shuttle."

## D. Calcium binding and tension response

Katz and Repke [32, 33] have identified two kinetically distinct microsomal transport processes: calcium-binding and calcium-uptake. Calcium-binding is thought to reflect the process of intracellular release of activator calcium, whereas calcium-uptake is postulated to reflect calcium uptake into storage sites.

The tension response to depolarization of heart muscle to a given level—the "clamp voltage"—consists of a rapid *twitch* and a secondary *slow* mechanical component. Since the threshold for calcium current is $-30$ to $-40$ mv [34] and the threshold for the twitch is nearly $-60$ mv,[35] it has been argued that the direct inward calcium current probably could not directly supply total activator $Ca^{++}$ for the twitch response. A regenerative type of internal calcium release, triggered by the inward calcium current, is probable.[36] It has been said that in Purkinje fibers a slower mechanical response is more closely linked to calcium entry.[37] These observations, and the kinetic data of Repke and Katz, also indicate that the source of depolarization-induced activator calcium release is different from the site(s) of uptake and storage. The physiologic muscle contraction may be a fusion of the twitch and slow responses mentioned.

Recently the voltage-clamp response of various myocardial tissues of differing species to short and long depolarizing pulses was reviewed extensively by Coraboeuf.[346] Long depolarizations of heart muscle produce a two component contraction composed of an initial component, termed $C_I$, which is similar to the phasic response triggered by short depolarizing pulses (5-50 ms in frog fibers). A later contracture, termed $C_{II}$, appears as a slower component after a delay of 150-200 ms. $C_{II}$ may not be observed in Purkinje fibers, and this component may also be impossible to separate from $C_I$ in particular myocardial tissues under given experimental conditions. $C_I$ mechanical response begins at a threshold of $-30$ to $-40$ mv, disappears at the potential where $I_{Ca^{++}}$ becomes zero, *i.e.*, at $\mathcal{E}_{Ca^{++}}$, and disappears in the presence of manganese, a $Ca^{++}$-free medium, or D-600, all of which reduce $I_{Ca^{++}}$. $C_I$, or the phasic component, is the mechanical response to the slow inward calcium current, activated by the catecholamines, to be further discussed in the next section.

The relationship between $C_{II}$ and voltage is different from the $C_I$-voltage curve. A large $C_{II}$ tension is observed when the membrane is depolarized beyond $\mathcal{E}_{Ca^{++}}$ at a time when $I_{Ca^{++}}$ is an *outward* current, and is not blocked by manganese or in a $Ca^{++}$-free solution. In frog atrial fibers exposed to a $Na^+$-free lithium Ringer's solution, $C_{II}$ is abolished within 10-15 minutes while $C_I$ is still present and prolonged. Upon returning to normal Ringer's solution, $C_{II}$ recovers in association with replenishment of $[Na^+]_i$. Further, substances which increase $[Na^+]_i$, such as ouabain, increase $C_{II}$ amplitude while $C_I$ remains unaltered.[347] Therefore it has been proposed that the $C_{II}$ mechanical component is dependent upon internal sodium competing for calcium sites when the membrane is depolarized.

## E. Calcium "spikes"

To recapitulate, there are two depolarizing inward currents contributing to the action potential in the heart cell—a "fast" and a "slow" current. The former is carried by $Na^+$ and has the following properties:

### FAST INITIAL CHANNEL

1. Current is carried by $Na^+$-influx through a "pure" channel
2. May be abolished by the removal of external $Na^+$
3. Selectively blocked by tetrodotoxin
4. Completely inactivated by a long-lasting offset of membrane potential to approximately $-50$ mv.

The "slow" channel has the contrasting properties:

### SLOW CHANNEL

1. Channel is "mixed" in the sense that both $Ca^{++}$ and $Na^+$ may carry current
2. In $Na^+$-free medium slow channel current is activated at a threshold potential of $-30$ to $-50$ mv
3. Affected very little by removal of external $Na^+$
4. Unaffected by tetrodotoxin
5. Very sensitive to changes in external $Ca^{++}$ concentration
6. Effect may be reproduced by strontium and barium ions
7. May be blocked by the lanthanides and by the transition metals Co, Ni, Mn, and by verapamil and D-600, a methoxy derivative of verapamil
8. Increased greatly by the catecholamines and by the methylxanthines, an effect somewhat mimicked by cyclic AMP and dibutyryl cyclic AMP
   a. depolarized myocardium is more sensitive to isoproterenol than to epinephrine or norepinephrine effect on slow channel
   b. response may be blocked by propranolol
   c. catecholamines do not affect the kinetics of the slow

$Ca^{++}$ channel, but they increase the maximal conductance of these channels.

Both slow and fast channel kinetics may be described by the Hodgkin-Huxley equations as a voltage- and time-dependent conductance system.[274, 275, 341] Since there is a strict relation between the amplitude of epinephrine-induced depolarization and $[Ca^{++}]_o$, such recordings have been termed "calcium spikes."[342] The propagation of such impulses have been carefully characterized by Cranefield, Hoffman and Wit.[234, 241-243, 283, 284, 343, 344] In Purkinje fibers depolarized by $K^+$ and treated with epinephrine, slow propagation may be associated with one- or two-way block, summation, inhibition, and reentry. The pathway for reentry and circus movement may be shorter than 1 cm. Particularly important is the potential significance of these data in an area of myocardial ischemia partially depolarized and under the influence of enhanced catecholamine levels. Such conditions would favor the development of reentrant arrhythmias.

In the experiments cited above [243] the slow responses were stimulus-dependent. However, under certain circumstances spontaneous (slow) activity in depolarized myocardium has been reported, occurring either repetitively [269] or singly.[345] The potential significance of such spontaneous depolarizations in the genesis of arrhythmias arising in ischemic myocardium is yet to be determined.

## F. Effect of ischemia and hypoxia on excitation-contraction coupling

### 1. *Acute ischemia*

Acute ischemia has been said not to grossly alter transmission of the action potential nor immediately affect transmembrane potential.[38] However, the plateau of the action potential is abbreviated in response to ischemia [39] and hypoxia,[40] possibly because of the inhibitory effect of acidosis on $Ca^{++}$ influx,[41] although the action potential may remain unaltered even when developed tension is negligible.[42] Prolonged ischemia eventually results in depolarization because failure of the $Na^+$, $K^+$-pump will result in intracellular $K^+$ depletion and inexcitability.

Acute ischemia, with attendant intracellular acidosis, also affects $Ca^{++}$-troponin binding. Direct measurement reveals that low pH inhibits the affinity of troponin for calcium [43] (Table III). Katz,[44, 45] stressing that the immediate effects of myocardial ischemia do not include any gross alteration in the myofibrillar proteins,[46] and reduction in ATP concentrations does not cause rigor,[47] has postulated that this

Table III   A decrease in coronary blood flow is thought to effect an immediate reduction in contractility via the accumulation of hydrogen ions intracellularly. Hydrogen ion lowers the affinity of troponin for Ca$^{++}$ and at the same time increases the affinity of the sarcoplasmic reticulum for Ca$^{++}$.

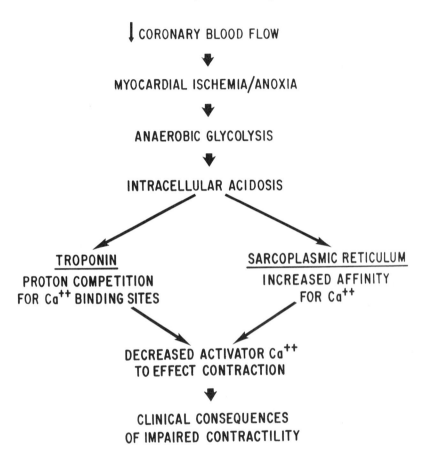

$\downarrow$ CORONARY BLOOD FLOW

$\Downarrow$

MYOCARDIAL ISCHEMIA/ANOXIA

$\Downarrow$

ANAEROBIC GLYCOLYSIS

$\Downarrow$

INTRACELLULAR ACIDOSIS

TROPONIN
PROTON COMPETITION
FOR Ca$^{++}$ BINDING SITES

SARCOPLASMIC RETICULUM
INCREASED AFFINITY
FOR Ca$^{++}$

DECREASED ACTIVATOR Ca$^{++}$
TO EFFECT CONTRACTION

$\Downarrow$

CLINICAL CONSEQUENCES
OF IMPAIRED CONTRACTILITY

inhibition of troponin-Ca$^{++}$ binding is primarily responsible for early pump failure.

Normally, cardiac relaxation is achieved by Ca$^{++}$ sequestration by the sarcoplasmic reticulum, thereby denying Ca$^{++}$ to the myofilaments for contraction. This process is greatly hastened by 3′,5′-(cyclic) AMP in the presence of the correct protein kinase.[48] The reaction is also pH-dependent: when protons are available sarcoplasmic reticulum binds Ca$^{++}$ avidly.[49, 50] Intracellular acidosis associated with ischemia and hypoxia would be expected to make less Ca$^{++}$ available to the contractile apparatus (Table IV). After ligation of the left circumflex

**Table IV**  The events leading to myocyte death. Connecting lines do not necessarily imply a cause-and-effect relationship.

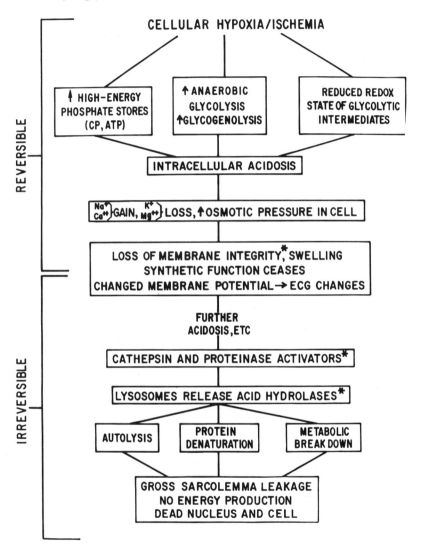

coronary artery in the dog, producing a 50-90 percent reduction in force development, calcium release by sarcoplasmic reticulum derived from ischemic muscle was lowered by 75 percent.[51] This applied to both spontaneous and pH-induced Ca++ release, and persisted for 14 days. The impairment occurred early, 12-60 min after ligation, when other membrane functions were normal.[52]

## 2. "Chronic" ischemia

In prolonged or "chronic" ischemia, not only was $Ca^{++}$ release by sarcoplasmic reticulum severely impaired, but $Ca^{++}$-binding was reduced as well during the first two weeks following left coronary arterial occlusion.[52] This correlated with the deficiencies in both mitochondria and the $Na^+$, $K^+$-ATPase system. In several other models of chronically-ischemic and failing hearts, the ability of sarcoplasmic reticulum to bind $Ca^{++}$ was impaired as well. Thus in the spontaneously failing heart-lung preparation,[53] the isolated failing rat heart,[54] the myopathic Syrian hamster,[55] and in human recipient cardiac tissue,[56] $Ca^{++}$-binding by sarcoplasmic reticulum was reduced. While such molecular "defects" have been classically considered detrimental,[57] they may be protective.[58] Since a reduction in activator $Ca^{++}$ diminishes the number of actomyosin cross-bridges reacting, a match between the (lowered) energy available to the ischemic myocardium and its energy demands are ensured. Since imbalance between energy supply and demand may initiate and/or further myocardial necrosis, the regulation of myocardial energy consumption by control of inotropic level by sarcoplasmic reticular $Ca^{++}$-binding would certainly be advantageous. Indeed, intracellular calcium overload appears to be harmful to the myocardial cell in a variety of circumstances.[59]

## G. Effects of potassium on contractility and excitation-contraction coupling

### 1. Positive inotropic action

A reduction in $[K^+]_o$ is positively inotropic and is associated with net $[Ca^{++}]_o$ uptake.[79] Some investigators hypothesized that an increase in $[K^+]_i/[K^+]_o$ could enhance $K^+$ efflux and $Ca^{++}$ influx through a coupling mechanism,[80] although the supporting evidence available is weak. However, when $[Ca^{++}]_o/[Na^+]^2$ was maintained to exclude any possible external $Na^+$-$Ca^{++}$ competition, this inotropic action depended upon $[Na^+]_o$ (see equation 10). Diminished $[Na^+]_o$ attenuated or abolished the inotropic action of $[K^+]_o$.[81] Another explanation offered was that lowered $[K^+]_o$ inhibited $Na^+$, $K^+$-pumping, a phenomenon previously described.[82, 83] This would lead to $[Na^+]_i$ accumulation, and augmented $Ca^{++}$ influx through a postulated $Na^+$, $Ca^{++}$-coupling mechanism.[5, 22, 84]

It appears that the effect of $[K^+]_o$ alterations on myocardial contractility are mediated by variation in $Ca^{++}$ influx and by increased $[Na^+]_i$.[328] The lack of direct inotropic properties of $K^+$ is rather supported by experiments in which $[K^+]_o$ was doubled without any changes in guinea pig papillary muscle force development.[85]

2. *Negative inotropic action*

The deleterious effects of potassium depletion and low serum and myocardial potassium concentrations was suggested by Harrison[86] in 1930 who reported low myocardial $K^+$ levels in patients with advanced congestive heart failure. Since that time this association has been confirmed in man,[87] and it appears that as much as 30 percent intracellular $K^+$ loss may be present in such patients.[88] In addition, prolonged potassium depletion may produce fine structural changes in the myocardium of laboratory animals [89-91] and man.[92] Potassium-deficient diets fed to the Syrian hamster who develops a spontaneous cardiomyopathy brought about earlier manifestations of poor left ventricular performance.[93] Therefore a causal relation was postulated between myocardial $K^+$ depletion and poor left ventricular contractility.[94, 95]

Recently Gunning and coauthors [96] studied the effects of chronic potassium deficiency on the right ventricular papillary muscle from kittens fed a $K^+$-deficient diet. After 25 to 44 days, lowered serum $K^+$ and myocardial $K^+$ contents accompanied the total body $K^+$ depletion. Sufficient depression of the velocity of contraction and extent of shortening was noted. Although the contractile state was severely impaired, myocardial oxygen consumption was equivalent to control values in both afterloaded and isometric contractions, suggesting that energy conversion was inefficient. Moreover, these abnormalities could be reversed with potassium repletion if done before irreversible structural change occurred.[97]

The potential depressant action of acute $K^+$ depletion are less clear. Poor left ventricular function was noted in a guinea pig heart-lung preparation by reducing perfusate potassium.[98] However, Gunning quoted Sonnenblick [96] as demonstrating no change in contractility in papillary muscles when potassium concentration was varied from 1.5-6.0 meq/L in the perfusate, leaving the problem unanswered.

## V. POTASSIUM AND METABOLISM

### A. Potassium and intermediary metabolism

Ion movements within the cell are intimately dependent upon metabolic reactions; at the same time, the activity of many metabolic pathways are affected by changes in ion concentrations. Potassium is an essential activator in several enzymatic reactions,[99] some leading directly to the synthesis of high energy phosphate compounds.[100] Specifically, the formation of acetylcoenzyme A is strongly activated by $K^+$.[101] AcetylCoA acetylates oxaloacetic acid to form citric acid in the tricarboxylic acid cycle, and also provides the acetyl moiety for acetylcholine, a substance which in turn increases $P_{K^+}$ in sinus node and atrial tissues during vagal stimulation. The transfer of phosphate from pyruvophosphate to ADP, catalyzed by pyruvic phosphokinase, requires $K^+$ for activation.[102]

Phosphorylase activity is markedly affected by ion concentrations;[103] glucagon-induced glycogenolysis is mediated by loss of cellular $K^+$ with phosphorylase activation.[104] It has been known for some time that in liver tissue, potassium and phosphate enter the cell during glucose uptake,[105] and $K^+$ promotes glycogen deposition.[106] Similar events occur in muscle: corticosteroid-induced $K^+$ depletion inhibits glycogen formation.[107] Muscle glycogen content and $K^+$ content correlate with each other.[108] Craig [109] postulated that $K^+$ leaves the cell in response to an increase in intermediary compounds of carbohydrate metabolism, with $K^+$ efflux regulating the formation of the intermediates. This no longer seems tenable, since the $K^+$-release response is also produced by exogenous cyclic AMP. Haugaard [110] showed that the complete oxidation of glucose in heart muscle requires $K^+$ and when $K^+$ is lacking changes in intermediary metabolism do occur.

## B. Potassium and mitochondrial function

The actions of $K^+$ upon mitochondrial respiratory control have received considerable attention. Mullins [111] demonstrated $^{42}K^+$ uptake by mitochondria, and Ulrich [112] showed preferential uptake of $K^+$ over $Na^+$ following addition of ATP and oxidizable substrate in low-$K^+$ media, which appeared to depend upon normal oxidation-phosphorylation coupling. While uncoupling by $K^+$-deficiency was hypothesized,[113] more recent work suggests that $K^+$ regulates cellular respiration directly by control of ADP production at the cell membrane with activation of ATPase(s).[114] Thus, stimulation of ATPase by $Na^+$ or $K^+$ effects parallel increases in oxygen consumption and ADP concentration. This view is supported by earlier experiments showing that the respiration rate in muscle increased markedly with increased $[K^+]_o$,[115] even when the concentrations were adjusted to eliminate the possibility of muscle contracture [116, 117]—the so-called "Solandt effect." It was demonstrated that specific inhibition of cation transport in other tissues was accompanied by a 30 to 40 percent reduction in respiration.[118] A specific oxygen cost of $Na^+$, $K^+$-pumping above the basal level was also reported.[119]

Recently it was reported that chemical K⁺-depletion of mitochondria resulted in greater oxygen consumption during state 4 respiration associated with a decrease in respiratory control.[120] Harrison and co-authors[91] also noted depressed mitochondrial ATPase activity with swelling of mitochondria in potassium-deficient rats. Other investigators reported abnormal respiratory control indices in failing myocardium and attributed the defects to muscle failure.[121] However, it has now been shown that chronic cardiac K⁺-depletion increases mitochondrial oxygen consumption in state 4 and decreases it in state 3 to decrease respiratory control nearly 20 percent.[97, 122] Since the association between failing heart muscle and K⁺ depletion is well known, it is entirely possible that inefficient oxygen metabolism of K⁺-depleted, failing heart muscle is due to changed mitochondrial respiratory control.

### C. Potassium as modulator of hormone action

Potassium may also affect the heart indirectly in its role as a modifier of hormone interactions. For instance, K⁺ may interfere with some actions of the catecholamines, increased in concentration as part of the generalized metabolic response to acute myocardial infarction. The nature of this effect varies from tissue to tissue. In the rat heart, K⁺ interferes with the ability of epinephrine to stimulate cyclic AMP formation,[123] while in other tissues K⁺ stimulates overall cyclic AMP activity. Thus it is unknown whether insulin release effected by increasing K⁺ concentrations are mediated by cyclic AMP.[124] Potassium may also interfere with cyclic AMP-induced reactions. The antilipolytic effect of ouabain is probably mediated through an action on K⁺ transport.[125, 126]

Early potassium efflux in response to glucagon- or catecholamine-induced glycogenolysis has already been mentioned. Following an initial increase in plasma K⁺ levels after administration of these agents, a sustained fall in [K⁺]$_o$ and phosphate levels may occur, probably secondary to the accompanying hyperglycemia.[127, 128] Glucagon may also stimulate insulin secretion, tending to drive K⁺ into cells. Therefore the effect of exogenous glucagon administration on [K⁺]$_o$ is unpredictable.[128-130]

On the other hand, the catecholamines may also modify K⁺ fluxes in cardiac tissues. Recently Borasio and Vassalle[286] reported on their studies of the stimulatory effect of norepinephrine on K⁺-uptake in Purkinje fibers. A stimulatory action of norepinephrine on Na⁺, K⁺-pump activity could account for enhanced automaticity. The augmented spontaneous rate and increased K⁺-uptake produced by norepinephrine was not altered by substituting $N_2$ for $O_2$, or by omitting glucose from their preparation.[286] Either or both of these actions were reduced or abolished by substitution of glucose with 2-deoxy-D-glucose, hypothermia, $Mg^{++}$-lack, substitution of $Na^+$ with choline, and tetrodotoxin, which blocks inward $Na^+$ current. Therefore norepinephrine increased $K^+$-uptake via a stimulation of active transport, which may be dissociated from enhanced automaticity.

## VI. MYOCARDIAL POTASSIUM DURING ISCHEMIA

### A. Effect of ischemia on $Na^+$, $K^+$-pumping

The anoxic and/or ischemic myocardium cannot metabolize free fatty acids, and depends upon inefficient anaerobic glycolysis for its energy production.[131-134] Under these circumstances FFA may accumulate in the myocardium, and may further depress myocardial function. Perhaps more important, while the normal myocardium extracts from 20 to 40 percent of the arterial lactate content, during hypoxia lactate is produced from glycogenolysis and anaerobic glucose metabolism.[135-144] Net lactate production is generally regarded as a satisfactory index of hypoxia in the human heart,[145] which in itself contributes to poor left ventricular performance.[146] It is therefore not surprising that lactate production is a function of glucose extraction (Fig. 13).

A large body of evidence now indicates that an adequate energy

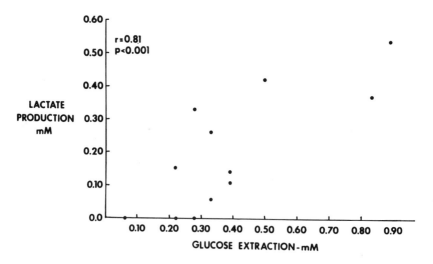

**Figure 13** Correlation between glucose extraction and lactate production during myocardial ischemia. Reproduced with permission from Gorlin.[145]

supply for membrane activity is necessary for maintenance of normal action potential duration.[320-324] Interference with the transduction of energy by $Na^+$, $K^+$-ATPase not only results in accumulation of $[Na^+]_i$ and lowers $[K^+]_i$ but also produces shortening of action potential duration, along with an increase in $[Ca^{++}]_i$ and contractility.[325, 326] ATPase inhibitors in the absence of $Ca^{++}$ may produce a shortening of the action potential duration without increasing the contractility, arguing against the model connecting $Ca^{++}$ influx and $K^+$ efflux presented in Figure 14A.[323, 327]

On the basis of an extensive series of investigations of many ionic interventions upon the action potential duration, another model of membrane events connecting $Na^+$, $K^+$-ATPase activity with $Na^+$, $K^+$, and $Ca^{++}$ movement was proposed by Prasad[328] (Fig. 14B). $Na^+$ and $Ca^{++}$ transport share the same carrier. At the outer surface of the cell membrane, $Na^+$ and $Ca^{++}$ combine with the carrier C and are carried to the inner surface of the cell membrane, where they are released inside the cell. The free carrier at the inner surface of the cell is then phosphorylated by $Na^+$, $K^+$-ATPase. This phosphorylated carrier is associated with an active transport of $Na^+$, $K^+$, and $Ca^{++}$. The carrier is free after it has released $K^+$ and $P_i$ inside the cell, and joins the common pool at the inner surface of the cell. The nonphosphorylated carrier at the inner surface of the cell carries $K^+$ outward, and after releasing $K^+$, carries $Na^+$ and $Ca^{++}$ inward. The phosphorylation of carrier depends upon the availability of ATP and ATPase. An inhibition of ATPase or a decrease in ATP would lead to a decrease in the number of phosphorylated carriers associated with carrier transport of $Na^+$, potassium, and $Ca^{++}$. An increase in the number of nonphosphorylated carriers would produce an increased efflux of $K^+$, leading to a shortening of the duration of action potential, and an increased influx of $Na^+$ and

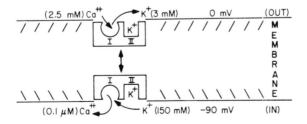

ONE NET CHARGE (+) ENTERS CELL

**Figure 14A**   Scheme illustrating one method by which $K^+$ and $Ca^{++}$ transport may be coupled. See text for details.[318]

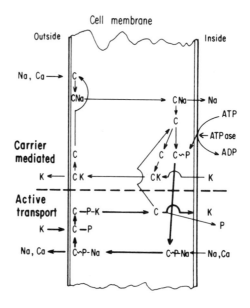

**Model for Ion movement**

**Figure 14B**   Proposed model for ion movement through the myocardial cell membrane. Part of the figure, below the broken line, depicts the active transport of ions, while the part above depicts the carrier-mediated ion transport. C, carrier; C~P, phosphorylated carrier, Na, sodium; K, potassium; Ca, calcium; P, inorganic phosphate (Pi). See text for explanation. Reproduced with permission.[328]

Ca⁺⁺, leading to an increase in contractility. A decrease in the phosphorylated carrier would lead to a decrease in the efflux of Na⁺ and Ca⁺⁺ and the influx of K⁺. An increased influx and a decreased efflux of Na⁺ and Ca⁺⁺ would produce an increase in the intracellular concentration of these two ions. A decreased influx and an increased efflux of K⁺ would produce a decrease in the $[K^+]_i$. If the decrease in the number of phosphorylated carriers were due to a decrease in the amount of ATP, all the ionic changes would occur, but contractility would not increase.

Although the models presented in Figures 14A and 14B are certainly possible, more recent data suggests that there are two separate pumps —one for Na⁺ and K⁺, and another for Na⁺ and Ca⁺⁺. When the terminal ~P of ATP is labelled and the "pump" is stimulated by $[Na^+]_i$, an E~P is formed which is a phosphoprotein with a molecular weight of 103,000 daltons. If K⁺ is added, E~P hydrolyzes to $P_i$ and E. If the same experiment is done with Ca⁺⁺ present, one may recover the same intermediate of 103,000 daltons, but the second stage is blocked when $K^+$ is added to the medium, *i.e.*, dephosphorylation does not occur. Simultaneously, another phosphoprotein may be identified, which has a molecular weight of about 150,000 daltons and which represents $Na^+$, $Ca^{++}$-ATPase. Exactly how $Ca^{++}$ blocks the first steps of $Na^+$, $K^+$-ATPase operation is still unknown.

These data tend to support the hypothesis of Langer and colleagues,[5, 7, 13, 22, 23, 29, 30, 332-335] who maintain that the inotropic action of digitalis depends upon secondary stimulation of the $Na^+$, $Ca^{++}$-pump after the $Na^+$, $K^+$-pump is inhibited. Recently Reuter[310] reviewed the evidence for a separate $Na^+$, $Ca^{++}$-pump in cardiac muscle as follows:

1. More than 80 percent of $Ca^{++}$ efflux depends upon the presence of external $Na^+$ and $Ca^{++}$, and the bulk of the exchange is $Ca^{++}$-for-$Na^+$, rather than $[Ca^{++}]_o$-for-$[Ca^{++}]_i$.

2. Two $Na^+$ and one $Ca^{++}$ appear to compete for one transport site (or "carrier") on both sides of the membrane.

3. The "carrier" does not have a high affinity for choline lithium, potassium, magnesium or lanthanum ions, but the affinity for strontium ions is about the same as that for $Ca^{++}$.

4. The temperature coefficient ($Q_{10}$) for $Ca^{++}$-efflux from 3°C to 35°C is low for an "uphill" transport.[135]

5. If $Ca^{++}$-efflux were direcly energy-dependent, such metabolic inhibitors as 2,4-dinitrophenol or cyanide should decrease $Ca^{++}$ transport; rather, these agents increase $Ca^{++}$-efflux.

6. $Ca^{++}$ efflux is unaffected by digitalis.

A hypothetical scheme which accounts for all the available experimental data appears in Figure 14C. A divalent anionic carrier, $X^=$, may be occupied competitively either by $2Na^+$ or $Ca^{++}$. The unloaded carrier is postulated to move slowly in comparison to the bound carrier. While the $Ca^{++}$-influx that occurs during the plateau of the action potential is electrogenic, the exchange system depicted here is electroneutral. If the affinities for $Na^+$ and $Ca^{++}$ were equal on both sides of the membrane, an exchange of $2Na^+$ for $1Ca^{++}$ leads to the following equilibrium distribution of ions:

$$\frac{[Ca^{++}]_i}{[Ca^{++}]_o} = \frac{[Na^+]_i^2}{[Na^+]_o^2}.$$

From this equation, any change in the $Na^+$ gradient will also affect the $Ca^{++}$ gradient. A decrease in $[Na^+]_o$ would increase $[Ca^{++}]_i$. Metabolic inhibitors which increase $[Na^+]_i$ also increase $[Ca^{++}]_i$. Calculations re-

outside                    inside

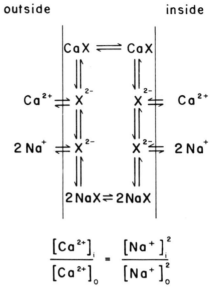

$$\frac{[Ca^{2+}]_i}{[Ca^{2+}]_o} = \frac{[Na^+]_i^2}{[Na^+]_o^2}$$

**Figure 14C** Carrier scheme for Na-Ca exchange across a membrane; two Na ions and one Ca ion compete for a carrier ($X^{2-}$) at the inside and outside surfaces of the membrane. The carrier can move as $Na_2X$ or as $CaX$ across the membrane, but the unloaded carrier cannot move. In such a transport scheme, a Ca gradient can be established across the membrane as a consequence of an existing Na gradient. The respective distribution ratios at equilibrium are given by the equation below the scheme. Reproduced with permission.[340] Copyright, 1974, American Heart Association, Inc.

veal that this relationship is qualitatively true, but that quantitative considerations predict the existence of either another energy source (in addition to the $Na^+$ gradient) or compartmentalization of $Ca^{++}$ in high concentrations near the sarcolemma.

Nonetheless, from the data discussed, there is little question that specific inhibition of membrane $Na^+$, $K^+$-ATPase significantly alters ion distribution and electrical properties of the myocardial cell. However, the extent to which $Na^+$, $K^+$-ATPase and $Na^+$, $Ca^{++}$-ATPase are affected by global ischemia of myocardium is unknown. According to classic theory, inhibition of the $Na^+$, $K^+$-pump, for instance by ouabain, results in net $[K^+]_i$ loss and $[Na^+]_i$ accumulation. Similarly, activation of $Na^+$, $K^+$-ATPase by diphenylhydantoin (at least in excitable tissues other than the myocardium) or increased $[Na^+]_i$ or $[K^+]_o$, effects changes in the opposite direction.[147, 148] Loss of energy supply to this pump may account for the early $[K^+]_i$ loss from ischemic/hypoxic myocardium.[149] However, it has been said that the pump only utilizes a minor fraction of the heart muscle cell's energy production and contractility ceases long before energy depletion approaches this order of magnitude. It should be mentioned that the entire question of whether ATP and membrane ATPase is the source of energy for "pumps" and whether the membrane potential is generated is unsettled and has sparked a heated interchange in the literature (351-357), (see discussion, pp. 176-177, and Chapter 4, pp. 290 and associated references). Actually, based upon revised values for $Na^+$, $K^+$-exchange, it is probably thermodynamically impossible for ATP production to power $Na^+$, $K^+$-pumps, which is the basis for the association-induction hypothesis. The "pump" interpretation of mechanism of action of ouabain mentioned above assumes that the rate of ATP hydrolysis determines the rate of $Na^+$-pumping. However, ouabain may be considered a cardinal absorbent and hence controls $K^+$ and $Na^+$ distribution. In fact, ouabain does shift the intrinsic equilibrium constant $K^{00}_{Na^+ \rightarrow K^+}$ from 100 to about 10,[227, 233] which, considering the concentrations of $Na^+$ and $K^+$ usually present in physiological media, may cause a virtually complete replacement of cell $K^+$ by $Na^+$.

## B. Recent data relating $Na^+$, $K^+$-exchange and ischemia

The connection between $[K^+]_i$ loss and depressed $Na^+$, $K^+$-ATPase activity during ischemic episodes has never been proven, although inferred. Recently, $Na^+$, $K^+$-ATPase activity was measured after "acute" and "chronic" ischemia of the canine myocardium.[52] One day after coronary artery ligation, there was no diminution in $Na^+$, $K^+$-ATPase activity, as judged by a normal $K_m$ for $Na^+$, $K^+$, and $I_{50}$ for ouabain ($K_m$ = concentrations of ion that produce half-maximal stimulation, $I_{50}$ = concentration of drug that inhibits the enzyme activity level by 50 percent). Since contractility was markedly reduced at the same time, these investigators concluded that the $Na^+$, $K^+$-ATPase system was not directly involved initially. However, seven days after ligation, $Na^+$, $K^+$-ATPase levels were impaired. Upon restoration of blood flow, $[K^+]_i$ was taken up by the myocardium again. Thus according to these data, while $K^+$-efflux may occur independently of pump activity immediately after ischemia, good $Na^+$, $K^+$-pump function is necessary to replenish $[K^+]_i$ after recovery of coronary blood flow.

Of interest is the work of Dhalla and associates [264, 265] who recently investigated $Na^+$, $K^+$-ATPase activity in the perfused rat heart made to fail by substrate-lack. No change in the $Na^+$, $K^+$-ATPase activity or contractile force occurred in hearts perfused with glucose in the medium. However, a decrease in $Na^+$, $K^+$-ATPase activity took place before a reduction in developed tension in hearts perfused with substrate-free medium which was reversible on further perfusion with

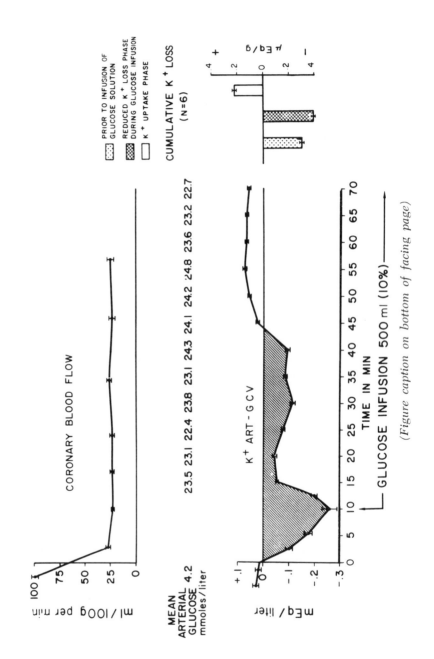

(*Figure caption on bottom of facing page*)

medium containing glucose. These investigators found that the sensitivities of the enzyme preparations from control and failing hearts with respect to the inhibitory effects of ouabain and calcium were not different. The decrease in $Na^+$, $K^+$-ATPase activity from hearts deprived of glucose was observed at different concentrations of $Na^+$, $K^+$, and $H^+$ in the incubation medium, and was due to a decrease in the maximal velocity of reaction ($V_{max}$), without any changes in the affinity of the substrate ($K_m$) (see appendix). These data show that $Na^+$, $K^+$-ATPase activity is sensitive to lack of substrate (glucose).

## C. Sequence of ion changes during ischemia and hypoxia

Myocardial hypoxia, whether it be secondary to systemic anoxia[150] or local oxygen deprivation, results in sodium retention[151] and potassium loss[152] from the heart. Potassium loss during anoxic incubation of both atrial and ventricular muscle results from a decrease in the rate of $K^+$-influx rather than from an increased rate of efflux.[152a] Similarly, reduced coronary blood flow also effects net myocardial $K^+$ loss,[153-155] which is a function of both the severity and duration of ischemia (Fig. 15A).[156] When coronary blood flow and myocardial oxygen supply meet myocardial oxygen demands, arteriovenous potassium difference across the heart is independent of coronary blood flow. However, loss of intracellular $[K^+]_i$ parallels lactate production when coronary blood flow is reduced: 1 meq $K^+$ is lost per 2 $\mu$mole of lactate produced (Figs. 15B and 15C). Restoration of coronary blood flow results in rapid $K^+$ uptake which is flow-dependent until myocardial $K^+$ is replenished.[157]

After myocardial infarction, myocardial $K^+$ loss may be delayed because of deficient coronary blood flow, but within 12 hours the $K^+$ in the infarcted area is equal to the $K^+$ in the extracellular fluid.[158, 159] Myocardial $K^+$ content of necrotic tissue is a function of the time

**Figure 15A** Effects of infusion of glucose solution on $K^+$ transfer during ischemia. Coronary blood flow (top panel) remained at ischemic levels during an infusion of 500 ml of 10% glucose, 40 mEq of KCl, and 20 U of insulin, beginning after 10 min of ischemia which increased arterial glucose concentrations sixfold (middle of figure). The bottom panel indicates the time course of the reversion of the $K^+$ loss consequent to ischemia in a group of six animals. The columns to the right indicate the cumulative ion loss during the initial 10 min of ischemia, the cumulative loss during the first 30 mm of glucose infusion indicating a reduced rate of loss, and the subsequent uptake of $K^+$. In contrast to animals not receiving GIK, none of these developed ventricular tachycardia and fibrillation despite a similar reduction of coronary blood flow. Reproduced with permission.[153]

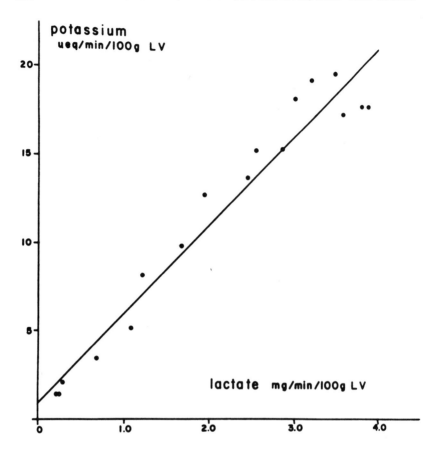

**Figure 15B**   Data relating rate of myocardial potassium efflux and rate of lactate production during ischemia. y=0.87+5.10x. Correlation coefficient −0.97. Reproduced with permission from Case.[156]

elapsed since myocardial infarction but approaches 30 percent of normal.[160, 161]

Concentrations of ions other than $K^+$ are altered by myocardial ischemia and anoxia. While coronary sinus blood pH is normally lower than arterial pH because of myocardial $CO_2$ production, there is a marked pH drop during ischemia. This may be accounted for in part by lactic acid production,[156] and by α-glycerol phosphate. Even more quickly—within 8-10 seconds—hydrogen ion accumulates enough to reduce intracellular $H^+$ acceptors such as methylene blue.[162] A negative redox potential occurs as the terminal electron transport system is reduced, corresponding with lactate production (Fig. 16).[163]

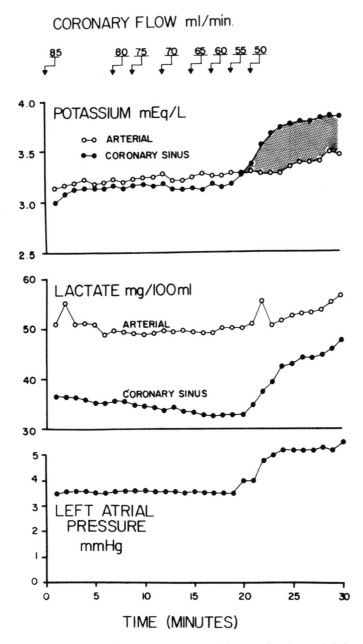

**Figure 15C** Coronary flow, potassium and lactate levels, and left atrial pressure in ischemic dog. Reproduced with permission from Case.[157]

Myocardial influx of sodium and calcium roughly parallel myocardial loss of magnesium and potassium after tissue damage.[159-169] A sequence of events: $Mg^{++}$ leaving the cell, $Ca^{++}$ influx, $Na^+$ influx and finally $K^+$ loss has been suggested.[168] A summary of events leading to myocyte death with the place of ion changes indicated appears in Table IV. During recovery from an acute myocardial infarction, myocardial [$Mg^{++}$], [$K^+$], [$Na^+$] may become normal, followed by changes in [$Ca^{++}$] and inorganic $P_i$.[287]

## D. Myocardial potassium loss and the electrocardiogram

After ligation of a coronary artery or production of a coronary thrombus, the associated ventricular irritability is related to the rate of rise and level of [$K^+$]$_o$.[153] Lowering of coronary sinus [$K^+_o$] by glucose and insulin infusion results in a diminution in frequency of ventricular premature beats. Application of $K^+$ to the myocardium and intracoronary injection of $K^+$ salts produce the "injury current" noted on the electrocardiogram, which is similar to the pattern observed after experimental ligation of a coronary artery.[170-178] S-T elevation during epicardial lead mapping is associated with subendocardial and epicardial ischemia, as evidenced by lactate production and high-energy phosphate depletion.[179] Two events are involved to produce ischemic S-T segment displacement on the scalar electrocardiogram. Increased

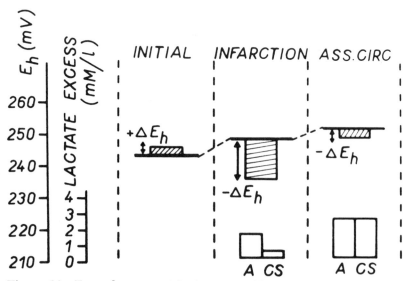

**Figure 16**  $E_h$ = redox potential; A = aorta; CS = coronary aorta. Reproduced with permission from Ziegelhoffer.[163]

slope of phase 2 of the action potential in ischemic myocytes render these cells relatively positive with respect to normal cells. This positive area of ischemic muscle thus raises the S-T-segment recorded during the plateau (Fig. 17B). Reduced resting transmembrane potential in ischemic cells also effects S-T-segment displacement. Some evidence indicates that the early S-T-segment elevation is due to changes in action potential duration, while S-T-displacement due to decreased resting membrane potential maintains the S-T-elevation.[179a]

When $[K^+]_o$ increases rapidly, ventricular fibrillation may be produced with even small doses of $K^+$: 15 mg/Kg in dogs injected intravenously over 2-3 seconds is sufficient.[180] Ventricular fibrillation may also be produced by injected $K^+$ directly into the coronary arteries.[172] If these results be applicable in man, approximately 6 gm of necrotic myocardium might release on the order of 0.5 meq $K^+$ and produce ventricular fibrillation. This situation, however, is quite different from the experimental setting discussed, for $K^+$ release from necrotic myocardium would be slower and be subject to washout by whatever perfusion remains in the area.

## VII. "ISCHEMIC ARRHYTHMIAS"

### A. Heterogeneous nature of myocardial ischemia and infarction

After total coronary artery occlusion, the reduction in perfusion in regions of acute ischemia are nonuniform,[289-292] sometimes with a disproportionate reduction in flow to the inner half of the ischemic zone.[293, 294] Outside the ischemic zone, a rim of hyperemia may be found.[290, 295] There is evidence suggesting that after coronary artery occlusion, the increase in blood supply to the border zone surrounding an infarct, and the biochemical gradients associated with this flow gradient may contribute to the genesis of ventricular fibrillation.[316] Not only is the extent and severity of ischemia patchy with respect to the zones surrounding a necrotic area of myocardium, but is nonuniform from endocardium to epicardium, the latter being favored during coronary occlusion. The subendocardium is more vulnerable to ischemia as compared to the subepicardium.[296, 297, 329] The reason proposed for this is the normal transmyocardial gradient in systolic coronary blood flow, resulting from greater systolic subendocardial intramural tension rising above perfusion pressure and inhibiting flow.[298] Experiments using tissue content of $^{42}K$ and $^{86}Rb$ to measure regional myocardial flow in normal and ischemic tissue also reveal that total coronary collateral flow exceeds retrograde flow, and suggest that the collateral pathways involve the microcirculation rather than the

larger epicardial arteries.[299] Diversion of retrograde flow in the ischemic preparation reduces radionuclide uptake to 25 percent of control
in subepicardial tissue, but only to 70 percent of the control value in
subendocardial tissue. These data support the existence of transmural
heterogeneity in collateral blood flow in ischemic tissue, which has
recently been reported after partial coronary occlusion as well.[300]

## B. S-T segment variation and heterogeneity of ischemia

Heterogeneity of ischemia also produces heterogeneity of the metabolic [307, 308] and electrical consequences of ischemia. For example, the
direction of the S-T segment elevation recorded at a site distal to the
site of injury depends upon the spatial orientation of the exploring
electrode in relation to the site of injury.[170, 175] More recent studies [301, 302] indicate that epicardial S-T segment *depression* occurs as a
primary event when subepicardial ischemia is mild. This view is somewhat supported by the data of Kjekshus [317] who notes S-T segment depression in the presence of normal blood flow in both the subendocardial and subepicardial layers after total coronary occlusion. The
data from Timogiannikis and associates [300] are also consistent with the
contention that S-T segment depression represents a lesser degree of
ischemia than S-T segment elevation, but the results fail to show a
clear relation between increasing flow and change in direction of S-T
segment vector. In the presence of patchy ischemia following partial
coronary occlusion, it may be technically more difficult to map the S-T
segment variations with coronary flow in a given muscle area.

However, whether S-T segment shifts actually reflect localized tissue
injury or whether they reflect net potential differences from within the
entire myocardial wall is unknown. Although Rakita and co-workers [203]
recorded an increasing S-T segment displacement from endocardium
to epicardium, there is more evidence to suggest that there is no simple
correlation between epicardial S-T segment shifts and associated intramyocardial electrical activity.[304, 305] A "certain independence" between
epicardial and subendocardial electrical activity was suggested by
Wendt and collaborators,[306] who reported marked regional differences
in the degree of intramural S-T segment shifts during coronary occlusion. Not only are these electrical events heterogeneous, but the
regional response to various pharmacologic agents capable of affecting
myocyte electrical responses may be equally as heterogeneous.

## C. The action potential and myocardial ischemia

Metabolic changes attending myocardial ischemia and hypoxia
disturb electrophysiology sufficiently to produce serious arrhythmias.

The spontaneous discharge rate of ischemic pacemaker tissue may be reduced, resulting in sinus bradycardia.[181, 182] Intraventricular conduction defects are not uncommon.[309] In atrial and ventricular muscle, acute ischemia and hypoxia shorten the action potential duration by abbreviating its plateau, phase 2, to increase the slope of the action potential downstroke while reducing peak amplitude,[39, 40, 183, 184] Purkinje fibers in a zone of myocardial infarction share in the diminished resting and action potentials, depressed upstroke velocity, enhanced automaticity and phase 4 depolarization.[256] Subsequently there is a loss in resting transmembrane potential and rate of rise in the action potential (Fig. 17A). There is also a significant conduction delay in affected fibers. Many of these resemble the changes observed after loss of cell potassium (Figs. 9 and 17B). However, the shortening of the action potential duration produced by various maneuvers interfering with cell metabolism has no widely accepted ionic mechanism. An increase in $g_{K^+}$ or a decrease in electrogenic $K^+$ uptake during the plateau have been offered as possible explanations. An alternative but unlikely, explanation is that depletion of ATP, a chelator of $Ca^{++}$, may raise intracellular $Ca^{++}$ beneath the sarcolemma and hence reduce the inward $Ca^{++}$ current.[276, 277] Since there is a direct relationship between increased $[Ca^{+2}]_i$ and $g_{K^+}$ in some extracardiac tissues, it is possible that elevations in both $g_{K^+}$ and $[Ca^{+2}]_i$ are responsible for the shortened action potential during ischemia and hypoxia.

Shortening of action potential duration in anoxic ventricular muscle is a function of ATP content and glycolytic rate.[185, 186] Resting membrane potential may be preserved in anoxic myocardium for up to 12 hours,[187] which has perplexed investigators who also record significant $K^+$ loss (see earlier discussion and Chapter 4 regarding the association-induction hypothesis).[188] Some data suggest that rather than compartmentalization of $K^+$ accounting for these findings, the resting

## EFFECTS OF ISCHAEMIA

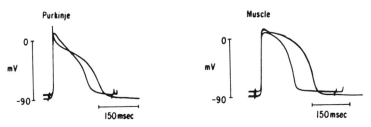

**Figure 17A** Effects of ischemia on Purkinje and ventricular muscle action potentials.

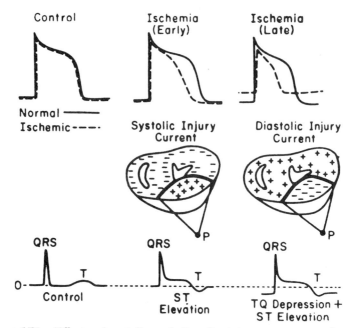

**Figure 17B** Effects of systolic and diastolic injury currents on the action potential and correlation with electrocardiographic changes.

membrane potential of anoxic myocardium is maintained by the activity of the electrogenic $Na^+$-pump.[189] According to these data, while glycolytic ATP may provide sufficient energy to drive this pump, it is insufficient to maintain the action potential duration and contractility, or prevent $K^+$ loss (contrast with other investigators who insist there is normally insufficient energy produced to fuel the $Na^+$, $K^+$-pump). Abbreviation of the action potential and the extent of $K^+$ loss is significantly less in anoxic atrial than in anoxic ventricular-muscle, probably because of higher atrial endogenous glycogen stores which confer protection.[190] The functional refractory period of acutely-ischemic myocardium is also shortened with important clinical consequences.[191] In contrast with the effects of acute ischemia, chronic ischemia of myocardial tissue is associated with prolongation of the refractory periods.[191-193] Overall conduction velocity is reduced in an irregular fashion in ischemic tissue,[194] thus facilitating the development and perpetuation of reentrant arrhythmias.[194a]

## D. Ventricular fibrillation threshold

Anoxia and ischemia of the myocardium disturb both impulse formation and conduction. Ischemia also results in nonuniform reduction of refractory periods to increase their degree of disparity, termed the "temporal dispersion."[195, 196] The ventricular fibrillation threshold is reduced during ischemia as well,[197-201] consistent with the increased risk of ventricular fibrillation during myocardial ischemia frequently observed.[201, 255] Greater electrical energy is also necessary to defibrillate the infarcted ventricle.[315] The increase in disparity of refractory periods is widely believed to increase the likelihood of reentrant arrhythmias after acute myocardial infarction.[194a, 202-204] When excitability and conductivity are depressed in an ischemic area, premature beats are slowly propagated through the area and may be slowed sufficiently to allow time in the surrounding normal area for recovery and reentry. Progression of this phenomenon initiates rapidly repetitive beats, and fibrillation may be induced as wave fronts are fragmented.[200, 201, 258, 259] Local hyperkalemia may also enhance ventricular vulnerability and simulates the changes noted during ischemia.[256, 257] Whether or not the regional hyperkalemia model is a true representation of the pathophysiologic changes that occur in the ischemic heart is a function of the extent of trapping of $K^+$ extracellularly, *i.e.*, failure of adequate "washout" in an inadequately perfused area of myocardium.

A number of studies associate bradycardia with an increase in disparity of refractory periods in nonischemic tissue.[196, 201] Recently it has also been shown that in fact bradycardia has the opposite effect in ischemic myocardium, and reduces disparity of refractory periods.[205, 206] Ventricular fibrillation threshold is also decreased at lower heart rates. While outside the scope of this review, it is interesting that decreased vagal tone increases electrical instability of acutely ischemic myocardium independently of heart rate.[205] Presumably, the augmented energy needs associated with increased heart rate account for these observations.[207] Since there is evidence that ventricular ectopia occurs during fast and slow rates, the concept of an optimal antiarrhythmic heart rate has been proposed.[207a]

The extent of involvement of cellular abnormalities of $K^+$ metabolism in the production of "ischemic arrhythmias" is unclear. Since $K^+$ is in fact the most important electrolyte, responsible for the maintenance of the resting transmembrane potential, and $K^+$ loss from ischemic myocytes is appreciable, a relation between $K^+$ loss and induction of arrhythmias has been strongly suspected for some time. While other ions and cellular events may certainly modify the electrophysiological properties of heart tissue leading to "ischemic arrhythmias," including acidosis,[208] and lactate[260] and possibly free fatty acids,[261, 262] it is reasonable to continue considering that a disturbance of $K^+$ metabolism and distribution is intimately involved in the production of "ischemic arrhythmias," recognizing that this is presently unsettled.

### E. Localization and mechanism of "ischemic" arrhythmias

Harris and Rojas [310] reported an early phase (first 20 min) of rapid paroxysmal ventricular tachycardia after major coronary artery ligation in the dog, followed by a late arrhythmia period beginning 12-15 hours after ligation, also characterized by ventricular ectopic activity. These investigators suggested that the mechanism for both periods of arrhythmias was enhanced automaticity of foci located at the borders of ischemic and noninfarcted myocardium. In order to further explore this hypothesis, Scherlag and associates [247, 311] recorded electrocardiograms and electrograms using plunge wire electrodes in the endocardium and epicardium of ischemic canine myocardium. Activation of Purkinje and muscle tissue was studied within the first 20-30 minutes and 24 hours after coronary artery ligation. The ventricular arrhythmias during the first 20 minutes during vagally-induced atrial arrest and ventricular automaticity was unchanged from the control period; the idioventricular escape rate averaged 30 beats/minute both before and 20 minutes after coronary occlusion. Temporal dispersion in recovery of excitability was demonstrated in ischemic myocardium which may account for reentry in this setting.[195, 196, 258, 259] However, the conduction times between the onset of ventricular activation (His bundle potential) and the endocardial recordings in normal and ischemic tissue are unchanged after coronary occlusion.[247]

The appearance of early ventricular arrhythmias coincided with marked diminution and delay of epicardial activation in the ischemic zone. Reentrant activation within ischemic myocardium could have been responsible for these early arrhythmias. Slowing of the heart rate reversed the delay in activation in association with the termination of the arrhythmia. Since the reentrant circuit was not explicitly defined and the possibility exists that a quiescent cell may become automatic under certain conditions,[311] enhanced automaticity may have played a role, but the data of Scherlag are more consistent with a reentry mechanism.

The ventricular arrhythmias noted 24 hours after coronary artery ligation were isolated by vagally-induced atrial slowing and were suppressed by rapid atrial pacing. These late arrhythmias were therefore a result of enhanced ventricular automaticity, and could have resulted from enhanced phase 4 depolarization of Purkinje cells in the infarcted myocardium [256] or may have arisen from the myocardium itself.

## F. Intracellular potassium loss and "early" *versus* "late" ischemic arrhythmias

While K$^+$ loss from ischemic myocardium could account for the marked delay and deterioration of epicardial activation leading to early ventricular arrhythmias, it is unlikely that local K$^+$-loss and accumulation is involved in the genesis of the late arrhythmias, since phase 4 depolarization is markedly slowed by increasing [K$^+$]$_o$.[312] In the early period after occlusion, the action potentials of Purkinje fibers are shortened and diastolic depolarization is minimum. One day after occlusion, action potentials are prolonged and diastolic depolarization is enhanced.[244, 313, 314] During both periods, the amplitudes of resting and action potentials are reduced. Some of these early changes may be due to K$^+$-egress, since the amplitude of the resting membrane potential, the amplitude and duration of the action potential and the rate of phase 4 (diastolic depolarization) are all inversely related to [K$^+$]$_o$. However, superfusion of the experimental preparation, which would be expected to remove [K$^+$]$_o$ rapidly, does not always reverse the observed electrophysiologic changes. Slow recovery could also be explained by a continuing flux of K$^+$ from deeper layers of the tissue to the endocardial surface.[316] Similar electrophysiologic changes—reduced resting and action potentials and shortened action potential duration—were observed in myocardial cells during the early post-occlusion period as well.[314] In contrast with Purkinje cells, which are relatively resistant to oxygen lack (perhaps because of their lesser energy needs), hypoxia may be more important in the genesis of these electrophysiological changes in working myocardial cells.

## G. Local action of K$^+$ alone

Cardiac arrhythmias are initiated and maintained by either disorders of impulse formation, impulse conduction or both occurring simultaneously.[234, 283, 284] Localized loss of intracellular K$^+$ during myocardial ischemia lowers the ratio [K$^+$]$_i$/[K$^+$]$_o$, with the following consequences:

1. Conduction velocity may first increase but then decreases due to the reduced $\acute{\mathcal{E}}_m$ (may reverse at higher K$^+$ levels and lowered $dV/dt$);
2. Excitability may increase;
3. Membrane responsiveness may increase due to lowered $dV/dt$;
4. Repolarization is accelerated because of increased potassium permeability, thereby shortening action potential duration and refractory period and predisposing to reentrant rhythms;

5. Automaticity is depressed secondary to decreased slope of phase 4 depolarization (may reverse at higher K$^+$ levels).

Since the effects of a change in potassium gradient at the cellular level are complex and may involve the above alterations simultaneously, the mechanisms of arrhythmia formation during regional hyperkalemia were investigated in the dog.[235] This technique reproduces the arrhythmias seen after acute myocardial infarction following experimental coronary artery ligation and may serve as a useful learning model.[236, 237] Two features of this model are of especial interest: (1) the relative changes in electrical properties of the inner and outer ventricular wall and the free-running fascicles monitored by extracellular electrodes, and (2) the associated changes in cation content. Isotonic KCl was infused at 0.5-2.0 ml/min into the left anterior descending or the left circumflex coronary artery of 37 anaesthetized dogs. Conduction was monitored with His and left bundle branch recording catheters and with bipolar electrodes at endocardial and epicardial levels in the perfused zone. RS-T segments rose progressively in the perfused area despite normal coronary blood flow, along with local shortening of the RS-T segment. These RS-T elevations were attributed both to a base-line shift due to differences in $\mathcal{E}_m$ between perfused and nonperfused areas, i.e., a diastolic injury current, and differences in amplitudes of action potential between ischemic and partially depolarized tissue and normally perfused tissue. "Unstable" ventricular extrasystoles arose, progressed to ventricular fibrillation within 20 minutes and were frequently coupled. His-Q and bundle branch conduction times were not altered by regional perfusion, but the QRS complex was locally prolonged. Attempts to induce repetitive ventricular responses with pacing stimuli delivered to either endocardium or epicardium were unsuccessful when applied during RS-T elevation just before arrhythmia, suggesting that enhanced excitability was not present. Intramural electrodes showed increasing conduction delay in the perfused regions, and epicardial depression—more severe than endocardial—preceded significant arrhythmias, especially ventricular fibrillation (Fig. 18). This disproportionate epicardial block was of the magnitude of 2:1 or greater of intramural block. The Q-T interval shortened in the perfused area, indicating that not only slowing of conduction but local earlier repolarization might have contributed to the production of unstable ventricular premature beats. Moreover, epicardial activation preceded endocardial activation during these extrasystoles in perfused regions, reversing the normal endocardial-epicardial activation route and identifying the ectopic com-

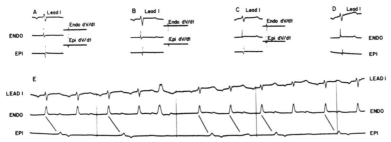

**Figure 18A** Epicardial and endocardial electrograms from the perfused region. A: Controls, showing dV/dt. B-D: RS-T elevation in lead I. Reduction in height of electrograms with reduction in maximum dV/dt. E: Onset of ventricular extrasystoles. Although lead I shows little change, slurring of electrograms is apparent. Delay from endocardial (ENDO) to epicardial (EPI) activation is accentuated with epicardial activation occurring during the T wave of the remainder of the heart. Additionally, the Q-T interval has shortened in comparison with control (rate unchanged). Only the first, third, sixth, seventh, eighth, and tenth beats result in epicardial activation. When the epicardium is allowed to recover (pause between third and sixth conducted beats), the conduction time from inner to outer wall shortens. Paper speed 200 mm/sec, time lines 1/sec. Reproduced with permission from Ettinger et al.[235]

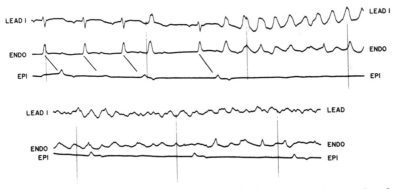

**Figure 18B** Onset of ventricular tachyarrhythmia several seconds after Figure 18A, panel E. Severe intramural block is present. When 1:1 conduction does occur at this heart rate, some of the epicardial (EPI) depolarizations are especially slurred. When tachyarrhythmia begins, the epicardial electrogram is an undulating line and may reflect irregular low-voltage activation or asystole. Bottom: Three seconds later. Ventricular fibrillation has begun and is reflected in the lead I ECG and in the endocardial (ENDO) potentials. Epicardium appears not to participate in fibrillation but instead depolarizes slowly. Epicardial depolarizations are probably conducted from deeper layers, but their origin cannot be determined with certainty. Paper speed 200 mm/sec, time lines 1/sec. Reproduced with permission from Ettinger et al.[235]

plexes as intramyocardial in origin (Fig. 19). Myocardial K⁺ and water content were determined, and, although water content was homogeneous throughout the ventricular wall, tissue concentrations of K⁺ were significantly higher in the epicardium than in the endocardium. While a specific reentrant pathway could not be identified with the use of needle electrode recordings in a three-dimensional electrical network, epicardial conduction delay was sufficient to allow reentry of the delayed impulse through normal areas in which repolarization had already been completed. Through such a reentrant mechanism, serious unwanted tachyarrhythmias may be precipitated (Fig. 20).[238]

Although the conduction delay in the outer wall was greatest where Purkinje fibers were absent,[239, 240] the role of the Purkinje network in the hypothesized reentry pattern could not be determined.[235] However, slowing of conduction in Purkinje fibers has been demonstrated when exposed to epinephrine and K⁺ together and to K⁺ alone.[241-243]

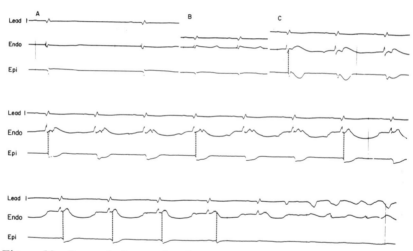

**Figure 19**    Reversal of normal endocardial-epicardial activation during extrasystoles. A: Control. RS-T elevation persisted in the endocardial electrogram in this instance. B: After 2 minutes of KCl perfusion, RS-T elevation is present in the lead I ECG. The shape of the epicardial (EPI) electrogram has been altered, with lower voltage and less rapid rise to the peak. C: Onset of coupled ventricular extrasystoles (second and fourth beats). Epicardial activation precedes endocardial (ENDO) activation during these extrasystoles and coincides with the beginning of the QRS complex of the extra beats. Since endocardial-epicardial conduction delay is not pronounced here, it is hypothesized that the electrodes are not located within the actual region generating these extra beats, the latter probably lying nearby. Paper speed 200 mm/sec. Reproduced with permission.[235]

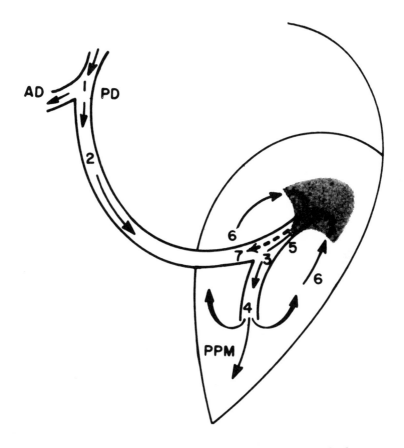

**Figure 20** Model for unidirectional block and reentrant arrhythmias: pictured are the anterior (AD) and posterior (PD) divisions of the left bundle branch. The posterior division supplies the posterior papillary muscle (PPM) where it arborizes into smaller branches, two of which are depicted here. Under normal conditions, depolarization (solid arrows) proceeds in anterograde fashion through the His-Purkinje system (1-3), resulting ultimately in a radial activation of the ventricular myocardium (4). In instances such as infarction which lead to cell injury and depolarization (shaded area) anterograde activation may be slowed or blocked (5). However, the wave front proceeding through the normal Purkinje system and propagating sequentially along the normal papillary muscle (6) may, to a variable degree, enter and activate the depressed segment (broken lines). If the resultant impulse propagates quite slowly and reaches adjacent more normal tissue after the end of the effective refractory period, it may reenter the cardiac conducting system (7) and, with subsequent propagation, result in an ectopic beat. It is conceivable that drugs might be effective in the treatment of such reentrant arrhythmias if they enhanced conduction to the point that anterograde activation proceeded normally or if they further depressed conduction, establishing bi-directional block in what was previously a reentrant loop. See text for further discussion. Reproduced with permission from Rosen and Hoffman.[238]

Recently, reduced action potential amplitudes, maximum diastolic potentials, and maximum depolarization velocities in association with prolonged action potential durations were reported in subendocardial Purkinje fibers surviving extensive myocardial infarction in dogs,[244] emphasizing that Purkinje fibers may participate in the genesis of ischemic arrhythmias. In other studies conducted during myocardial ischemia, intramural block [245] and nonhomogeneous variation in electrical properties of the ventricular wall [246] have been considered important. Arrhythmias arising in an injured, ischemic area of myocardium may be suppressed with vagal stimulation, suggesting that such arrhythmias are of reentrant origin.[247] Finally, epicardial conduction delay during a prearrhythmic phase in ischemic myocardium has been linked to reentry in a manner similar to that observed in the regional hyperkalemia model.[245, 248]

During ischemia, not only the perfusion but cation content of the left ventricle is heterogeneous from endocardium to epicardium.[249, 250] In the regional hyperkalemic model, nonuniform $K^+$ increases in the epicardium are associated with epicardial conduction slowing. Since catecholamines augment myocardial $K^+$ uptake,[251] and $K^+$ may accelerate release of stored norepinephrine in the myocardium,[252] it has been suggested that the catecholamines may play a part in the transmural heterogeneity of $K^+$ during ischemia.[235] In the ischemic animal, hypoxia is greatest in the endocardium rather than in the epicardium, making the direct actions of hypoxia an unlikely responsible mediator for the observed cation distribution.

During acute systemic hyperkalemia, $K^+$-increments and conduction delay in the left ventricle are uniform from endocardium to epicardium; RS-T elevation and ventricular arrhythmias are not characteristically observed. At high plasma $K^+$ levels during systemic infusion, progressive H-Q and QRS delays are seen and *asystole* occurs.[285] On the His-bundle electrogram, hyperkalemia may cause an A wave followed by prolongation of the H-Q interval, reflecting continued supraventricular conduction with conduction delay in the atrioventricular node.[288] At levels of plasma $K^+$ greater than 12 meq/L prior to asystole, double those achieved during regional hyperkalemia, no similar pattern of conduction slowing from inner to outer wall is noted.[263] These data further support the notion that *local* $K^+$ infusions decrease the ratio $[K^+]_i / [K^+]_o$, since the $K^+$ presented does not enter the myocyte to any appreciable extent.[253, 254]

## VIII. POTASSIUM ADMINISTRATION

The antiarrhythmic properties of $K^+$ are now well recognized and have recently been reviewed.[76, 209] Only a few milliequivalents of $K^+$

may be necessary to effect a change of rhythm. However, the rate of administration must be judged according to renal function, the plasma $K^+$ concentration, effect on the electrocardiogram, and bowel loss. In patients with congestive heart failure, hyperkalemia may occur readily.[210] Sodi-Pallares grades $K^+$ administration after myocardial infarction according to the serum $K^+$ value, in conjunction with a high $K^+$ diet and glucose-insulin infusion.[219] However, the indications for $K^+$-therapy are unclear, as is the dosage schedule and the anticipated results. Moreover, $K^+$-loading may result in unexpected ventricular tachycardia and/or fibrillation. Many investigators consider parenteral potassium therapy hazardous and frequently with little benefit despite the fact that $K^+$-depletion is clinically common.[67, 211]

The administration of $K^+$ salts in order to "replace" intracellular $K^+$ represents a somewhat different problem. Whether intracellular $K^+$ in ischemic myocardium may be appreciably altered by extracellular $K^+$-loading is uncertain. *In vitro*, $[K^+]_i$ of normal heart muscle is nearly unchanged even when $[K^+]_o$ is increased five-fold.[212] From data in other tissues, Surawicz[213] suggested that $K^+$ may be compartmentalized in "anaerobic myocardium" and emphasized that the nonexchangeable $K^+$ is itself independent of $[K^+]_o$.[214] Based upon $^{42}K$ efflux data and other considerations, intracellular compartmentalization of $K^+$ does in fact appear likely.[188, 189, 215-218]

## IX. SUMMARY

Potassium is an important electrolyte in heart cells, and manifests the greatest membrane permeability in the unexcited state; hence it is responsible for the generation of the resting membrane potential. Clinical disorders of conduction and impulse formation occur within physiological values of serum potassium.

Potassium is indirectly involved in excitation-contraction coupling, and its relation to intracellular calcium metabolism is reviewed. While potassium movements within the cell are metabolic-dependent, it is also true that the activity of many metabolic pathways are affected by changes in potassium concentration.

During anoxia and ischemia, sodium and calcium are gained by the myocyte, and potassium and magnesium are lost by the cell. At the same time, the action potential duration is abbreviated, the slope of the action potential downstroke (phase 2) is increased, and the resting membrane potential may be reduced. A relationship between disturbances in intracellular potassium and ischemic arrhythmias appears likely.

## References

1. Kones, R. J.: Topics in biological transport. I. Ionic and particular diffusion. *J Mol Cell Cardiol* 3:179-192, 1971.
2. Bonting, S. L., Simon, K. A., Hawkins, N. M.: Studies on sodium, potassium activated adenosine triphosphatase. I. Quantitative distribution in several tissues of the cat. *Arch Biochem* 95:416-423, 1961.
3. Besch, H. R., Jr., Schwartz, A.: On a mechanism of action of digitalis. *J Mol Cell Cardiol* 1:195-199, 1970.
4. Page, E.: The actions of cardiac glycosides on heart muscle cells. *Circulation* 30:237-251, 1964.
5. Langer, G. A.: Myocardial K+ loss and contraction frequency. *J Mol Cell Cardiol* 4:85-86, 1972.
6. Bigger, J. T., Jr.: Antiarrhythmic drugs in ischemic heart disease. *Hosp Practice* 7:69-80, 1972.
7. Langer, G. A.: Ion fluxes in cardiac excitation and contraction and their relation to myocardial contractility. *Physiol Rev* 48:708-757, 1968.
8. Weidmann, S.: The effect of the cardiac membrane potential on the rapid availability of the sodium-carrying system. *J Physiol* 127:213-224, 1955.
9. Fozzard, H. A., Gibbons, W. A.: Action potential and contraction of heart muscle. *Amer J Cardiol* 31:182-192, 1973.
10. Kones, R. J.: The equivalent electric circuit of the heart cell membrane. *Medikon* (Belgium): in press.
11. Armstrong, C. M., Bezanilla, F.: Currents relating to movement of the gating particles of the sodium channels. *Nature* 242:459-461, 1973.
12. Beeler, G. W., Jr., Reuter, J.: Membrane calcium current in ventricular myocardial fibers. *J Physiol* 207:191-209, 1970.
13. Langer, G. A., Serena, S. D.: The effects of strophanthidin upon contraction and ionic exchange in rabbit ventricular myocardium: relation to control of active state. *J Mol Cell Cardiol* 1:65-90, 1971.
14. Nayler, W. G., Merrillees, N. C. R.: Cellular exchange of calcium in *Calcium and the Heart*, edited by Harris, P. and Opie, L., Academic Press, New York, 1971, pp. 24-65.
15. Reuter, H.: Dependence of slow current in Purkinje fibers on the extra-cellular calcium concentration. *J Physiol* (London) 207:479-492, 1967.
16. New, W., Trautwein, W.: The ionic nature of slow inward current and its relation to contraction. *Pflueg Arch Physiol* 334:24-38, 1972.
17. Wood, E. H., Heppner, R. L., Weidmann, S.: Inotropic effects of electric currents. I. Positive and negative effects of constant electric currents or current pulses applied during cardiac action potentials. II. Hypothesis: calcium movements, excitation-contraction coupling and inotropic effects. *Circ Res* 24:409-445, 1969.
18. Kaufman, R. L., Antoni, H., Hennekes, R., et al.: Mechanical response of of the mammalian myocardium to modifications of the action potential. *Cardiovasc Res:* 5 (supplement 1) 64-70, 1971.
19. Gibbs, C. L., Gibson, W. R.: Isoprenaline, propranolol, and the energy output of rabbit cardiac muscle. *Cardiovasc Res* 6:508-515, 1972.
20. Brutsaert, C. L., Claes, V. A., Goethais, M. A.: Effect of calcium on force-velocity-length relations of heart muscle of the cat. *Circ Res* 32:385-392, 1973.
21. Ueba, Y., Ito, Y., Chidsey, C. A., III: Intracellular calcium and myocardial contractility. I. Influence of extracellular calcium. *Amer J Physiol* 22:1553-1557, 1971.
22. Langer, G. A.: The intrinsic control of myocardial contraction-ionic factors. *New Eng J Med* 285:1065-1071, 1971.

23. Langer, G. A.: Sodium exchange in dog ventricular muscle, relation to frequency of contraction and its possible role in the control of myocardial contractility. *J Gen Physiol* **50**:1221-1239, 1967.

24. Lee, K. S., Klaus, W.: The subcellular basis for the mechanism of inotropic action of cardiac glycosides. *Pharm Rev* **23**:193-261, 1971.

25. Shigenobu, K., Sperelakis, N.: Calcium current channels induced by catecholamines in chick embryonic hearts whose fast sodium channels are blocked by tetrodotoxin or elevated potassium. *Circ Res* **31**:932-953, 1972.

26. Visscher, M. B., Lee, Y. C. P.: Calcium ions and the cardiotonic action of glucagon. *Proc Natl Acad Sci US* **69**:463-465, 1972.

27. Singh, B. N., Williams, M. V. A.: A fourth class of antidysrhythmic action? Effect of verapamil on ouabain toxicity, on atrial and ventricular intracellular potentials, and on other features of cardiac function. *Cardiovasc Res* **6**:109-119, 1972.

28. Seaman, P.: The membrane actions of anesthetics and tranquilizers. *Pharm Rev* **24**:583-655, 1972.

29. Shine, K. I., Serena, S. D., Langer, G. A.: Kinetic localization of contractile calcium in rabbit myocardium. *Amer J Physiol* **221**:1408-1417, 1971.

30. Sanborn, W. G., Langer, G. A.: Specific uncoupling of excitation and contraction in mammalian cardiac tissue by lanthanum. *J Gen Physiol* **56**:191-217, 1970.

31. Bailey, L. E., Ong, S. D., Queen, C. M.: Calcium movement during contraction in the cat heart. *J Mol Cell Cardiol* **4**:121-138, 1972.

32. Repke, E. I., Katz, A. M.: Calcium-binding and calcium-uptake by cardiac microsomes. A kinetic analysis. *J Mol Cell Cardiol* **4**:401-416, 1972.

33. Katz, A. M., Repke, E. I.: Calcium-membrane interactions in the myocardium: Effects of ouabain, epinephrine and 3',5'-cyclic adenosine monophosphate. *Amer J Cardiol* **31**:193-201, 1973.

34. Ochi, R.: The slow inward current and the action of manganese ions in guinea-pig's myocardium. *Pflueg Arch Physiol* **316**:81-94, 1970.

35. Ochi, R., Trautwein, W.: The dependence of cardiac contraction upon depolarization and slow inward current. *Pflueg Arch Physiol* **323**:187-203, 1971.

36. Ford, L. E., Podolsky, R. J.: Regenerative calcium release within muscle cells. *Science* **167**:58-59, 1970.

37. Gibbons, W. R., Fozzard, H. A.: Voltage dependence and time dependence of contraction in sheep cardiac Purkinje fibers. *Circ Res* **28**:446-460, 1971.

38. Katz, A. M.: Myocardial metabolism in ischemic heart disease, in *Atherosclerosis and Coronary Heart Disease* edited by Likoff, W., Segal, B. L., Insull, W., Jr., Grune and Stratton, New York, 1972, pp. 190-199.

39. Kardesch, M., Hogencamp, C. E., Bing, R. J.: The effect of complete ischemia on the intracellular electrical activity of the whole mammalian heart. *Circ Res* **6**:715-720, 1958.

40. Trautwein, W., Dudel, J.: Aktions-potential und Kontraktion des Herzmuskels im Sauerstoffmangel. *Pfluegers Arch* **263**:23-32, 1956.

41. Bielecki, K.: The influence of changes in pH of the perfusion fluid on the occurrence of the calcium paradox in the isolated rat heart. *Cardiovasc Res* **3**:268-271, 1969.

42. Coraboeuf, E., Gargouil, Y.-M., Lapaud, J., et al.: Action de l'anoxie sur les potentiels électriques des cellules cardiaques de mammifères actives et inertes. (Tissu ventriculaire isolé de Cobaye). *C R Acad Sci* **246**:3100-3103, 1958.

43. Fuchs, F., Reddy, Y. S., Briggs, F. N.: Effect of pH and ionic strength on calcium binding to troponin. *Biophys J* **9**:A11, 1969.

44. Katz, A. M., Hecht, H. H.: The early "pump" failure of the ischemic heart. *Amer J Med* **47**:497-502, 1969.
45. Katz, A. M.: Effects of ischemia and hypoxia upon the myocardium, in *Coronary Heart Disease*, edited by Russek, H. I., Zohman, B. L., J. B. Lippincott Co., Philadelphia, 1971, pp. 45-56.
46. Jennings, R. B.: Early phase of myocardial ischemic injury and infarction. *Amer J Cardiol* **24**:753-765, 1969.
47. Katz, A. M., Tada, M.: The "stone heart": a challenge to the biochemist. *Amer J Cardiol* **29**:578-588, 1972.
48. Kirchberger, M. A., Tada, M., Repke, D. I., et al.: Cyclic adenosine 3',5'-monophosphate-dependent kinase stimulation of calcium uptake by canine cardiac microsomes. *J Mol Cell Cardiol* **4**:673-680, 1972.
49. Nakamaru, Y., Schwartz, A.: The influence of hydrogen ion concentration on calcium-binding and release by skeletal muscle sarcoplasmic reticulum. *J Gen Physiol* **39**:22-32, 1972.
50. Nakamaru, Y., Schwartz, A.: Possible control of intracellular calcium metabolism by [$H^+$]: sarcoplasmic reticulum of skeletal and cardiac muscle. *Biochem Biophys Res Commun* **41**:830-836, 1970.
51. Entman, M. L., Lewis, R. M., Schwartz, A.: Cardiac sarcoplasmic reticulum: an early lesion in myocardial ischemia. *Clin Res* **21**:81, 1973.
52. Schwartz, A., Wood, J. M., Allen, J. C., et al.: Biochemical and morphologic correlates of cardiac ischemia. I. Membrane systems. *Amer J Cardiol* **32**: 46-61, 1973.
53. Gertz, E. W., Hess, M. L., Lain, R. F., et al.: Activity of the vesicular calcium pump in the spontaneously failing heart-lung preparation. *Circ Res* **20**:477-484, 1967.
54. Miur, J. R., Dhalla, N. S., Orteza, J. M., et al.: Energy-linked calcium transport in subcellular fractions of the failing rat heart. *Circ Res* **26**:429-438, 1970.
55. McCollum, W. B., Crow, C., Harigaya, S., et al.: Calcium binding by cardiac relaxing system isolated from myopathic Syrian hamsters (strains 14.6, 82.62, and 40.54). *J Mol Cell Cardiol* **1**:445-457, 1970.
56. Lindenmayer, G. E., Sordahl, L. A., Harigaya, S., et al.: Some biochemical studies on subcellular systems isolated from fresh recipient human cardiac tissue obtained during transplantation. *Amer J Cardiol* **27**:277-283, 1971.
57. Kones, R. J.: The molecular and ionic basis for altered myocardial contractility. *Res Commun Chem Path Pharmacol* **5** (suppl 1): 1-84, 1973.
58. Katz, A. M.: Biochemical "defect" in the hypertrophied and failing heart. Deleterious or compensatory? *Circulation* **47**:1076-1079, 1973.
59. Fleckenstein, A.: The key role of Ca in the production of non-coronarogenic myocardial necrosis. Proc VI Ann Meeting Int Study Group for Research in Cardiac Metabolism, Freiburg, Germany, 28 Sept. 1973.
60. Weidmann, S.: The effect of the cardiac membrane potential on the rapid availability of the sodium-carrying system. *J Physiol* **127**:213-224, 1955.
61. Carmeliet, E. E.: Effets des ions potassium sur la résistance membranaire et la mouvement del'ion [42]K dans les fibres de Purkinje de mouton. *Arch Int Physiol* **68**:857-859, 1960.
62. Fisch, C., Knoebel, S. B., Feigenbaum, H., et al.: Potassium and the monophasic action potential, electrocardiogram, conduction and arrhythmias. *Progr Cardiovasc Dis* **8**:387-418, 1966.
63. Weidmann, S.: Shortening of the cardiac action potential due to brief injections of KCl following the onset of activity. *J Physiol* **132**:157-163, 1956.
64. Gettes, L. S., Surawicz, B.: Effects of low and high concentrations of

potassium on the simultaneously recorded Purkinje and ventricular action potentials of the perfused pig moderator band. *Circ Res* **23**:717-729, 1968.

65. Gettes, L. S., Surawicz, B., Shine, J. C.: Effect of high K, low K, and quinidine on QRS duration and ventricular action potential. *Amer J Physiol* **203**:1135-1140, 1962.

65a. Greenspan, K., Elizari, M. V.: The pharmacological effects of potassium: the occurrence of sino-ventricular conduction. *J Clin Pharm* **14**:155-162, 1974.

66. Surawicz, B., Gettes, L. S.: Two mechanisms of cardiac arrest produced by potassium. *Circ Res* **12**:415-421, 1963.

67. Surawicz, B., Logic, J. R.: Effect of electrolytes on cardiac automaticity and conduction, in *Pre and Postoperative Management of the Cardiopulmonary Patient*, edited by Oaks, W. W., Moyer, J. H., Grune and Stratton, New York, 1970, pp. 268-276.

68. Surawicz, B.: Relationship between electrocardiogram and electrolytes. *Amer Heart J* **73**:814-834, 1967.

69. Surawicz, B.: Arrhythmias and electrolyte disturbances. *Bull N Y Acad Med* **43**:1160-1180, 1967.

70. Surawicz, B.: Arrhythmias and electrolyte disturbances, in *Cardiac Arrhythmias*, edited by Han, J., Charles C Thomas, Springfield, Illinois, 1972, pp. 211-232.

71. Ten Eick, R. E., Singer, D. H.: Human cardiac arrhythmias: mechanisms and models, *ibid*, pp. 3-37.

72. Pick, A.: Arrhythmias and potassium in man. *Amer Heart J* **72**:295-306, 1966.

73. Watanabe, Y., Dreifus, L.: Arrhythmias: mechanisms and pathogenesis, in *Cardiac Arrhythmias*, edited by Dreifus, L. S., Likoff, W., Grune and Stratton, New York, 1973, pp. 35-54.

74. Zipes, D. P.: Electrolyte derangements in the genesis of arrhythmias, *ibid*, pp. 55-69.

75. Fisch, C.: Relation of electrolyte disturbances to cardiac arrhythmias. *Circulation* **47**:408-419, 1973.

76. Zipes, D. P., Fisch, C.: Potassium et troubles du rythme. *Coeur Med Intern* **11**:277-291, 1972.

77. Surawicz, B., Gettes, L. S.: Effect of electrolyte abnormalities on the heart and circulation, in *Cardiac and Vascular Diseases*, edited by Conn, H. L., Jr., Gorwitz, O., Lea and Fébiger, Philadelphia, 1971, Vol. 1, pp. 539-567.

78. Kones, R. J.: Topics in biological transport. II. Electrical properties of cardiac membranes and the cardiac action potential: ion conductance, membrane impedance, capacitance and rectification. In preparation.

79. Thomas, L. J., Jr.: Increase of labelled calcium uptake in heart muscle during potassium lack contracture. *J Gen Physiol* **43**:1193-1206, 1960.

80. Fleckenstein, A., Kaufman, R.: Über den Einfluss der extracellulären $K^+$-Konzentration auf das mechanische Verhalten des isolierten Warmblüter-Myokards (Papillarmuskel von Rhesus-Ayen). *Pfluegers Arch Physiol* **298**: R17-R18, 1966.

81. Reiter, M., Seibel, K., Stickel, F. J.: Sodium dependence of the inotropic effect of a reduction in extracellular potassium concentrations. *Arch Pharmakol Exp Pathol* **268**:361-378, 1971.

82. Whittam, R.: The asymmetrical stimulation of a membrane triphosphatase in relation to active cation transport. *Biochem J* **84**:110-118, 1962.

83. Page, E., Goerke, R. J., Storm, S. R.: Cat heart muscle in vitro. IV. Inhibition of transport in quiescent muscles. *J Gen Physiol* **47**:531-543, 1964.

84. Langer, G. A.: Effects of digitalis on myocardial ionic exchange. *Circulation* **45**:180-187, 1972.

85. Reiter, M., Stickel, F. J.: Der Einfluss der Kontraktionsfrequenz auf das

Aktions potential des Meerschweinchen-Papillarmuskels. *Arch Pharmakol Exp Pathol* **260**:342-365, 1968.

86. Harrison, T. R., Pilcher, C., Ewing, G.: Studies in congestive heart failure. IV. The potassium content of skeletal and cardiac muscle. *J Clin Invest* **8**:325-335, 1930.

87. Harrison, C. E., Novak, L. P.: Total body fluids and electrolytes in cardiac failure. *Amer J Cardiol* **26**:636-637, 1970.

88. Novak, L. P., Harrison, C. E., Jr.: Abnormalities of cellular potassium concentration in uncompensated and compensated congestive heart failure. *Mayo Clin Proc* **48**:107-113, 1973.

89. Harrison, C. E., Jr., Brown, A. L., Jr.: Myocardial digoxin-³H content in experimental hypokalemic cardiomyopathy. *J Lab Clin Med* **72**:118-128, 1968.

90. Molnar, Z., Larsen, K., Spargo, B.: Cardiac changes in the potassium-depleted rat. *Arch Pathol* **74**:339-347, 1962.

91. Harrison, C. E., Jr., Novak, L. P., Connolly, D. C., et al.: Adenosine triphosphatase activity of cellular organelles in experimental potassium depletion cardiomyopathy. *J Lab Clin Med* **75**:185-196, 1970.

92. Keye, J. D., Jr.: Deaths in potassium deficiency: report of a case including morphologic findings. *Circulation* **5**:766-770, 1951.

93. Bajusz, E.: Concluding remarks. *Ann N Y Acad Sci* **156**:620-629, 1965.

94. Bajusz, E.: *Nutritional Aspects of Cardiovascular Disease*, J. B. Lippincott Co., Philadelphia, 1965.

95. Raab, W.: Myocardial electrolyte derangement. Crucial feature of pluri-causal, so-called coronary heart disease (dysionic cardiomyopathy). *Ann N Y Acad Sci* **156**:629-634, 1969.

96. Gunning, J. F., Harrison, C. E., Jr., Coleman, H. N., III: The effects of chronic potassium deficiency on myocardial contractility and oxygen consumption. *J Mol Cell Cardiol* **4**:139-153, 1972.

97. Harrison, C. E., Jr., Cooper, G., IV, Zujko, K. J., et al.: Myocardial and mitochondrial function in potassium depletion cardiomyopathy. *J Mol Cell Cardiol:* in press.

98. Hochrein, H., Zaqqa, Q., Petschellies, B., et al.: Experimental studies on the hemodynamics and myocardial metabolism of electrolytes in hypo- and hyperpotassemia and under the influence of digitalis. *Acta Cardiologica* **20**:148-156, 1965.

99. Ussing, H. H.: The alkali metal ions in isolated systems and tissues, in *Handbuch der Experimentellen Pharmakologie*, edited by Eichler, O., Springer-Verlag, Berlin, 1960.

100. Dixon, M., Webb, E. C.: *Enzymes*, Academic Press, New York, 1964, pp. 448-452.

101. van Korff, R. W.: The effect of alkali metal ions on the acetate activating enzyme system. *J Biol Chem* **203**:265-271, 1953.

102. Boyer, P. D., Lardy, H. A., Phillips, P. H.: Further studies on the role of potassium and other ions in the phosphorylation of the adenylic acid system. *J Biol Chem* **149**:529-533, 1943.

103. Haugaard, N., Hess, M. E.: Actions of autonomic drugs on phosphorylase activity and function. *Pharm Rev* **17**:27-69, 1965.

104. Finder, A. G., Boyme, T., Shoemaker, W. C.: Relationship of hepatic potassium efflux to phosphorylase activation induced by glucagon. *Amer J Physiol* **206**:738-742, 1964.

105. Fenn, W. O.: The deposition of potassium and phosphate with glycogen in rat livers. *J Biol Chem* **128**:297-307, 1939.

106. Buchanan, J. M., Hastings, A. B., Nesbett, F. B.: The effect of ionic environ-

ment on the synthesis of glycogen from glucose in rat liver slices. *J Biol Chem* **180**:435-445, 1949.

107. Niedermeier, W., Carmichael, E. B.: Action of desoxycorticosterone acetate on glycogen. *Proc Soc Exp Biol NY* **111**:777-780, 1962.

108. Drahota, Z., Gutman, E.: Long term regulatory influence of the nervous system on some metabolic differences in muscles of different function. *Physiol Bohem* **12**:339-348, 1963.

109. Craig, A. B.: Observations on epinephrine and glucagon-induced glycogenolysis and potassium loss in the isolated perfused frog liver. *Amer J Physiol* **193**:425-430, 1958.

110. Haugaard, N., Istkovitz, H.: Hexose oxidation by rat heart homogenate: Properties of a multienzyme system. *Arch Biochem Biophys* **65**:229-242, 1956.

111. Mullins, L. J.: Radioactive ion distribution in protoplasmic granules. *Proc Soc Exp Biol N Y* **45**:856-858, 1940.

112. Ulrich, F.: Ion transport by heart and skeletal muscle mitochondria. *Amer J Physiol* **197**:997-1004, 1959.

113. Pressman, B. D., Lardy, H. A.: Influence of potassium and other alkali cations on respiration in mitochondria. *J Biol Chem* **197**:547-556, 1952.

114. Bond, D. M., Whittam, R.: Effects of sodium and potassium ions on oxidative phosphorylation in relation to respiratory control by cell membrane adenosine triphosphatase. *Biochem J* **97**:523-531, 1965.

115. Hegnauer, A. H., Fenn, W. D., Cobb, D. M.: The cause of the rise in oxygen consumption of frog muscle in excess of potassium. *J Cell Comp Physiol* **4**:505-526, 1934.

116. Keynes, R. D., Maisel, C. W.: Energy requirement for sodium ion excretion from a frog muscle. *Proc Roy Soc Lon* B**142**:383-387, 1954.

117. Solandt, D. V.: The effect of potassium on the excitability and resting metabolism of frog's muscle. *J Physiol* **86**:162-170, 1936.

118. Elshove, A., Van Rossum, D. V.: Net movements of sodium and potassium and their relation to respiration in slices of rat liver incubated *in vitro*. *J Physiol* **168**:531-553, 1963.

119. Whittam, R., Willis, J. S.: Ion movement and oxygen consumption in kidney cortex slices. *J Physiol* **168**:158-177, 1963.

120. Gomey-Puyon, A., Sandoval, F., Tuena, M., et al.: Induction of respiratory control by K+ in mitochondria. *Biochem Biophys Res Commun* **36**:316-321, 1969.

121. Lindenmayer, G. E., Sordahl, L. A., Schwartz, A.: Re-evaluation of oxidative phosphorylation in cardiac mitochondria from normal aniamls in heart failure. *Circ Res* **23**:439-450, 1968.

122. Harrison, P. E., Zujko, K., Coleman, H. N.: Mitochondrial function in potassium (K) depletion cardiomyopathy. *J Lab Clin Med* **75**:185-196, 1970.

123. Namm, D. H., Mayer, S. E.: Effects of epinephrine on cardiac cyclic 3',5'-AMP, phosphorylase kinase, and phosphorylase. *Mol Pharm* **4**:61-69, 1968.

124. Grodsky, G. M., Bennett, L. L.: Cation requirements for insulin secretion in the isolated perfused pancreas. *Diabetes* **15**:910-913, 1966.

125. Fain, J. N.: Effect of K+, valinomycin, tetraphenylborate and ouabain on lipolysis by white fat cells. *Mol Pharm* **4**:349-357, 1968.

126. Kypson, J., Triner, L., Nahas, G. G.: Effects of ouabain and K+-free medium on activated lipolysis and epinephrine-stimulated glycogenolysis. *J Pharm Exp Ther* **159**:8-17, 1968.

127. Cahill, G. F., Zottu, S., Earle, A. S.: In vivo effects of glucagon on hepatic glycogen, phosphorylase and glucose-6-phosphatase. *Endocrinology* **60**:265-272, 1957.

238 GLUCOSE, INSULIN, POTASSIUM, AND THE HEART

128. Kones, R. J., Phillips, J. H.: Glucagon: present status in cardiovascular disease. *Clin Pharm Ther* 12:427-444, 1971.
129. Kones, R. J., Phillips, J. H.: Glucagon in congestive heart failure. *Chest* 59:392-397, 1971.
130. Kones, R. J., Dombeck, D. H., Phillips, J. H.: Glucagon in cardiogenic shock. *Angiology* 23:525-535, 1972.
131. Ballinger, W. F., Vallen weider, H.: Anaerobic metabolism of the heart. *Circ Res* 11:681-685, 1962.
132. Braasch, W., Gudbjarnason, S., Puri, P. S., et al.: Early changes in energy metabolism in the myocardium following acute coronary artery occlusion in anesthetized dogs. *Circ Res* 23:429-438, 1968.
133. Neill, W. A., Krasnow, N., Levine, H. J., et al.: Myocardial anaerobic metabolism in intact dogs. *Amer J Physiol* 204:427-432, 1963.
134. Owen, P., Thomas, M., Young, V., et al.: Comparison between metabolic changes in local venous and coronary sinus blood after acute experimental coronary arterial occlusion. *Amer J Cardiol* 25:562-579, 1970.
135. Michal, G., Naegle, S., Danforth, W. H., et al.: Metabolic changes in heart muscle during anoxia. *Amer J Physiol* 197:1147-1151, 1959.
136. Gorlin, R.: Evaluation of myocardial metabolism in ischemic heart disease. *Circulation* 40 (suppl IV): 155-163, 1969.
137. Clark, A. I., Gaddie, R., Stewart, C. P.: Anaerobic activity of the isolated frog's heart. *J Physiol* 75:321-331, 1932.
138. Huckabee, W. E.: Relationships of pyruvate and lactate during anaerobic metabolism. V. Coronary adequacy. *Amer J Physiol* 200:1169-1176, 1961.
139. Shea, T. M., Watson, ?. M., Piotrowski, S. F., et al.: Anaerobic myocardial metabolism. *Amer J Physiol* 203:463-469, 1962.
140. Krasnow, N., Gorlin, R.: Myocardial lactate metabolism in coronary insufficiency. *Ann Int Med* 59:781-787, 1963.
141. Parker, J. O., Chiong, M. A., West, R. O., et al.: Sequential alterations in myocardial lactate metabolism, S-T segments, and left ventricular function during angina induced by atrial pacing. *Circulation* 40:113-131, 1969.
142. Mueller, H., Gregory, J., Ayers, S., et al.: Myocardial metabolic adaptations to coronary and non-coronary cardiogenic shock. *Circulation* 38 (suppl VI): 143, 1968.
143. Mueller, H., Ayres, S. M., Giannelli, S., Jr., et al.: Cardiac performance and metabolism in shock due to acute myocardial infarction in man: response to catecholamines and mechanical cardiac assist. *Trans N Y Acad Sci* 34: 309-333, 1972.
144. Mueller, H., Ayres, S. M., Grace, W. J.: Principle defects which account for shock following acute myocardial infarction in man: implications for treatment. *Crit Care Med* 1:27-38, 1973.
145. Gorlin, R.: Assessment of hypoxia in the human heart. *Cardiology* 57:24-34, 1972.
146. Wildenthal, K., Mierzwiak, D. S., Myers, R. W., et al.: Effects of acute lactic acidosis on left ventricular performance. *Amer J Physiol* 214:1352-1359, 1968.
147. Siegel, G. J., Goodwin, B. B.: Sodium-potassium-activated adenosine triphosphatase of brain microsomes: modification of sodium inhibition by diphenylhydantoins. *J Clin Invest* 51:1164-1169, 1972.
148. McCans, J. L., Brennan, F. J., Chiong, M. A., et al.: Effects of ouabain and diphenlhydantoin on myocardial potassium balance in man. *Amer J Cardiol* 31:320-326, 1973.
149. Obeid, A., Smulyan, H., Gilbert, R., et al.: Regional metabolic changes in the myocardium following coronary artery ligation in dogs. *Amer Heart J* 83:189-196, 1972.

150. Kones, R. J.: Oxygen therapy for acute myocardial infarction: basis for a practical approach. *Southern Med J* **67**: 1322-1328, 1974.
151. Hercus, U. M., McDowell, R. J. S., Mendel, D.: Sodium exchanges in cardiac muscle. *J Physiol* **129**:177-184, 1955.
152. Conn, H. L., Jr.: Effects of digitalis and hypoxia on potassium transfer and distribution in the dog. *Amer J Physiol* **184**:548-552, 1966.
152a. McDonald, T. F., MacLoed, D. P.: The effect of 2',4'-dinitrophenol on the electrical and mechanical activity, metabolism and ion movements in guinea-pig ventricular muscle. *Brit J Pharmacol* **44**:711-722, 1972.
153. Regan, T. J., Harman, M. A., Lehan, P. H., et al.: Ventricular arrhythmias and K⁺ transfer during myocardial ischemia and intervention with procaine amide, insulin, or glucose solution. *J Clin Invest* **46**:1657-1668, 1967.
154. Gerlings, E. D., Miller, D. T., Gilmore, J. P.: Oxygen availability: a determinant of myocardial potassium balance. *Amer J Physiol* **216**:559-562, 1969.
155. Case, R. B., Roselle, M. A., Crampton, R. S.: Relation of ST depression to metabolic and hemodynamic events. *Cardiologia* **48**:32-41, 1966.
156. Case, R. B., Nasser, M. G., Crampton, R.: Biochemical aspects of early myocardial ischemia. *Amer J Cardiol* **24**:766-774, 1969.
157. Case, R. B.: Myocardial potassium loss during ischemia, in *Myocardiology*, edited by Bajusz, E., Rona, G., University Park Press, Baltimore, 1972, Vol. 1, pp. 665-672.
158. Jennings, R. B., Crout, J. R., Smitters, G. W.: Studies on distribution and localization of potassium in early myocardial ischemic injury. *Arch Path* **63**:586-592, 1957.
159. Jennings, R. B., Sommers, H. M., Kaltenbach, J. P., et al.: Electrolyte alterations in acute myocardial ischemic injury. *Circ Res* **14**:260-269, 1964.
160. Iseri, L. T., Alexander, L. C., McCaughey, R. S., et al.: Water and electrolyte content of cardiac and skeletal muscle in heart failure and myocardial infarction. *Amer Heart J* **43**:215-227, 1952.
161. Dittrich, H.: Untersuchungen über den Kalium-Natrium- and Wassergehalt an Leichenherzen bei Herzinsuffizienz und Myocarinfarkt. *Beitr Path Anat* **121**:426-436, 1959.
162. Jennings, R. B., Kaltenbach, J. P., Sommers, H., et al.: Studies of the dying myocardial cell, in *Etiology of Myocardial Infarction*, edited by James, T. N., Keyes, J. W., Little Brown, Boston, 1963, pp. 189-204.
163. Ziegelhoffer, A., Siska, K., Holec, V., et al.: Influence of assisted circulation on cardiac metabolism, in *Myocardiology*, edited by Bajusz, E., Rona, G., University Park Press, Baltimore, 1972, Vol. 1, pp. 484-491.
164. Jennings, R. B., Shen, A. C.: Calcium in experimental ischemia, *ibid*, pp. 639-655.
165. Seelig, M. S.: Myocardial loss of functional magnesium. I. Effect on mitochondrial integrity and potassium retention. II. In cardiomyopathies of diverse etiology. *Ibid*, pp. 615-638.
166. Vasku, J. E., Urbanek, L., Chary, Z., et al.: The nonspecific changes in the heart muscle after various cardiotoxic interventions and their efficient experimental prevention. *Arzneim-Forsch (Drug-Res)* **19**:660-663, 1969.
167. Klein, R., Haddow, J. E., Kind, C., et al.: Effect of cold on muscle potentials and electrolytes. *Metabolism* **17**:1094-1103, 1968.
168. Lehr, D.: Tissue electrolyte alteration in disseminated myocardial necrosis. *Ann N Y Acad Sci* **156**:344-378, 1969.
169. Vasku, J., Bednarik, B., Urbanek, E., et al.: A new type of mechanical heart assistance: a combined pump for bypass and counterpulsation. *Ann N Y Acad Sci* **34**:58-83, 1972.
170. Wolferth, C. C., Bellet, S., Liveszy, M. M., et al.: Negative displacement

of the RS-T segment in the electrocardiogram and its relationships to positive deplacement; an experimental study. *Amer Heart J* **29**:220-245, 1945.

171. Soloff, L., De los Santos, G. A., Oppenheimer, J. M.: Electrocardiographic changes produced by potassium and other ions injected into the coronary arteries of intact dogs. *Circ Res* **8**:479-484, 1960.

172. Logic, J. R., Krotkiewski, A., Koppius, A., et al.: Negative inotropic effect of K+: Its modification by Ca++ and acetylstrophanthidin in dogs. *Amer J Physiol* **215**:14-22, 1968.

173. Wiggers, C. J.: Monophasic and deformed ventricular complexes resulting from surface applications of potassium salts. *Amer Heart J* **5**:346-350, 1930.

174. Nahum, L. H., Hamiton, W. F., Hoff, H. E.: Injury current in the electro-cardiogram. *Amer J Physiol* **139**:202-207, 1943.

175. Hellerstein, H., Katz, L.: Electrical effect of injury at various myocardial locations. *Amer Heart J* **36**:184-220, 1948.

176. Salmanovich, V. S.: Ionic nature of the shift of the S-T segment in myo-cardial ischemia and infarction, in *Electrolytes and Cardiovascular Disease*, edited by Bajusz, E., Vol. II, S. Karger, New York and Basel, 1966, pp. 100-122.

177. Diver, G. A., Ziegler, W. G., Geddes, M. A., et al.: Depolarizing electrode monophasic curves and myocardial infarction ST shift. *Amer J Physiol* **202**: 35-40, 1962.

178. Roselle, H. A., Crampton, R. S., Case, R. B.: Alterations of the depressed S-T segment during coronary insufficiency: Its relation to mechanical events. *Amer J Cardiol* **18**:200-207, 1966.

179. Karlsson, J., Templeton, G. H., Willerson, J. T.: Relationship between epi-cardial S-T segment changes and myocardial metabolism during acute coronary insufficiency. *Circ Res* **32**:725-730, 1973.

179a. Samson, W. E., Scher, A. M.: Mechanism of S-T segment alteration during acute myocardial injury. *Circ Res* **8**:780-787, 1960.

180. Gordon, A. S., Jones, J. C.: The mechanism of ventricular fibrillation and cardiac arrest during surgery. *J Thorac Cardiov Surg* **38**:618-629, 1959.

181. Imai, S., Riley, A. L., Berne, R. A.: Effect of ischemia and adenyl nucleo-tides in cardiac and skeletal muscles. *Circ Res* **15**:443-450, 1964.

182. Billette, J., Elharrar, V., Porlier, G., et al.: Sinus slowing produced by experimental ischemia of the sinus node in dogs. *Amer J Cardiol* **31**:331-335, 1973.

183. Trautwein, W., Gottstein, U., Dudel, J.: Der Aktionsstrom der Myokardfaser im Sauerstoffmangel. *Pfluegers Arch Ges Physiol* **260**:40-60, 1954.

184. Webb, J. L., Hollander, P. B.: Metabolic aspects of the relationship between the contractility and membrane potentials of the rat atrium. *Circ Res* **4**:618-626, 1956.

185. McDonald, T. F., Hunter, E. G., MacLeod, D. P.: Adenosine triphosphate partition in cardiac muscle with respect to Arans-membrane electrical activ-ity. *Pflüger's Arch* **322**:95-108, 1971.

186. McDonald, T. F., MacLeod, D. P.: Anoxia-recovery cycle in ventricular muscle: action potential duration, contractility and ATP content. *Pflüger's Arch* **325**:305-322, 1971.

187. MacLeod, D. P., Prasad, K.: Influence of glucose on the transmembrane action potential of papillary muscle. Effects of concentration, phlorizin and insulin, nonmetabolizable sugars, and stimulators of glycolysis. *J Gen Physiol* **53**:792-815, 1969.

188. Hunter, E. G., McDonald, T. F., MacLeod, D. P.: Metabolic depression and myocardial potassium. *Pflüger's Arch* **335**:266-278, 1972.

189. McDonald, T. F., MacLeod, D. P.: Maintenance of resting potential in

anoxic guinea pig ventricular muscle: electrogenic sodium pumping. *Science* 172:570-572, 1971.

190. McDonald, T. F., MacLeod, D. P.: Anoxic atrial and ventricular muscle electrical activity, cell potassium, and metabolism: a comparative study. *J Mol Cell Cardiol* 5:149-159, 1973.

191. Mandell, W. J., Burgess, M. J., Neville, J., et al.: Analysis of T-wave abnormalities associated with myocardial infarction using a theoretic model. *Circulation* 38:178-188, 1968.

192. Wilson, F. N., Johnston, F. D., Hill, I. G. W.: Form of the electrocardiogram in experimental myocardial infarction. IV. Additional observations on the later effects produced by ligation of the anterior descending branch of the left coronary artery. *Amer Heart J* 10:1025-1041, 1935.

193. Gelband, H., Bassett, A. L.: Depressed transmembrane potentials during experimentally induced ventricular failure in cats. *Circ Res* 32:625-634, 1973.

194. Durrer, D., Van Lier, A. A. W., Buller, J.: Epicardial and intramural excitation in chronic myocardial infarction. *Amer Heart J* 68:765-776, 1964.

194a. Boineau, J. P., Cox, J. L.: Slow ventricular activation in acute myocardial infarction. A source of re-entrant premature ventricular contractions. *Circulation* 48:702-713, 1973.

195. Han, J., Moe, G. K.: Nonuniform recovery of excitability in ventricular muscle. *Circ Res* 14:44-60, 1964.

196. Han, J., Millet, D., Chizzouitti, B., et al.: Temporal dispersion of recovery of excitability in atrium and ventricle as a function of heart rate. *Amer Heart J* 71:481-487, 1966.

197. Wiggers, C. J., Wegria, R.: Quantitative measurement of fibrillation thresholds of the mammalian ventricle with observation on the effect of procaine. *Am J Physiol* 131:296-308, 1940.

198. Shumway, N. E., Johnson, J. A., Stish, R. J.: The study of ventricular fibrillation by threshold determinations. *J Thorac Surg* 34:643-653, 1957.

199. Han, J., Garcia de Jalon, P. D., Moe, G. K.: Fibrillation threshold of premature ventricular responses. *Circ Res* 18:18-25, 1966.

200. Sugimoto, T., Schaal, S. F., Wallace, A. G.: Factors determining vulnerability to ventricular fibrillation induced by 60-CPS alternating current. *Circ Res* 21:601-608, 1967.

201. Han, J.: Ventricular vulnerability during acute coronary occlusion. *Amer J Cardiol* 24:857-864, 1969.

202. Han, J.: The concepts of reentrant activity responsible for ectopic rhythma. *Amer J Cardiol* 28:253-262, 1971.

203. Scherlag, B. J., Helfant, R. H., Haft, J. I., et al.: Electrophysiology underlying ventricular arrhythmias due to coronary litigation. *Amer J Physiol* 219:1665-1671, 1970.

204. Kerzner, J., Wolf, M., Kosowsky, B. D., et al.: Ventricular ectopic rhythms following vagal stimulation in dogs with acute myocardial infarction. *Circulation* 47:44-50, 1973.

205. Kent, K. M., Smith, E. R., Redwood, M. B., et al.: Electrical stability of acutely ischemic myocardium. Influence of heart rate and vagal stimulation. *Circulation* 47:291-298, 1973.

206. Epstein, S. E., Goldstein, R. E., Redwood, D. R., et al.: The early phase of acute myocardial infarction: pharmacologic aspects of therapy. *Ann Int Med* 78:918-936, 1973.

207. Kones, R. J.: Cardiogenic shock—therapeutic implications of altered myocardial energy balance. *Angiology* 25:317-333, 1974.

207a. Chadda K. D., Banka, V. S., Helfant, R. H.: Rate dependent ventricular ectopia following acute coronary occlusion. The concept of an optimal anti-antiarrythmic heart rate. *Circulation* **44**:654-658, 1974.

208. Rogers, R. M., Spear, J. F., Moore, E. N., et al.: Vulnerability of canine ventricle to fibrillation during hypoxia and respiratory acidosis. *Chest* **63**: 986-994, 1973.

209. Soffer, A., (ed.): *Potassium Therapy*, Charles C Thomas, Springfield, Illinois, 1968.

210. Brown, H., Tanner, G. L., Hecht, H. H.: Effect of potassium salts in subjects with heart disease. *J Lab Clin Med* **37**:506-514, 1951.

211. Burchell, H. B.: Dilemmas in potassium therapy. *Circulation* **47**:1144-1146, 1973.

212. Page, E., Solomon, A. K.: Cat heart muscle in vitro. I. Cell volumes and intracellular concentrations in papillary muscle. *J Gen Physiol* **44**:327-344, 1960.

213. Surawicz, B.: Evaluation of treatment of acute myocardial infarction with potassium, glucose and insulin. *Prog Cardiovasc Dis* **10**:545-560, 1968.

214. Mudge, G. H.: Cellular mechanisms of potassium metabolism. *Lancet* **73**: 166-168, 1953.

215. Vick, R. L., Hazlewood, C. F., Nichols, B. L.: Distribution of potassium, sodium, and chloride in canine Purkinje and ventricular tissue. *Circ Res* **27**:159-169, 1970.

216. Page, E., Page, E. G.: Distribution of ions and water between tissue compartments in the perfused left ventricle of the rat heart. *Circ Res* **22**:435-446, 1968.

217. Page, E., Power, B., Borer, J. S., et al.: Rapid exchange of cellular or cell surface potassium in the rat's heart. *Proc Natl Acad Sci US* **60**:1323-1329, 1968.

218. Polimeni, P. I., Vasselle, E.: Potassium fluxes in Purkinje and ventricular muscle fibers during rest and activity. *Amer J Physiol* **218**:1381-1388, 1970.

219. Hutter, O. F., Noble, D.: Rectifying properties of heart muscle. *Nature* **188**:495, 1960.

220. Carmeliet, E.: L'influence de la concentration extracellulaire du K+ sur la permeabilitie de la membrane des fibres de Purkinje de mouton pour les ions 42K. *Helvet Physiol Acta* **18**:C15-C16, 1960.

221. Noble, D.: Electrical properties of cardiac muscle attributable to inward going (anomalous) rectification. *J Cell Comp Physiol* **66**:127-135, 1965.

222. Carmeliet, E. E.: Chloride ions and the membrane potential of Purkinje fibres. *J Physiol* **156**:375-388, 1961.

223. Hall, A. E., Hutter, O. F., Noble, D.: Current-voltage relations of Purkinje fibres in sodium-deficient solutions. *J Physiol* **166**:225-240, 1963.

224. Hazlewood, C. F.: Pumps or no pumps. *Science* **177**:815-816, 1972.

225. Ling, G. N.: *A Physical Theory of the Living State: The Association-Induction Hypothesis*, Blaisdell, New York, 1962.

226. Ling, G. N.: Studies on ion permeability. I. What determines the rate of Na+ ion efflux from frog muscle cells? *Physiol Chem Phys* **2**:242-248, 1970.

227. Ling, G. N.: The physical state of solutes and water in living cells according to the Association-Induction Hypothesis. *Ann N Y Acad Sci* **204**:6-50, 1973.

228. Minkoff, L., Damadian, R.: Energy requirements of bacterial ion exchange. *Ann N Y Acad Sci* **204**:249-260, 1973.

229. Hazlewood, C. F., Nichols, B. L., Chamberlain, N. F.: Evidence for the existence of a minimum of two phases of ordered water in skeletal muscle. *Nature* **222**:747-750, 1969.

230. Ling, G. N., Cope, F. W.: Potassium ion: Is the bulk of intracellular K+ adsorbed? *Science* **163**:1335-1336, 1969.

231. Vick, R. L., Chang, D. C., Nichols, B. L., et al.: Sodium, potassium, and water in cardiac tissues. *Ann N Y Acad Sci* **204**:575-592, 1973.
232. Ling, G. N.: Physiology and anatomy of the cell membrane: the physical state of water in the living cell. *Fed Proc* **24**:103-112, 1965.
233. Ling, G. N., Bohr, G.: Studies on ion distribution in living cells. II. Cooperative interaction between intracellular potassium and sodium ions. *Biophys J* **10**:519-538, 1970.
234. Cranefield, P. F., Wit, A. L., Hoffman, B. F.: Genesis of cardiac arrhythmias. *Circulation* **42**:190-204, 1973.
235. Ettinger, P. O., Regan, T. J., Oldewurtel, H. A., et al.: Ventricular conduction delay and arrhythmias during regional hyperkalemia in the dog. *Circ Res* **33**:521-531, 1973.
236. Logic, J. R.: Electrophysiologic effects of regional hyperkalemia in the canine heart. *Proc Soc Exp Biol Med* **141**:725-730, 1972.
237. Logic, J. R.: Enhancement of the vulnerability of the ventricle to fibrillation (VF) by regional hyperkalemia. *Cardiovasc Res* **7**:501-507, 1973.
238. Rosen, M. R., Hoffman, B. F.: Mechanisms of action of antiarrhythmic drugs. *Circ Res* **32**:1-8, 1973.
239. Scher, A. M., Young, A. C.: Ventricular depolarization and the genesis of QRS, in *Electrophysiology of the Heart*, edited by Hecht, H., *Ann N Y Acad Sci* **65**:768-778, 1957.
240. Scher, A. M.: Excitation of the heart: progress report, in *Advances in Electrocardiography*, edited by Schlant, R. C., Hurst, J. W., Grune and Stratton, New York, 1972, pp. 61-71.
241. Wit, A. L., Hoffman, B. F., Cranefield, P. F.: Slow conduction and reentry in the ventricular conducting system. I. Return extrasystole in canine Purkinje fibers. *Circ Res* **30**:1-10, 1972.
242. Wit, A. L., Hoffman, B. F., Cranefield, P. F.: Slow conduction and reentry in the ventricular conducting system. II. Single and sustained circus movement in networks of canine and bovine Purkinje fibers. *Circ Res* **30**:11-22, 1972.
243. Cranefield, P. F., Wit, A. L., Hoffman, B. F.: Conduction of the cardiac impulse. III. Characteristics of very slow conduction. *J Gen Physiol* **59**:227-246, 1972.
244. Friedman, P. L., Stewart, J. R., Fenoglio, J. J., Jr., et al.: Survival of subendocardial Purkinje fibers after extensive myocardial infarction in dogs. *Circ Res* **33**:597-611, 1973.
245. Scherlag, B. J., Lazzara, R., Abelleira, J. L., et al.: Mechanisms of early and late arrhythmias due to myocardial ischemia and infarction. *Circulation* **46**:II-59, 1972.
246. Cox, J. L., Daniel, T. M., Boineau, J. P.: The electrophysiologic time-course of acute myocardial ischemia and the effects of early coronary artery reperfusion. *Circulation* **48**:971-983, 1973.
247. Scherlag, B. J., Helfant, R. H., Haft, J. I., et al.: Electrophysiology underlying ventricular arrhythmias due to coronary ligation. *Am J Physiol* **219**:1665-1671, 1970.
248. Waldo, A. L., Kaiser, G. A., Castany, R. J., et al.: Study of arrhythmias associated with acute myocardial infarction. *Circulation* **38**:VI-200, 1968.
249. Regan, T. J., Markov, A., Khan, M. I., et al.: Myocardial ion and lipid changes during ischemia and catecholamine induced necrosis: Relation to regional blood flow, in *Myocardiology: Recent Advances in Studies on Cardiac Structure and Metabolism*, Vol. 1, edited by Bajusz, E. and Rona, G., University Park Press, Baltimore, 1972, pp. 656-664.
250. Griggs, D. M., Nakamura, Y.: Effect of coronary constriction on myocardial distribution of iodoantiphyrine-1311. *Amer J Physiol* **215**:1082-1088, 1968.

251. Regan, T. J., Moschos, C. B., Lehan, R. H., et al.: Lipid and carbohydrate metabolism of myocardium during the biphasic inotropic response to epinephrine. *Circ Res* **19**:307-316, 1966.

252. Bogdanski, D. F., Brodie, B. B.: Effects of inorganic ions on the storage and uptake of H³-norepinephrine by rat heart slices. *J Pharmacol Exp Ther* **165**:181-189, 1969.

253. Page, E., Solomon, A. K.: Cat heart muscle in vitro. I. Cell volumes and intracellular concentrations in papillary muscle. *J Gen Physiol* **44**:327-344, 1960.

254. Mobley, B. A., Page, E.: Effect of potassium and chloride ions on the volume and membrane potential of single barnacle muscle cells. *J Physiol* **215**:19-70, 1971.

255. de Soyza, N., Kane, J., Bissett, J., et al.: Factors predisposing to ventricular tachycardia in acute myocardial infarction. *Clin Res* **22**:4A, 1974.

256. Lazzara, R., El-Sherif, N., Scherlag, B. J.: Electrophysiological properties of canine Purkinje cells in one-day-old myocardial infarction. *Circ Res* **33**:722-734, 1973.

257. Wellens, H. J. J., Lie, K. I., Durrer, D.: Further observations on ventricular tachycardia as studied by electrical stimulation of the heart. Chronic recurrent ventricular tachycardia and ventricular tachycardia during acute myocardial infarction. *Circulation* **44**:647-653, 1974.

258. Han, J.: Ventricular vulnerability in myocardial ischemia, in *Effect of Acute Ischemia on Myocardial Function*, edited by Oliver, M. F., Julian, D. G., Donald, K. W., Williams and Wilkins Co., Baltimore, 1972, pp. 141-156.

259. Han, J.: Ventricular vulnerability to fibrillation, in *Cardiac Arrhythmias*, edited by Dreifus, L. S., Likoff, W., Grune and Stratton, New York, 1973, pp. 87-95.

260. Wissner, S. B.: The effect of excess lactate upon the excitability of the sheep Purkinje fiber. *J Electrocardiol* **7**:17-26, 1974.

261. Kostis, J. B., Mavrogeorgis, E. A., Horstmann, E., et al.: Effect of high concentrations of free fatty acids on the ventricular fibrillation threshold of normal dogs and dogs with acute myocardial infarction. *Cardiology* **58**:89-98, 1973.

262. Oliver, M. F., Kurien, V. A., Greenwood, T. W.: Relation between serum free-fatty-acids and arrhythmias and death after acute myocardial infarction. *Lancet* **1**:710-714, 1968.

263. Ettinger, P. O., Regan, T. J., Oldewurtel, H. A., et al.: Ventricular conduction delay and asystole during systemic hyperkalemia. *Amer J Cardiol* **33**:876-886, 1974.

264. Dhalla, N. S., Sulakhe, P. V., Khandelwal, R. L., et al.: Adenyl cyclase activity in the perfused rat heart muscle made to fail by substrate-lack. *Cardiovasc Res* **6**:344-352, 1972.

265. Dhalla, N. S., Singh, J. N., Fedelesova, M., et al.: Biochemical basis of heart function. XII. Sodium-potassium stimulated adenosine triphosphatase activity in the perfused rat heart made to fail by substrate-lack. *Cardiovasc Res* **8**:227-236, 1974.

266. Lieberman, M.: Electrophysiological studies of a synthetic strand of cardiac muscle. *The Physiologist:* in press.

267. Polimeri, P. I.: Choline substitution for extracellular Na in cardiac Purkinje fibers: effects on K fluxes, in *Research in Physiology*, edited by Kao, F. F., Koizumi, K., Vassale, M., Aulo Gaggi, Bologna, 1971, pp. 45-57.

268. Soustre, H.: Electrogenese cardiaque du rate surrenalectomise, interpretation en fonction des variations de gradients ioniques et de permeabilities membranaires. *Pfluegers Arch* **333**:111-125, 1972.

269. Imanishi, S.: Calcium-sensitive discharges in canine Purkinje fibers. *Jap J Physiol* 21:443-461, 1971.
270. Kohlhardt, M., Bauer, B., Krause, H., et al.: New selective inhibitors of the transmembrane Ca conductivity in mammalian myocardial fibers. Studies with the voltage clamp technique. *Experientia* 28:288-289, 1972.
271. Kohlhardt, M., Bauer, B., Krause, H., et al.: Differentiation of the transmembrane Na and Ca channels in mammalian cardiac fibers by the use of specific inhibitors. *Pfluegers Arch* 335:309-322, 1972.
272. Rougier, O., Vassort, G., Garnier, D., et al.: Existence and role of slow inward current during the frog atrial action potential. *Pfluegers Arch* 308: 91-110, 1969.
273. Shigeto, N., Irisawa, H.: Slow conduction in the atrioventricular node of the cat: A possible explanation. *Experientia* 28:1442-1443, 1972.
274. Trautwein, W.: Membrane currents in cardiac muscle fibers. *Physiol Rev* 53:793-835, 1973.
275. Reuter, H.: Divalent cations as charge carriers in excitable membranes. *Progr Biophys Mol Biol* 26:3-43, 1973.
276. Girardier, L.: Dynamic energy partition in cultured heart cells. *Cardiology* 56:88-92, 1971/72.
277. Hyde, A., Cheneval, J.-P., Blondel, B., et al.: Electrophysiological correlates of energy metabolism in cultured rat heart cells. *J Physiol Paris* 64:269-292, 1972.
278. Johnson, E. A., Lieberman, M.: Heart: excitation and contraction. *Ann Rev Physiol* 33:479-532, 1971.
279. Weidmann, S.: Effect of current flow on the membrane potential of cardiac muscle. *J Physiol* 115:227, 1951.
280. Trautwein, W.: Generation of the cardiac action potential, in: *Electrical Activity of the Heart*, edited by Manning, G. W., and Ahuja, S. P., Charles C Thomas, Springfield, Illinois, 1969, pp. 9-22.
281. McAllister, R. E., Noble, D.: The time and voltage dependence of the slow outward current in cardiac Purkinje fibers. *J Physiol* 186:632, 1968.
282. Noble, D., Tsien, R. W.: The repolarization process of heart cells, in *Electrical Phenomena in the Heart*, edited by DeMello, W. C., Academic Press, New York, 1972, pp. 133-161.
283. Rosen, M. R., Wit, A. L., Hoffman, B. F.: Electrophysiology and pharmacology of cardiac arrhythmias. I. Cellular electrophysiology of the mammalian heart. *Amer Heart J* 88:380-385, 1974.
284. Wit, A. L., Rosen, M. R., Hoffman, B. F.: Electrophysiology and pharmacology of cardiac arrhythmias. II. Relationship of normal and abnormal electrical activity of cardiac fibers to the genesis of arrhythmias. *Amer Heart J* 88:515-524, 1974.
285. Ettinger, P. O., Regan, T. J., Eldewurtel, H. A.: Hyperkalemia, cardiac conduction, and the electrocardiogram: a review. *Amer Heart J* 88:360-371, 1974.
286. Borasio, P. G., Vassalle, M.: Effects of norepinephrine on active K transport and automaticity in cardiac Purkinje fibers, in *Myocardial Biology: Recent Advances in Studies on Cardiac Structure and Metabolism*, edited by Dhalla, N. S., University Park Press, Baltimore, 1974, Vol. 4, pp. 41-57.
287. Lehr, D., Chau, R.: Changes in the cardiac electrolyte content during development and healing of experimental myocardial infarction, in *Myocardial Metabolism: Recent Advances in Studies on Cardiac Structure and Metabolism*, edited by Dhalla, N. S., Rona, G., Baltimore, University Park Press, 1973, pp. 721-751.
288. Gould, L., Reddy, C. V. R., Gomprecht, R. F.: His bundle electrograms in a patient with hyperkalemia. *J Amer Med Assn* 230:87-88, 1974.

289. Griggs, D. M., Jr., Nakamura, Y.: Effect of coronary constriction on myocardial distribution of iodoantipyrine-¹³¹I. *Amer J Physiol* **215**:1082-1088, 1968.

290. Becker, L. C., Ferreira, R., Thomas, M.: Mapping of left ventricular blood flow with radioactive microspheres in experimental coronary artery occlusion. *Cardiovasc Res* **7**:391-400, 1973.

291. Moir, T. W., DeBra, D. W.: Effect of left ventricular hypertension, ischemia and vasoactive drugs on the myocardial distribution of coronary flow. *Circ Res* **21**:65-74, 1967.

292. Winbury, M. M., Howe, B. B., Weiss, H. R.: Effect of nitroglycerin and dipyridamole on epicardial and endocardial oxygen tension—further evidence for redistribution of myocardial blood flow. *J Pharm Exp Therap* **176**: 184-199, 1971.

293. Buckberg, G. D., Fixler, D. E., Archie, J. P., et al.: Experimental subendocardial ischemia in dogs with normal coronary arteries. *Circ Res* **30**: 67-81, 1972.

294. Becker, L. C., Fortuin, N. J., Pitt, B.: Effect of ischemia and antianginal drugs on the distribution of radioactive microspheres in the canine left ventricle. *Circ Res* **28**:263-269, 1971.

295. Rees, J. R., Redding, V. J.: Experimental myocardial infarction in the dog. Comparison of myocardial blood flow within, near, and distant from the infarct. *Circ Res* **25**:161-170, 1969.

296. Griggs, D. M., Jr., Tchokoev, V. V., DeClue, J. W.: Effect of beta-adrenergic receptor stimulation on regional myocardial metabolism: Importance of coronary vessel patency. *Amer Heart J* **82**:492, 1971.

297. Griggs, D. M., Jr., Tchokoev, V. V., Chen, C. C.: Transmural differences in ventricular tissue substrate levels due to coronary constriction. *Am J Physiol* **222**:705, 1972.

298. Kirk, E. S., Honig, C. R.: An experimental and theoretical analysis of myocardial tissue pressure. *Amer J Physiol* **207**:361-367, 1964.

299. Downey, H. F., Bashour, F. A., Stephens, A. J., et al.: Transmural gradient of retrograde collateral blood flow in acutely ischemic canine myocardium. *Circ Res* **35**:365-371, 1974.

300. Timogiannakis, G., Amende, I., Martinez, E., et al.: ST segment deviation and regional myocardial blood flow during experimental partial coronary artery occlusion. *Cardiovasc Res* **8**:469-477, 1974.

301. Ekmekei, A., Toyoshima, H., Kwoczynski, J. K., et al.: Angina Pectoris. IV. Clinical and experimental difference between ischaemia with S-T elevation and ischaemia with S-T depression. *Amer J Cardiol* **7**:412-426, 1961.

302. Prinzmetal, M., Toyoshima, H., Ekmekci, A., et al.: Myocardial ischemia. Nature of ischemic electrocardiographic patterns in the mammalian ventricles as determined by intracellular electrographic and metabolic changes. *Am J Cardiol* **8**:493-503, 1961.

303. Rakita, L., Borduas, J. L., Rothman, S., et al.: Studies on the mechanism of ventricular activity. XII. Early changes in the RS-T segment and QRS complex following acute coronary artery occlusion: Experimental study and clinical applications. *Amer Heart J* **48**:351-372, 1954.

304. Kennamer, R., Bernstein, J. L., Maxwell, M. H., et al.: Studies on the mechanism of ventricular activity. V. Intramural depolarization potentials in the normal heart with a consideration of currents of injury in coronary artery disease. *Amer Heart J* **46**:379-400, 1953.

305. Sayen, J. J., Peirce, G., Katcher, A. H., et al.: Correlation of intramyocardial electrocardiograms with polarographic oxygen and contractility in the non-ischemic and regionally ischemic left ventricle. *Circ Res* **9**:1268-1279, 1961.

306. Wendt, R. L., Canavan, R. C., Michalah, R.: Effects of various agents on

regional ischemic myocardial injury: electrocardiographic analysis. *Amer Heart J* **87**:468-482, 1974.

307. Corday, E., Lang, T.-W., Mierbaum, S., et al.: Closed chest model of intracoronary occlusion for study of regional cardiac function. *Amer J Cardiol* **33**:49-59, 1974.

308. Meerbaum, S., Lang, T.-W., Corday, E., et al.: Progressive alterations of cardiac hemodynamic and regional metabolic function after acute coronary occlusion. *Amer J Cardiol* **33**:60-68, 1974.

309. Rizzon, P., DiBiase, M. D., Baissus, C.: Intraventricular conduction defects in acute myocardial infarction. *Brit Heart J* **36**:660-668, 1974.

310. Harris, A. S., Rojas, A. G.: Initiation of ventricular fibrillation due to coronary occlusion. *Exp Med Surg* **1**:105-133, 1943.

311. Scherlag, B. J., El-Sherif, N., Hope, R., et al.: Characterization and localization of venticular arrhythmias resulting from myocardial ischemia and infarction. *Circ Res* **35**:372-383, 1974.

312. Cranefield, P. F.: Ventricular fibrillation. *N Eng J Med* **289**:732-736, 1973.

313. Friedman, P. L., Stewart, J. R., Wit, A. L.: Spontaneous and induced cardiac arrhythmias in subendocardial Purkinje fibers surviving extensive myocardial infarction in dogs. *Circ Res* **33**:612-625, 1973.

314. Lazzara, R., El-Sherif, N., Scherlag, B. J.: Early and late effects of coronary artery occlusion on canine Purkinje fibers. *Circ Res* **35**:391-399, 1974.

315. Tacker, W. A., Jr., Geddes, L. A., Cabler, P. S., et al.: Electrical threshold for defibrillation of canine ventricles following myocardial infarction. *Amer Heart J* **88**:476-481, 1974.

316. Lubbe, W. F., Peisach, M., Pretorius, R., et al.: Distribution of myocardial blood flow before and after coronary artery ligation in the baboon. Relation to early ventricular fibrillation. *Cardiovasc Res* **8**:478-487, 1974.

317. Kjekshus, J. K., Maroko, P. R., Sobel, B. E.: Distribution of myocardial injury and its relation to epicardial ST-segment changes after coronary artery occlusion in the dog. *Cardiovasc Res* **6**:490-499, 1972.

318. Schwartz, A.: Active transport in mammalian myocardium, in *The Mammalian Myocardium*, edited by Langer, G. A., Brady, A. J., John Wiley & Sons, New York, 1973, pp. 81-104.

319. Garrahan, P. J., Glynn, I. M.: The incorporation of inorganic phosphate into adenosine triphosphate by reversal of the sodium pump. *J Physiol* **192**:237-256, 1967.

320. Macleod, D. P., Prasad, K.: Influence of glucose on the transmembrane action potential and contraction of papillary muscle. Effects of concentration, phlorizin and insulin, nonmetabolized sugars, and stimulation of glycolysis. *J Gen Physiol* **53**:792-815, 1969.

321. Prasad, K., Callaghan, J. C.: Effects of glucose metabolism on the transmembrane action potential and contraction of human papillary muscle during surgical anoxia. *Ann Thorac Surg* **7**:571-581, 1969.

322. Prasad, K., MacLeod, D. P.: Influence of glucose on the transmembrane action potential of papillary muscle. Metabolic inhibitors, ouabain, $CaCl_2$ and their interaction with glucose, sympathomimetic amines, and aminophylline. *Circ Res* **24**:939-950, 1969.

323. Prasad, K.: Influence of energy supply and calcium on the low-sodium-induced changes in the transmembrane potential and contraction of guinea pig papillary muscle. *Can J Physiol Pharmacol* **48**:241-253, 1970.

324. Prasad, K., Callaghan, J. C.: Influence of glucose metabolism on the ouabain-induced changes in the transmembrane potential and contraction of human heart in vitro. *Can J Physiol Pharmacol* **48**:801-812, 1970.

325. Prasad, K.: Transmembrane potential, contraction, and ATPase activity of human heart in relation to ouabain. *Jap Heart J* **13**:59-72, 1972.

326. Prasad, K., Singh, S., Callaghan, J. C.: Transmembrane potential and contraction of human heart in relation to potassium and ouabain. *Jap Heart J* **12**:290-304, 1971.
327. Prasad, K.: Substrate and Ca$^{++}$ dependent effects of low potassium-induced changes in the transmembrane potential and contraction of human heart in vitro. *Proc Internat Congr Pharmacol* **4**:277, 1968.
328. Prasad, K.: Membrane Na$^+$-K$^+$-ATPase and electromechanics of human heart, in *Recent Advances in Studies on Cardiac Structure and Metabolism, Myocardial Biology*, edited by Dhalla, N. S., University Park Press, Baltimore, 1974, Vol. 4, pp. 91-105.
329. Brazier, J., Cooper, N., Buckberg, G.: The adequacy of subendocardial oxygen delivery. The interaction of determinants of flow, arterial oxygen content and myocardial oxygen need. *Circulation* **49**:968-977, 1974.
330. Pilla, A. A.: Electrochemical information transfer at living cell membranes. *Ann NY Acad Sci* **238**:149-169, 1974.
331. Hoffman, J.: Ionic transport across the plasma membrane. *Hosp Practice* **9**:119-127 (Oct.), 1974.
332. Langer, G. A.: Effects of digitalis on myocardial ionic exchange. *Circulation* **46**:180-187, 1972.
333. Langer, G. A.: Calcium in mammalian myocardium. Localization, control, and the effects of digitalis. *Circ Res* **34-35** (suppl III): 91-98, 1974.
334. Tillesch, J. H., Langer, G. A.: Myocardial mechanical responses and ionic exchange in high-sodium perfusate. *Circ Res* **34**:40-50, 1974.
335. Langer, G. A.: Ionic movements and the control of contraction, in *The Mammalian Myocardium*, edited by Langer, G. A., Brady, A. J., John Wiley & Sons, New York, 1974, pp. 193-217.
336. Vassort, G.: Existence of two components in frog cardiac mechanical activity. Influence of Na ions. *Europ J Cardiol* **1**:163-168, 1973.
337. Trautwein, W.: The slow inward current in mammalian myocardium. Its relation to contraction. *Europ J Cardiol* **1**:169-175, 1973.
338. Narahashi, T.: Chemicals as tools in the study of excitable membranes. *Physiol Rev* **54**:813-889, 1974.
339. Morad, M., Goldman, Y.: Excitation-contraction coupling in heart muscle: membrane control of development of tension. *Progr Biophys Mol Biol* **27**: 257-313, 1974.
340. Reuter, H.: Exchange of calcium ions in the mammalian myocardium. Mechanisms and physiological significance. *Circ Res* **34**:599-605, 1974.
341. Hodgkin, A. L., Huxley, A. F.: Currents carried by sodium and potassium ions through the membrane of the giant axon of *Loligo*. *J Physiol* **116**:449-472, 1952.
342. Surawicz, B.: Calcium responses ("calcium spikes"). *Amer J Cardiol* **33**: 689-690, 1974.
343. Cranefield, P. F., Klein, H. O., Hoffman, B. F.: Conduction of the cardiac impulse. I. Delay, block and one-way block in depressed Purkinje fibers. *Circ Res* **28**:199-219, 1971.
344. Cranefield, P. F., Hoffman, B. F.: Conduction of the cardiac impulse. II. Summation and inhibition. *Circ Res* **28**:220-233, 1971.
345. Arita, M., Surawicz, B.: Depolarization and action potential duration in cardiac Purkinje fibers. *Circ Res* **33**:39-47, 1973.
346. Coraboeuf, E.: Membrane electrical activity and double component contraction in cardiac tissue. *J Mol Cell Cardiol* **6**:215-222, 1974.
347. Coraboeuf, E., Deroubaix, E.: Phasic and tonic components of contraction in mammalian myocardium. In preparation.

CHAPTER 4

# GLUCOSE, INSULIN, POTASSIUM THERAPY FOR HEART DISEASE

## I. INTRODUCTION AND OVERVIEW

In 1963 Laborit and Huguenard noted that treatment of rabbits with glucose and insulin prevented KCl-induced ventricular fibrillation.[1] GIK was then used to improve survival following cardiac arrest [2] and in cardiogenic shock.[1] GIK solution was termed "repolarizing" because of an anticipated restoration of cardiac membrane potential via a raise in intracellular potassium ($K^+$) concentration. The electrocardiographic pattern of myocardial infarction receded after exposure to a solution of $K^+$ and magnesium ($Mg^{++}$) aspartate, presumably also supporting the notion that repolarization of ischemic myocardium was necessary and beneficial.[3]

Harris [4] had suggested that ventricular automaticity might be increased when myocardial cells with a lower excitability threshold were stimulated by a current of injury produced by a potassium gradient at the boundary between an infarcted and noninfarcted area of muscle. Ventricular fibrillation followed production of experimental myocardial infarction.[5, 6] Since enhanced perfusion of infarcted myocardium protected against arrhythmias, possibly by clearance of a toxic agent,[7, 8] a substance released by the injured tissue was suspected as the etiologic agent. Presence of arrhythmias correlated well with increases in $K^+$-release from areas of myocardial infarction.[9, 10] Finally, infusion of large amounts of insulin and glucose or of sodium bicarbonate prevented ventricular ectopic activity in association with decreased $K^+$ in the coronary sinus effluent.[11] Thus, while some evidence existed that myocardial $K^+$ loss contributed to the genesis of arrhythmias, the precise mechanism of initiation and maintenance of such postulated $K^+$-loss-induced arrhythmias remained unknown. $K^+$ involvement in local boundary currents remained to be proved. A potential gradient between infarcted and noninfarcted myocardium would have to be considerable and the contact area between them wide in order to produce

249

an effective stimulating current,[12] the infarcted tissue acting as an anode with respect to the adjacent excited tissue.[13]

The "necrotizing cardiomyopathies" in animal models were characterized by early and spotty loss of intracellular $K^+$ before structural change was apparent.[14, 15] Such $K^+$ loss was also attended by disappearance of glycogen granules and phosphorylase activity in the same muscle fibers. In these experiments, $K^+$- and $Mg^{++}$-deficiency predisposed myocardium to toxic degeneration and the administration of salts of these cations was preventive. Hence both Selye and Mishra concluded that $[K^+]_o/[K^+]_i$ balance influenced the course of potentially cardiotoxic events and could be modified by manipulation of ion concentrations outside the cell.[16, 17]

Larcan and associates reported that 40 patients with acute myocardial infarction treated with a complex "polarizing solution" had less morbidity, mortality, and earlier regression of electrocardiographic changes than a control group.[18] Sodi-Pallares, following his initial report of the benefits of increased oral water and KCl intake in patients with all sorts of heart disease,[19, 20] directed his attention to the treatment of acute myocardial infarction with intravenous polarizing solutions. Daily infusion of 100 ml 5 to 10 percent glucose solution containing 40 meq KCl and 40 units regular (CZI) insulin at rates of 40 to 60 drops/min decreased the severity and duration of electrocardiographic abnormalities. Arrhythmias were suppressed, chest pain was relieved,[21-23] and symptoms of congestive heart failure improved,[24] while the probability of a residual anginal syndrome was diminished.[25] More recently, in reply to objections to the use of his polarizing solution, Sodi-Pallares has detailed his latest formula for this therapy as follows:

(i)    300-600 mg $Na^+$, 3900 Mg $K^+$ diet,

(ii)  24 hour infusion of polarizing solution with a) 10 percent glucose and 20 u CZI insulin b) 20 percent glucose and 40 u CZI insulin c) 50 percent glucose and 60 u CZI insulin

(iii) $K^+Cl^-$ addition graded to the serum $K^+$ ($[K^+]_p$) value (60 meq for $[K^+]_p = 3$-4 meq/L; 40 meq for $[K^+]_p = 4$-5 meq/L; 20 meq for $[K^+]_p = 4$-5.5 meq/L; 0 for $[K^+]_p = 5.5$);

(iv)  total water intake $\geq 3L/24$ hr,

(v)  modification of the above according to the electrocardiogram and clinical status; and

(vi)  avoidance of "unnecessary" depolarizing and inotropic agents.

Sodi-Pallares further outlined his experimental work buttressing his approach to the use of polarizing solution and claimed the following benefits accompanied its use: [26]

1. diminution of RS-T segment displacement, suppression of ectopic rhythms and better conduction, suggesting improvement of the transmembrane potentials,[28]
2. increased contractility,[28]
3. "improvement" of the metabolic pathways in the Krebs cycle,[30]
4. lessening of the electrolyte imbalance, exemplified by reversal of retention of $Na^+$ and loss of $K^+$, reflecting improved function of the altered pump mechanisms,[28]
5. increase in the retrograde coronary flow.

According to Sodi-Pallares, partially injured myocardial fibers surrounding an area of myocardial infarction lose part of their intracellular $K^+$ but retain the ability to restore it under the influence of polarizing solution. Insulin permits cellular entry of $K^+$ and glucose which is held to activate oxidative phosphorylation and hence augment ATP and glycogen stores.[30]

## II. EFFECT OF GIK ON MYOCARDIAL INFARCT SIZE

### A. Jeopardized myocardium in a "twilight zone"

The potential limitation of myocardial infarct size is an important, fresh approach to an old problem of left ventricular "pump" or "power" failure. Cardiogenic shock is now the major cause of death in patients being treated for acute myocardial infarctions. Despite careful management of this syndrome with pharmacologic agents, mechanical circulatory assistance and surgery, its mortality has not changed significantly. The difficulty in managing the fully developed syndrome of cardiogenic shock suggests that prevention may be a more fruitful area to explore than variations of presently employed therapeutic techniques. Patients with "power failure" have over 40-70 percent of their left ventricular muscle mass destroyed, and the muscle loss is additive.[31-35] Therefore, some means of controlling the extent of myocardial infarction may have a preventive impact upon the subsequent development of cardiogenic shock.

Successful limitation of irreversible ischemic myocadial injury would be impossible if it were not for the recent appreciaton of the progression of necrosis surrounding an area of myocardial infarction. Jennings and associates [36] established that architectural changes in mitochondria occur after 20 minutes of ischemia, and a proportionally greater number of myocytes undergo irreversible damage after that period of time.

However, the necrosis actually observed after experimental coronary artery ligation is not uniform, and the existence of a zone of muscle surrounding necrotic myocardium whose fate is yet to be determined at the time of the insult has been demonstrated.[37-41] Progressive deterioration of hemodynamic and metabolic parameters are also not uniform, and although they are related, do not bear a simple relation with one another.[318]

An area of infarcted myocardium may be visualized as a central, necrotic zone surrounded by patches of still potentially viable muscle, called the "twilight zone." This ischemic zone may continue to change up to eighteen hours after coronary occlusion, as the necrotic zone enlarges at the expense of the intermediate zone.[37] The ischemic zone has been further divided into two categories by Sobel and Shell,[42] who distinguish "blighted" and "jeopardized" tissues. Blighted myocardium is irreparably damaged and is doomed regardless of any subsequent event. Jeopardized muscle is reversibly damaged and may either become blighted or recover if the ischemia is reversed. Significant metabolic alterations occur in noninfarcted areas of myocardium. Elevation in serum or creatine phosphokinase levels provide an index of the extent and severity of ischemic injury, proportional to the size of necrotic and blighted areas and the extent of reduction in coronary blood flow.[42-44, 73]

## B. Myocardial oxygen and energy balance

Certain lines of evidence suggested that the fate of the ischemic zone might be altered by a more favorable oxygen balance, either by an increase in myocardial oxygen supply or decrease in its demand (Fig. 1). Over the past fifteen years, studies conducted by Braunwald and collaborators,[45-47] have identified the major and minor determinants of myocardial oxygen consumption. The important variables increasing myocardial oxygen needs are intramyocardial tension, heart rate and inotropic state. Ventricular wall stress in turn directly depends upon intraventricular pressure and radius by the LaPlace equation. Therefore, wall tension is a function of both afterload and preload. However, the myocardial oxygen cost of work against a pressure load is considerably higher than the cost of work against a volume load. Tachycardia and increases in myocardial contractility significantly augment myocardial oxygen consumption. Norepinephrine, isoproterenol, paired pacing, calcium, glucagon, digitalis, and other positive inotropic agents may increase the imbalance between oxygen supply and demand by increasing the latter.[48] Negative inotropic

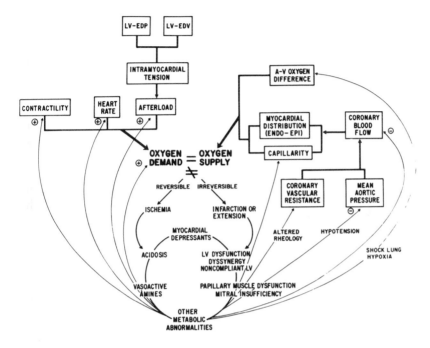

**Figure 1**   The central role of balance between myocardial oxygen supply and demand and their determinants are shown. Improvement of myocardial oxygenation increases chances for survival of marginally viable tissue in the ischemic zone of a myocardial infarction. The variables determining myocardial oxygen supply (right side) are altered by negative feedback loops from complications of poor left ventricular function (center cycle). Those factors affecting myocardial oxygen demand (left side) are altered by positive feedback loops from these events perpetuating the syndrome. Both the negative feedback on oxygen supply and the positive feedback on oxygen demand tend to further the inequality between the two and may jeopardize poorly perfused myocardial tissue.

maneuvers make this relationship more favorable by reducing myocardial oxygen consumption.[49] Thus, propranolol is capable of elevating intramyocardial oxygen tensions.[50]

Recognition of the determinants of myocardial oxygen consumption and balance has had important consequences. The survival of the ischemic zone of a myocardial infarction may depend upon the balance between oxygen supply and demand. Interventions which make this balance unfavorable may endanger ischemic myocardium, or even possibly extend the infarction by expanding the jeopardized zone. While small elevations in myocardial oxygen extraction may occur, the most important determinants of oxygen demand in ischemic myocardium are those governing the mechanical performance of the heart.[51] Despite other "compensatory" mechanisms which tend to reduce myocardial oxygen need,[52] the ischemic zone is sensitive to changes in myocardial oxygen demand effected by lowering heart rate, inotropic state, and afterload. Thus the size of a myocardial infarction, as judged by total creatine phosphokinase analysis, is increased by tachycardia, produced by ventricular pacing or atropine or isoproterenol administration.[53] Similarly, reductions in arterial pressure, or more complex changes in several determinants of myocardial oxygen consumption making oxygen balance more favorable, may lessen the degree of myocardial ischemia.[54, 55] The investigation of therapeutic maneuvers to reduce the zone of ischemia had led to important new approaches to the problem of left-ventricular "power" failure, as mentioned (Table I).

## C. Epicardial and precordial mapping of S-T segment elevations

### 1. History

The localization of a myocardial infarction has been determined clinically from the pattern of S-T segment elevations in the standard electrocardiogram.[56-62] This time-honored practice dates from Wilson and associates [63, 64] who postulated that the electrical potential recorded from the exploring precordial electrode accurately reflected the epicardial potential beneath.

There is ample and convincing experimental evidence showing that direct epicardial open-chest recording of S-T segment elevation reflects ischemia in the underlying myocardium.[65-69] Wegria and collaborators confirmed the close relationship between S-T segment elevation and reduction in coronary blood flow,[65] which was later correlated with the degree of anaerobic metabolism produced.[66, 72] More recently, Prinzmetal and coauthors [67, 68] and Case and associates [69] have reemphasized the accurate reflections of the degree of ischemia by abnormal S-T segments recorded from an electrode overlying the injured myocardium.

### 2. Recent techniques

Extending these observations, Maroko and associates developed a method of mapping epicardial S-T segments to delineate the borders of zones of myocardial ischemia.[70, 71] In this technique, 10-14 epicardial leads are recorded on the anterior surface of the left ventricle in the distribution and area of the site of occlusion of a branch of the left anterior descending coronary artery. The average S-T segment eleva-

**Table I**   For some time following myocardial ischemic injury, as drawing suggests, affected heart tissue served by occluded coronary arteries consists of a relatively small, patchy necrotic zone surrounded by a zone of abnormal yet still viable tissue at high risk of further irreversible damage or possibly amenable to salvage through medical or surgical interventions. The goal of limiting infarct size in man and thus influencing both the immediate and long-term prognosis in acute infarction is now being actively pursued. It has already been learned (table) that certain interventions have a positive, others a negative, effect on infarct size. Reproduced with permission from *Hospital Practice* 8:61, 1973.

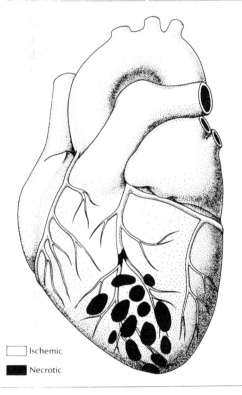

☐ Ischemic

■ Necrotic

**Interventions that reduce myocardial injury**

A. *By decreasing myocardial oxygen demands*
   1. Propranolol
   2. Practolol
   3. Ouabain in the failing heart
   4. Intra-aortic balloon counterpulsation

B. *By increasing myocardial oxygen supply*
   1. Directly
      a. Coronary artery reperfusion
   2. Through collaterals
      a. Elevation of coronary perfusion pressure
      b. Intra-aortic balloon counterpulsation

C. *By enhancing anaerobic metabolism*
   1. Glucose-insulin-potassium
   2. Hypertonic glucose (also acts by increased osmolarity)

D. *By enhancing transport to the ischemic zone of substrates utilized in energy production (presumed)*
   1. Hyaluronidase

E. *By protecting against autolytic and heterolytic processes (presumed)*
   1. Hydrocortisone

**Interventions that increase myocardial injury**

A. *By increasing myocardial oxygen requirements*
   1. Isoproterenol
   2. Glucagon
   3. Ouabain
   4. Bretylium tosylate
   5. Tachycardia

B. *By decreasing myocardial oxygen supply*
   1. Reduction of coronary perfusion pressure

tion for each animal is determined at intervals after occlusion. S-T segment elevation of over 2 mV fifteen minutes after ligation of the coronary artery branch signifies ischemic injury in the area supplied. The number of sites with S-T elevation further defines the ischemic area (Fig. 2).

The usefulness of maps of S-T segment elevation is underscored by the correlation of epicardial maps with the creatine phosphokinase (CPK) content of corresponding tissue segments.[70, 74] S-T segment ele-

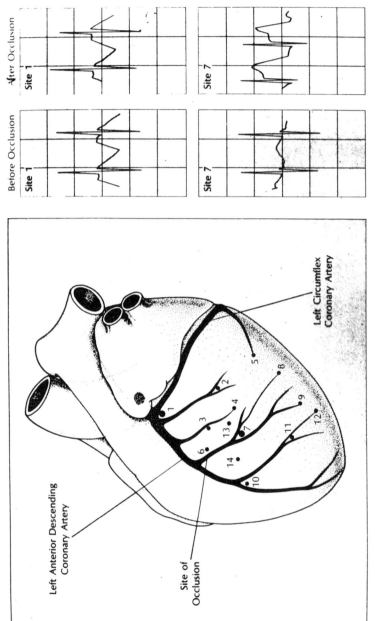

**Figure 2** Ischemic injury is revealed in epicardial ECG's obtained shortly after induced occlusion from sites on anterior surface of dog heart, as shown schematically at the left. Whereas ECG from a site in the area distal to the occluded vessel (lower right) shows marked S-T segment changes, none are seen in tracing from a site that is remote from the injured zone (upper right). Reproduced with permission.[70]

vation in excess of 2 mV is associated with a decrease in myocardial CPK activity (Fig. 3), and also correlates with histologic signs of necrosis twenty-four hours later.[70, 75] The decrease in myocardial CPK activity reflects the mass of dead tissue after coronary occlusion.[42, 76]

### 3. *Effect of agents altering contractility*

Positive inotropic agents, such as isoproterenol, glucagon, and bretylium, given prior to a repeated occlusion of a branch of a coronary artery increased the severity and extent of ischemic injury [70] (Fig. 4). Digitalis in the nonfailing heart increased ischemic injury, whereas in the depressed heart it diminished the extent of ischemic injury.[77] Tachycardia also increased the severity of ischemic injury [70] and this has been repeatedly confirmed.[53, 71] When heart rate was increased by electrical stimulation, the S-T segment elevation observed was less than was achieved with isoproterenol, showing that the effects of this agent were partly due to the resultant tachycardia and partly mediated by augmented contractility. Elevation in arterial pressure produced by methoxamine infusion decreased the severity of ischemic injury, whereas a reduction in blood pressure was associated with increased ischemic injury.[70] It was felt that in the experimental setting used, the increase in total coronary artery flow effected by the rise in arterial pressure outweighed the deleterious effect of augmented myocardial oxygen consumption. However in the pharmacologically depressed heart, elevations in arterial pressure caused small but significant increases in ischemic injury, postulated to occur because myocardial oxygen requirements rose to a greater extent than coronary perfusion.[77]

The administration of propranolol decreased ischemic injury as judged by S-T segment elevations and the area of depression in myocardial CPK activity [70, 71, 78, 79] (Figs. 5 and 6). Not only was the extent and severity of the ischemic injury reversible for up to three hours after experimental coronary occlusion, but an increase in injury could be counteracted by the subsequent and/or simultaneous use of propranolol. Propranolol might therefore be of value in limiting ischemic injury. Other properties of this agent—reduction in platelet adhesiveness, bradycardic effect, diminution in renin secretion, and improvement of myocardial contractility in the presence of compromised coronary flow—may well also be desirable during ischemic episodes.[80, 81] Indeed, with the use of total CPK measurements, propranolol was recently again reported to decrease infarct size in the conscious dog.[82] A preliminary report of a small series of patients with uncomplicated myocardial infarctions suggests that propranolol may be useful in

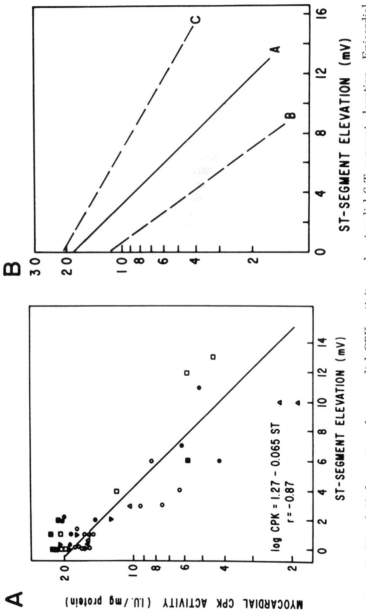

Figure 3 (Panel A) depression of myocardial CPK activity and epicardial S-T segment elevation. Epicardial recordings were obtained 15 min after coronary artery occlusion from readily identifiable sites. CPK activity was

(*Figure caption continued on following page.*)

reducing the size of myocardial infarctions.[83] Other techniques, such as the use of intra-aortic balloon counterpulsation, have been investigated and found to diminish the area of ischemic injury.[84] As sometimes noted with propranolol, sequential combination of intra-aortic balloon counterpulsation with another agent may reduce the extent of ischemic injury (Fig. 4).

As mentioned, the beneficial or deleterious effects of the agents discussed and intra-aortic balloon counterpulsation on extent and severity of ischemic injury are closely related to their effect on myocardial oxygen consumption. An unfavorable influence of a maneuver on myocardial oxygen balance increases the area of ischemic injury.

## 4. *Effect of coronary reperfusion*

These concepts were extended to a consideration of myocardial energy balance, including the delivery and fate of substrate to the myocardium, and to factors influencing the death of tissue other than energy supply. Restoration of coronary blood flow, by releasing a previously tied ligature on a branch of a canine coronary artery, was found to be effective in preventing myocardial injury,[85, 86, 319] although accelerated necrosis was reported recently in one study.[320] Fifty-seven percent of sites showing S-T segment elevation were histologically normal twenty-four hours later. The extent of myocardial necrosis was

---

(*Figure 3 continued from preceding page.*)
measured in homogenates from full wall specimens obtained from the same sites 24 hrs later, and is expressed on a logarithmic scale. Multiple samples were obtained from six dogs. Corresponding symbols represent samples from the same dog. (Panel B) depression of myocardial CPK activity after administration of isoproterenol and propranolol in animals with coronary artery occlusion. Data from multiple samples from six animals given isoproterenol and from six animals given propranolol: Line A: regression line for control study (see panel A), (log CPK = 1.269-0.065 ST; r = −0.87). Line B: regression line relating S-T segment elevation after coronary artery occlusion before isoproterenol was given, and log CPK from myocardial sites that showed increased S-T segment elevation during isoproterenol infusion (log CPK = 1.080-0.076 ST; r = −0.80). Thus, in animals that had received isoproterenol, depression of myocardial CPK activity was greater than that which would be expected from S-T-segment elevation occurring prior to isoproterenol infusion. Line C: regression line for S-T segment elevation after coronary artery occlusion before the propranolol was given and low CPK from corresponding sites 24 hr later (log CPK = 1.302-0.035 ST; r = −0.53). Thus, in animals that had received propranolol, depression of myocardial CPK activity was less than that which would be expected from S-T segment elevation occurring prior to drug administration. Reproduced with permission.[70]

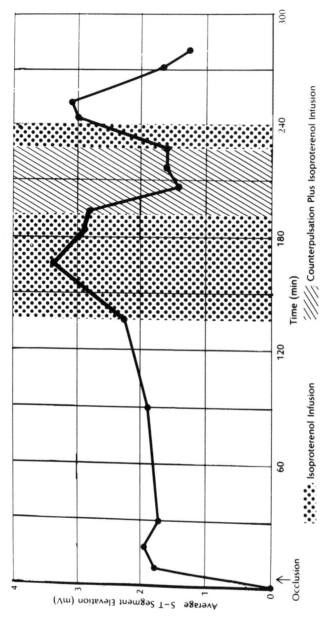

**Figure 4** Counterpulsation begun after three hours of maintained occlusion consistently reduced area of injury, as shown by decrease in average S-T segment elevation; moreover, extension of injury produced by isoproterenol could be offset by counterpulsation. The response of one treated dog (above) suggests a possible clinical combination in suitable infarction cases: isoproterenol to elevate cardiac output plus counterpulsation to counteract the increase in myocardial oxygen consumption isoproterenol induced. Reproduced with permission from Braunwald, E., Maroko, P. R.: *Hosp Practice* 8:68, 1973.

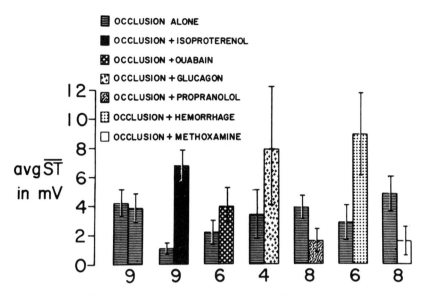

**Figure 5** Influence of repeated coronary artery branch occlusions under the changes induced by isoproterenol, ouabain, glucagon, propranolol, hypotension, and hypertension on the average S-T segment elevation (S-T) after an occlusion. Bars represent standard errors of the mean. Figures below columns indicate number of experiments. Reproduced with permission.[70]

assessed one week later and indeed was strikingly reduced in animals in which such coronary reperfusion was accomplished.

### 5. *Effect of corticosteroids*

The effect of hydrocortisone 50 mg/Kg given intravenously on myocardial infarct size was also studied.[87] Again, epicardial S-T segment elevation 15 minutes after coronary occlusion was compared to myocardial CPK activity and histological appearance twenty-four hours later in each site. In the treated groups, hydrocortisone was given either at thirty minutes after coronary occlusion, or at six hours after occlusion. A supplementary dose of hydrocortisone 25 mg/Kg was given twelve hours after occlusion. The two treated groups of animals showed less CPK depression than was anticipated from the S-T segment elevation at each site. Sites with S-T segment elevations greater than 2 mV in the control group were associated with histologic changes of necrosis in 96 percent of specimens taken from underlying tissue,

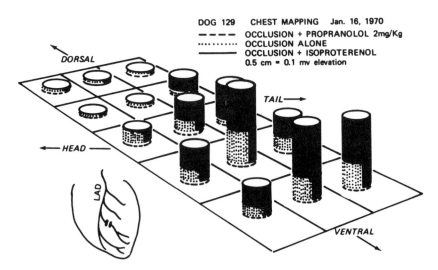

**Figure 6A**  Schematic representation of S-T segment elevation in each of the 15 precordial sites after occlusion alone, occlusion during the infusion of isoproterenol and occlusion after administration of propranolol. Insert is schematic representation of the heart showing occlusion of the apical branch. Reproduced with permission.[70]

whereas this occurred in 61 and 63 percent of specimens taken from tissue in the treated groups. Since over one-third of the sites were prevented from undergoing necrosis, it was concluded that the intervening hydrocortisone treatment was protective even when it was initiated six hours after coronary occlusion. Decreased autolysis due to hydrocortisone-induced stabilization of lysosomal membranes was thought to be the mechanism of action of the corticosteroid.[88]

6. *Effect of inhibiting lipolysis*

Recent studies have shown that catecholamines are released after acute myocardial infarction, that free-fatty acidemia results from the enhanced lipolytic activity and that free fatty acids may be harmful to the heart. Myocardial concentrations of both free fatty acids and myocardial catecholamine levels are high following coronary occlusion. Increased delivery of free fatty acids to the heart of itself augments myocardial oxygen needs, independent of any associated change in contractility.[89] Perhaps 30 percent of the increase in myocardial oxygen consumption caused by the catecholamines is attributable to the energy needs of free fatty acid-induced metabolic stimulation.[90] Moreover,

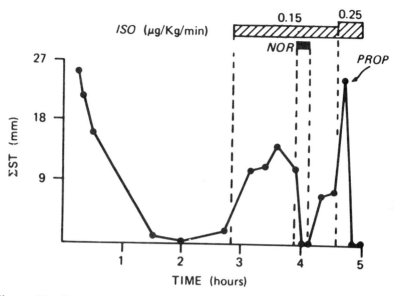

**Figure 6B** Experiment from group of animals with permanent coronary occlusion. The S-T segment elevation decreased spontaneously but reappeared with infusion of isoproterenol (ISO). This S-T segment elevation could be reversed by infusion of norepinephrine (NOR) (0.01 mg/kg per min), which increased mean arterial pressure from 104 to 125 mm Hg (4 hours after occlusion) or by administration of propranolol (PROP) (1 mg/kg) 4½ hours after occlusion. Reproduced with permission.[70]

free fatty acids, quite apart from a potential arrhythmogenic role, depress myocardial contractility,[91, 92] a property that may be related to the increased energy demands dictated by free fatty acidemia.[93] Indeed, using epicardial lead mapping, the S-T segment elevation observed after coronary occlusion was raised by free fatty acidemia.[94] Isoproterenol given before a repeated occlusion increased the severity and extent of the ischemic injury, which was reduced in the presence of β-pyridyl-carbinol, an inhibitor of lipolysis. Not only does β-pyridyl-carbinol effectively reduce the extent and severity of myocardial ischemic changes as reflected by S-T segment mapping, but recent studies indicate the amount of muscle tissue salvaged is sufficient to improve ventricular performance and hemodynamics after acute coronary occlusion.[317] Thus the use of β-pyridyl-carbinol experimentally may provide a means of conserving energy from dissipation in noncritical metabolic pathways to help protect ischemic myocardium.

### 7. Effect of hyaluronidase, cobra venom factor and other agents

Finally, the possibility of increasing the delivery of energy-producing substrates to myocardial cells during ischemia with the use of hyaluronidase was also investigated.[95] Epicardial S-T segment elevations were mapped in animals given hyaluronidase thirty minutes after coronary artery ligation, and subsequently tissue beneath the sites of S-T segment elevation was analyzed for enzymatic and histologic changes. A significant reduction in the extent and severity of ischemic damage was observed (Fig. 7 and Table I), consistent with the view that depolymerization by hyaluronic acid improved substrate delivery to cells. Experimentally, even an apparently unrelated agent such as cobra venom factor may also reduce the extent and severity of myocardial necrosis after coronary occlusion.[324] This substance destroys C-3 activity and hence may protect ischemic myocardium by removing the immunologic component of tissue necrosis mediated by the complement system. Other substances, including inosine, retabolil, orotic acid with vitamin $B_{12}$ and "P-132" a long-chain fatty acid were recently reported to hasten recovery from myocardial ischemia.[325] The actions of metabolites of cardiac nucleotides are particularly interesting. Ischemia and hypoxia cause a rapid release of all adenine breakdown products.[326, 327] These observations leave the possibility open that an alteration in the size or nature of the nucleotide pools may deter deterioration of nucleotide function. For instance, the actions of allopurinol on the ischemic and hypoxic heart may be significant and deserve consideration. The various methods of reducing the size of experimental myocardial infarctions are summarized in Table II.

### 8. Precordial mapping

Recently the epicardial mapping technique was modified by recording S-T segments from precordial sites.[71] In this way, a noninvasive method for assessing myocardial injury was developed using fifteen recording sites in dogs (Fig. 8) and thirty-five sites in man (Fig. 9). This technique may prove to be a valuable clinical tool, although the precise role it may play is not yet clearly defined.[96] Stimulated by their work in laboratory animals,[321] Maroko, Braunwald and associates[322, 323] successfully employed the precordial mapping technique to show a reduction in S-T segment elevation after acute myocardial infarction in man after treatment with hyaluronidase.

### D. GIK reduces infarct size

A number of studies suggest that the combination of glucose-insulin-potassium might improve myocardial energy balance. As mentioned,

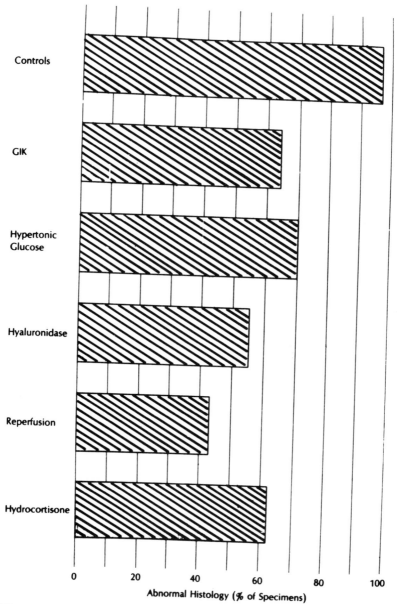

**Figure 7** Graph shows percentage of myocardial specimens having S-T segment elevation 15 minutes following occlusion that showed necrosis 24 hours later. In the control group most specimens (97%) were necrotic. In animals treated by a variety of interventions a substantial percentage of the myocardium was spared. Reproduced with permission from Braunwald, E., Maroko, P. R.: *Hosp Practice* 8:73, 1973.

Table II　Prevention of heart cell death—current methods.

## PREVENTION OF HEART CELL DEATH

I. REDUCE MYOCARDIAL ENERGY DEMAND

　　DECREASE AFTERLOAD: Vasodilator drugs, IABP
　　DECREASE INOTROPIC STATE: Beta-adrenergic blockade
　　DECREASE HEART SIZE: Digitalis in failing heart.

II. METABOLIC INTERVENTION

　　ENHANCE ANAEROBIC METABOLISM: Glucose-insulin-potassium
　　INHIBITION OF LIPOLYSIS: B-pyridyl-carbinol

III. INCREASE MYOCARDIAL SUBSTRATE SUPPLY

　　AUGMENT CORONARY BLOOD FLOW: Reperfusion, revascularization,
　　IABP
　　AUGMENT OXYGEN DELIVERY: ↑2, 3-diphosphoglycerate,
　　hyperbaric oxygen
　　FACILITATE SUBSTRATE TRANSPORT: Hyaluronidase

IV. PROTECT CELLULAR INTEGRITY

　　DECREASE AUTOLYSIS
　　STABILIZE LYSOSOMES: Corticosteroids
　　BLOCK COMPLEMENT SYSTEM: Cobra venom factor
　　MAINTAIN CELL VOLUME: Hyperosmolar solutions

the myocardium normally produces energy for contraction from oxidation of free fatty acids. During oxygen deprivation, anaerobic glycolysis may produce some energy for myocardial function.[97-99] Accordingly,
the effects of increasing the availability of glucose and potentially the
activity of anaerobic pathways was studied with the epicardial mapping technique.[100] Studies were undertaken in thirty-seven dogs
divided into four groups treated as follows:

　　group 1—control infusion of normal saline begun thirty minutes
　　　　　　after experimental coronary occlusion (11 dogs), and
　　　　　　epicardial electrocardiograms recorded periodically fif-
　　　　　　teen minutes thereafter. Twenty-four hours later trans-
　　　　　　mural specimens analyzed for CPK concentration, and
　　　　　　histologic examination by light and electron microscopy
　　　　　　performed on tissue sections;
　　group 2—GIK infusion of 500 g glucose/L, 210 mEq KC1/L and
　　　　　　10 units regular insulin/L begun 30 minutes after coro-

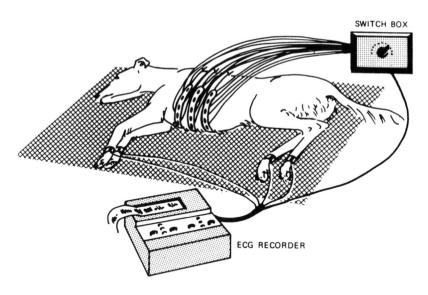

**Figure 8** Placement of the 15 precordial electrodes in the dog. Reproduced with permission.[71]

nary occlusion at 40 ml/Kg/24 hours (14 dogs) and examination performed as in group 1;

group 3—glucose infusion containing 500 mg/L, begun 30 minutes after coronary occlusion at 40 ml/Kg/24 hours (6 dogs), and examinations as in group 1;

group 4—GIK infusion as in group 2, but begun three hours after coronary occlusion, and administered with 1 mg/Kg propranolol intravenously (repeated at 9, 15 and 21 hours after occlusion). Examinations performed as in group 1.

In group 1, postocclusion tachyarrhythmias were frequent. S-T segment elevation bore a constant relation to depressed myocardial CPK values from the same sites twenty-four hours later (Figs. 6 and 10). Ninety-five percent of the sites examined with normal S-T segments showed normal histology, whereas 97 percent of sites with abnormal S-T segment elevation showed abnormal histology compatible with ischemic necrosis. On electron microscopic examination, these sites showed depletion of glycogen granules, mitochondrial swellings, disruption of mitochondrial membranes and dilatation of the cristae, separation and hyperextension of sarcomeres, karyorrhexis, and margination of nuclear chromatin.

In group 2 that received GIK solution, the heart rate and mean

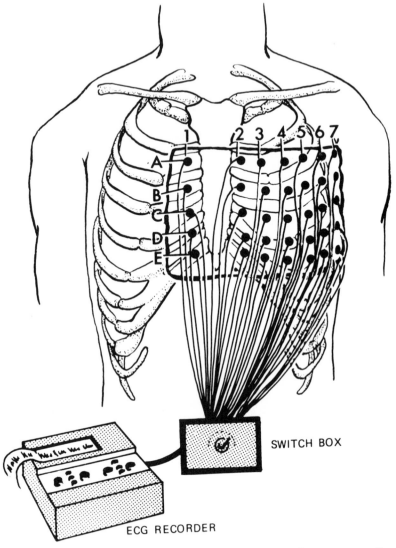

**Figure 9** Schematic representation of the 35 electrode set on a patient's chest. Reproduced with permission.[71]

arterial pressure were no different than observed in the control group. There was no reduction in the incidence of arrhythmias, and glucose and $K^+$-levels were higher than in the control group. Sites with the same S-T segment elevations showed less CPK depression than did the control group, *i.e.*, the slope of the regression line between CPK and S-T segment elevation was lowered.

EXP 298

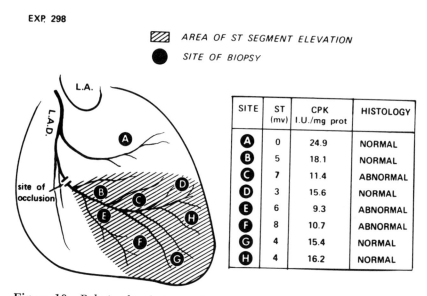

AREA OF ST SEGMENT ELEVATION

SITE OF BIOPSY

| SITE | ST (mv) | CPK I.U./mg prot | HISTOLOGY |
|------|---------|------------------|-----------|
| Ⓐ | 0 | 24.9 | NORMAL |
| Ⓑ | 5 | 18.1 | NORMAL |
| Ⓒ | 7 | 11.4 | ABNORMAL |
| Ⓓ | 3 | 15.6 | NORMAL |
| Ⓔ | 6 | 9.3 | ABNORMAL |
| Ⓕ | 8 | 10.7 | ABNORMAL |
| Ⓖ | 4 | 15.4 | NORMAL |
| Ⓗ | 4 | 16.2 | NORMAL |

**Figure 10** Relationship between S-T segment elevation 15 min after occlusion with CPK activity and histologic changes 24 hours later in an experiment in control group. (Left) Schematic representation of the anterior surface of the heart. L.A.—left atrial appendage; L.A.D.—left anterior descending coronary artery. The shaded area represents the area of S-T segment elevation after occlusion. The circles represent sites from which specimens were obtained. (Right) Comparison between S-T segment elevation with CPK activities and histologic analysis 24 hours later in the same sites. Reproduced with permission.[100]

Histologic examination showed that only 64 percent of sites with abnormal S-T segment elevations were associated with myocardial necrosis (Fig. 11). In the GIK-treated dogs 36 percent of sites were prevented from undergoing necrosis and glycogen depletion was spared. In addition, electron microscopy documented a decrease in frequency of such changes as was observed in group 1.

In group 3, treated with glucose solution alone, depletion of CPK activity was less than in the controls, but greater than in the GIK-treated group (Fig. 7). Thirty percent of sites in which S-T segment elevation was observed were protected from subsequent necrosis. Glycogen depletion was also less than observed in the control group, but more than noted in the GIK-treated animals. Thus, the protection conferred by glucose alone was intermediate between normal saline infusion (control) and GIK infusion.

In group 4, GIK infusion and propranolol were begun three hours after experimental coronary occlusion. Seventeen percent of the speci-

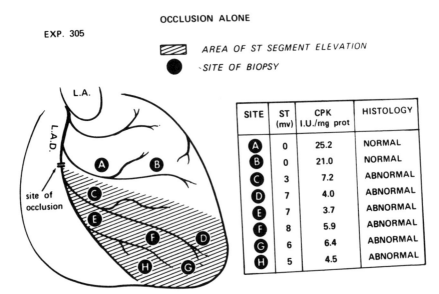

**Figure 11** Example of an experiment in group given GIK infusion. (Left) Schematic representation of the heart. The shaded area represents the area of S-T segment elevation 15 min after occlusion; circles represent the sites from which specimens were obtained. (Right) Comparison between S-T segment elevation 15 min following coronary occlusion and CPK activity and histologic changes 24 hours later (GIK infusion was started 15 min after the ECG recordings). Note that sites B, D, G and H exhibited S-T segment elevations but only slightly reduced CPK activity and normal histology. Reproduced with permission.[100]

mens with S-T segment elevation prior to the infusion were histologically normal 24 hours later, illustrating that as late an intervention as three hours after coronary occlusion may be beneficial.

From these data, it is clear that GIK significantly reduces the degree of myocardial damage resulting from experimental coronary occlusion. However, in Maroko's study there was no significant difference in the slope of the CPK regression line between the glucose- and GIK-treated groups. The number of sites at which S-T segment elevations did not exhibit histologic signs of early infarction in the glucose-treated group (30 percent) was closer to the GIK-treated group (36 percent) than the control (3 percent). Although 500 gm of glucose was used over twenty-four hours and the effect of hypertonicity was not directly assessed, GIK was not less effective than glucose, despite the lower blood glucose levels in the GIK-treated group.

### E. Effects of GIK on myocardial contractility during ischemia

Improvement in overall myocardial energy balance by GIK would also be expected to enhance contractility. Substantial work in preparations from laboratory animals does in fact reflect this action of GIK.[243, 244] Some years ago Bajusz[329] reported than $K^+$-aspartate and $K^+$-aspartate-glucose-insulin could accelerate healing in the cardiomyopathic hamster, *Mesocricetus auratus*.

Lochner and associates[330] restudied the effects of GIK on the mechanical effect as well as the histological appearance of the isolated perfused hamster heart. Both glucose-insulin and GIK significantly increased the healing of the myocardial lesions. Protein synthesis, as measured by the rate of incorporation of $[4,5\text{-}^3H]$ leucine and $[U\text{-}^{14}C]$ lysine into heart muscle, was significantly increased by glucose-insulin for seven days and by GIK for twenty-one days. However, there was no significant alteration in the mechanical activity of this heart preparation. Variation in other determinants of cardiac performance, possibly decreased stress-relaxation, could account for these data. Weissler and associates[303] showed that insulin increases glucose utilization and concentrations of high energy intermediates in association with improved ventricular performance in the anoxic heart, although this is unsettled.[306, 311] Lolley, Hewitt, and Drapanas[304] reported that left ventricular contractility increased during retroperfusion of the anoxic-arrested heart with GIK. Recently a preliminary report appeared which confirmed a positive inotropic action of GIK during acute ischemia in association with reduction in both extent of S-T segment elevation and number of sites so affected.[308]

## III. EFFECT OF GIK ON MYOCARDIAL ELECTRICAL PROPERTIES

### A. Introduction

The early proponents of GIK solution for the treatment of heart disease stressed the need for "repolarizing" the injured myocardium to prevent arrhythmias.[1-30] Repolarization was thought to effect improvement not only in the electrocardiogram but also in the pathophysiology and pathologic anatomy of several myocardial lesions.[101] Whether this is actually true has certainly not been proved as yet. While the evidence reviewed in Chapter 2 and in the first section of this chapter establishes that myocardial $K^+$ is indeed lost during ischemia, it is the result of the biochemical defect rather than the cause. Similarly, while resultant membrane hypopolarization may be reflected in S-T segment shifts in the surface electrocardiogram, its relation to the initiation and maintenance of lethal arrhythmias is less clear. To assume that intracellular myocardial $K^+$-loss is a critical factor in patient survival, and that its "replacement" by intravenous GIK solution will ameliorate this situation remains premature and neglects important unproven intervening relationships. There is some evidence that GIK will result in overall $K^+$-uptake by the heart, but the extracellular vs. intracellular distribution and the circumstances under which this may occur need to be defined.[304, 305] For instance, the functional and pathological changes associated with chronic myocardial $K^+$-deficiency in the presence of adequate oxygenation are entirely different from those observed in studies of $K^+$-depleted ischemic and hypoxic myocardium.[102, 103] The electrocardiographic changes noted by advocates of GIK solution may reflect changes in $[K^+]_i/[K^+]_o$ (intracellular and extracellular potassium activities respectively) and may not closely mirror changes in myocardial redox state. As mentioned, the instantaneous value of $[K^+]_i/[K^+]_o$ at each sarcolemmal point is not only a function of $[K^+]_i/[K^+]_o$ before an ischemic episode, but is also a function of time and washout efficiency, and is further dependent upon many intracellular and extracellular metabolic parameters. Indeed, although regional hyperkalemia in the adequately perfused heart can reproduce "ischemic" electrocardiographic changes and increase myocardial vulnerability to ventricular fibrillation,[104, 105] there is no direct evidence showing that GIK solutions reverse these electrical changes in the twilight zone surrounding a myocardial infarction. This is especially true when one considers the probable nonhomogeneous nature of $K^+$-loss with respect to myocardial site and passage of time. Recently, based upon voltage clamp data and analogical computations, mechanisms for the induction of arrhythmias other than disturbances in $K^+$ flux were shown to be possible.[106] In addition, patient mortality (or the incidence of arrhythmias in seriously-ill patients with advanced heart disease and multiple system involvement) remains an insensitive method of assessing either the efficacy of GIK therapy or its molecular mechanism of action.

In this section, various effects of the GIK combination on electrical properties of ischemic myocardium will be discussed, and some problems requiring further experimental data will be identified. Finally, the evidence for and against a possible reduction in the incidence of "ischemic arrhythmias" will be reviewed.

## B. Effect of GIK on transmembrane action potential

A substantial literature now documents a shortening of the action potential duration associated with anoxia and/or ischemia in heart muscle of laboratory animals,[107-111] and of man.[112-114] This is accompanied by a decrease in muscle contractility which has been attributed to potassium efflux during anoxia,[108, 110] possibly during repolarization, at which time potassium carries outward repolarization current during the action potential. Substrate-free media and the metabolic inhibitors iodoacetate, 2,4-dinitrophenol, and sodium cyanide also shorten the action potential duration as well as depress contractility. For this reason, the relationship between glucose metabolism and shortening of the action potential duration was investigated in human papillary muscles excised during open heart surgery.[113] The transmembrane action potential was recorded in media containing 0, 5, 20, and 30 mM glucose, 0.5 to 5.0 mU/ml insulin, and either equilibrated with 95 percent $O_2$ and 5 percent $CO_2$ or 95 percent $N_2$ and 5 percent $CO_2$. After exposure to a glucose-free and anoxic solution, papillary muscle force of contraction diminished within 15 minutes and the action potential shortened 15 to 20 minutes later (Fig. 12). When exposed to increasing concentrations of glucose, depression of contractility and reduction in action potential duration were progressively lessened (Fig. 13). After equilibration in glucose-free anoxic medium, the addition of glucose proportionally lengthened the action potential duration and increased the depressed overshoot and resting membrane potential (Fig. 14). The addition of insulin alone to the depressed preparation, in the absence of glucose, could not restore any of the electrophysiological parameters (Fig. 15). However, when insulin was added to the anoxic preparation in the presence of glucose, the electrophysiological effects of anoxia were abolished (Fig. 16).

These studies suggest that when glycogen and ATP stores are depleted in the hypoxic heart muscle, a low glucose concentration in the bath cannot provide enough energy via anaerobic pathways to maintain the action potential or sustain contraction. The studies of Morgan *et al.*[115-118] demonstrate that during anoxia-induced anaerobic glycolysis, heart-muscle uptake of glucose is a function of external glucose and insulin concentrations. Certain glycolytic enzymes are stimulated during anoxia,[118] allowing greater energy production via anaerobic metabolism. These data are also in agreement with the improvement in both electrical and mechanical performance of an anoxic Langendorf heart preparation.[119] It appears that the ability of the heart to survive anoxia depends upon its glycogen content, which may be increased by glucose and insulin.[98, 115, 120-122, 124-126] Finally, oxidative phosphorylation is stimulated along with heart performance by glucose-insulin -potassium in combination.[30]

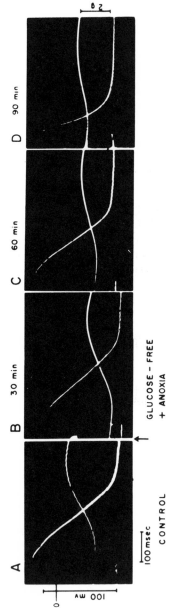

**Figure 12** Effect of glucose-free Krebs-Ringer solution and anoxia on the simultaneously recorded transmembrane action potential and contraction of human papillary muscle. (A) Control in oxygenated Krebs-Ringer solution containing 20 mM glucose. Arrow marks the start of the exposure of the muscle to glucose-free solution and anoxia. The subsequent tracings (B, C, D) are in glucose-free solution and anoxia at intervals shown at the top of each tracing. Calibration is indicated. Note the shortening of the action potential duration and contraction in glucose-free solution and anoxia. Reproduced with permission from Prasad and Callaghan.[113]

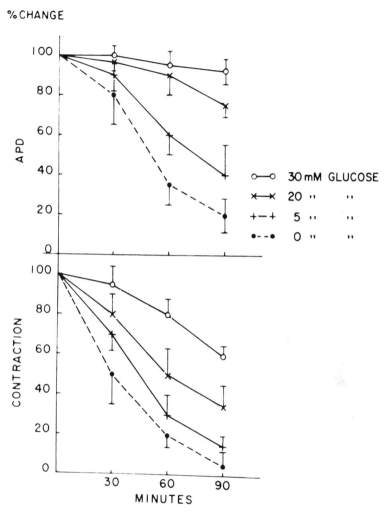

**Figure 13** The effects of various concentrations of glucose in the presence of anoxia on the action potential duration (APD) and contraction of human papillary muscle with respect to time. The values are expressed as percentage change from the control in 20 mM glucose, with $O_2$ taken as 100 percent. Note the marked reduction in the APD and contraction in the absence of glucose, as compared to less marked changes in the presence of glucose. Vertical bars represent standard error. Reproduced with permission.[113]

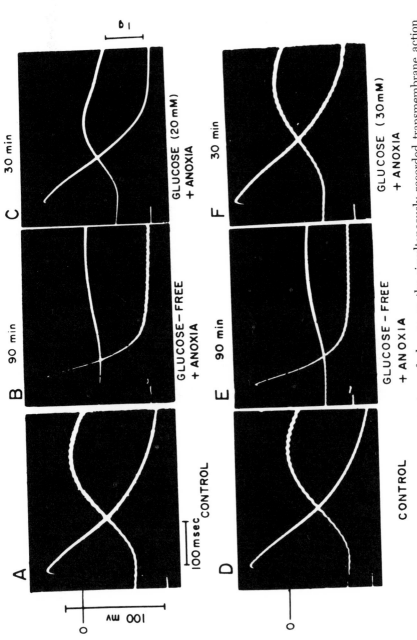

**Figure 14**   Effects of various concentrations of glucose on the simultaneously recorded transmembrane action potential and contraction of human papillary muscle from a single experiment. (A, D) Control in oxygenated Krebs-Ringer solution containing 20 mM glucose; (B, E) after 90 minutes in glucose-free solution and anoxia; (C, F) after 30 minutes in 20 and 30 mM glucose, respectively, under anoxia. Note the reversal of the effect of glucose-free solution and anoxia on the APD and contraction by glucose. Calibration is indicated. Reproduced with permission 113

## C. Specific relation of GIK-induced changes in action potential to metabolism in anoxic heart muscle

The association of anoxic changes of the action potential with substrate-free media and metabolic inhibitors, reversal with glucose (concentration-dependent) and glucose-insulin, and lack of beneficial effect of insulin in substrate-free bath pointed toward a stimulation of anaerobic metabolism by glucose thus providing additional energy for maintenance of myocellular function, sufficient to maintain the action potential. However, since individual enzyme activities and concentrations of intermediary substrates were not measured, direct proof of this mechanism was lacking. In early experiments, the effect of glucose could be partially duplicated by similar concentrations of 2-deoxyglucose and xylose but not by sucrose, thus eliminating an osmotic effect as a possible mechanism in these investigations. On the other hand, since 2-deoxyglucose and xylose were not metabolized, their actions did not seem to be related to intermediary metabolism. However, because these sugars were transported by the glucose transport system,[127, 128, 131] the possibility arose that activation of the glucose transport system might reduce the rate of potassium efflux and thereby exert an effect on the action potential.[107] The decrease in action potential duration during anoxia was proposed to be a result of rapid repolarization from an increase in the rate of potassium efflux during repolarization.[110, 129, 130] Glucose was thought to reduce the rate of potassium efflux and thereby widen the action potential. For this to occur, the "carrier" transporting glucose through the sarcolemma and potassium out of the cell would have to be identical. If this were so, when the glucose concentration in the medium was low all glucose entering the myocyte would be metabolized and the empty "carrier" would be available at the inner surface of the sarcolemma. In the presence of high glucose concentrations, glucose might accumulate intracellularly. Similarly, nonmetabolizable sugars might accumulate within the cell when present in the extracellular medium. In both instances, a back transport of sugar would occupy a finite number of "carriers," reducing those available for outward potassium flux. This view was supported by the finding that epinephrine increased action potential duration, and, from simultaneous inhibition of hexokinase, could increase intracellular "free" glucose.[127] In order to further delineate the relationship

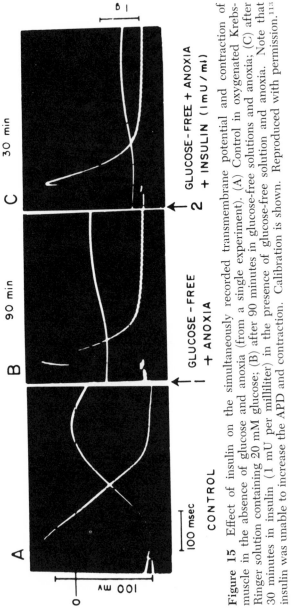

**Figure 15** Effect of insulin on the simultaneously recorded transmembrane potential and contraction of muscle in the absence of glucose and anoxia (from a single experiment). (A) Control in oxygenated Krebs-Ringer solution containing 20 mM glucose; (B) after 90 minutes in glucose-free solutions and anoxia; (C) after 30 minutes in insulin (1 mU per milliliter) in the presence of glucose-free solution and anoxia. Note that insulin was unable to increase the APD and contraction. Calibration is shown. Reproduced with permission.[113]

between the electrophysiological actions of glucose and insulin, an extended series of experiments with the nonmetabolizable sugars D-xylose, 2-deoxyglucose, arabinose, 3-0-methylglucose, D-galactose, L-glucose, and α-methyl-D-glucoside were performed.[123] None of the sugars could duplicate the effect of glucose on the abbreviated action potential. Moreover, the action potential duration was directly related to the glucose concentration in the medium regardless of the level of oxygenation. In fact, the action potential could be maintained for many hours by a glucose concentration of 50 mM in the complete absence of oxygen. Following reduction of the action potential duration in the presence of 5 mM glucose, increasing the concentration to 50 mM uniformly restored the action potential length. Interestingly, the sensitivity of a given papillary muscle to the actions of the low glucose concentrations increased with repeated incubation periods in media containing 5 mM glucose, most likely from a number of factors progressively reducing metabolic activity. Phlorizin, a specific inhibitor of glucose transport,[132, 133] competitively interfered with the effect of glucose on the action potential duration, while insulin prevented or reversed the effect of phlorizin.

Norepinephrine, epinephrine, and isopropylnorepinephrine increased the shortened action potential duration in media containing 5 mM glucose coincident with an increase in contractility. When iodoacetate and 2-deoxyglucose were added, isopropylnorepinephrine increased contractile force but failed to restore the abbreviated action potential duration. This is consistent with the view that the effect of the catecholamines on the action potential is more dependent upon glycolysis than is the positive inotropic action in this experimental setting. However, it is now appreciated that the electrophysiological changes effected by the catecholamines are mediated in a complex fashion.[134] Both the availability of intracellular cyclic adenylate calcium ion in the interstitium are involved in the lengthening of the plateau of the action potential.[135, 136] Indeed, even oscillation of intracellular cyclic AMP concentration during the contraction cycle has been recently described.[137] Aminophylline produces changes in the reduced action potential duration similar to those caused by the catecholamines.

These data support the proposal that anaerobic metabolism utilizing either glycogen or exogenous glucose is capable of maintaining normal transmembrane electrical activity in papillary muscles. Since the energy

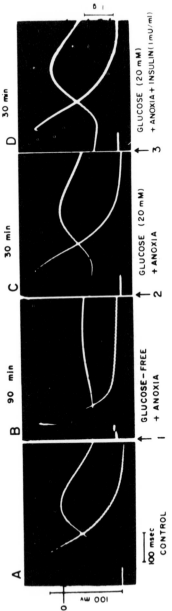

**Figure 16**   The effect of insulin on APD and contraction of the muscle in the presence of glucose and anoxia. (A) Control tracing in oxygenated Krebs-Ringer solution containing 20 mM glucose (at arrow 2, glucose was added in the bath to make a concentration of 20 mM); (C) 30 minutes later (at arrow 3, insulin was added in the bath); (D) 30 minutes later. Note the increase in APD and contraction with insulin in the presence of glucose and anoxia. Reproduced with permission.[113]

requirements of myocardial electrical activity are relatively small, this is not surprising.[138] The sympathomimetic amines—by stimulation of adenyl cyclase and elevating cyclic AMP levels—would promote phosphorylase activity and glycogenolysis. Similarly, aminophylline— by phosphodiesterase inhibition and consequent elevation in cyclic AMP levels—would be expected to produce a similar effect on the action potential duration, which is actually the case. This evidence indirectly supports the notion that the effect of the catecholamines on action potential duration is mediated at some level by glycolysis.

Unfortunately, insulin had little or no effect on the abbreviated action potential duration in the absence of oxygen, or on the effect of glucose on the action potential duration.[123] In the light of the studies previously cited showing that insulin in fact augments glucose transport,[115-118] this lack of insulin effect was disturbing. Possibly, the fact that insulin-induced glucose uptake was associated with glycogen synthesis,[139-141] whereas augmented glucose uptake from an increased extracellular concentration was directly metabolized, may provide an explanation. More likely, however, glucose transport was not rate-limiting at the time when insulin was employed.

Recently, these results have been amply confirmed,[112, 142, 143] and the effects of ouabain and calcium on the action potential duration of human papillary muscles studied. Glucose was able to lengthen the anoxia-induced abbreviated action potential duration as described, and the effect could be increased or decreased by low or high doses of ouabain respectively.[112] This phenomenon was thought to be related to a stimulation and depression of membrane ATPase by ouabain. Further, the shortening of the action potential duration brought about by ouabain alone was maximized by non-oxygenated glucose-free media and metabolic inhibitors.[142] In the presence of these inhibitors of glycolysis, however, no positive inotropic effect of ouabain was observed. These data show that energy is required for the ouabain effect on contractility, but also supports the interpretation of data on actions of glucose and insulin previously discussed. In reviewing these data it is important to note that the electrophysiological actions of digitalis are not simple and involve primary alterations in the sarcolemmal $Na^+$, $K^+$-ATPase.[138, 144] As such, potassium, sodium, calcium, and electrical properties of the sarcolemma, T-tubules, and sarcoplasmic reticulum are necessarily involved. The binding of digitalis to ATPase,[145] the uptake of digitalis by myocardium [146] and the onset of its inotropic action [146, 147] are slowed by elevated extracellular potassium activities. Therefore, the possibility exists that some interaction between altered potassium metabolism by the papillary muscle in nonoxygenated, glucose free media and ouabain modified the recorded data to some extent.

## D. Relation of GIK-induced changes in action potential of anoxic muscle to potassium efflux

Hypoxia [148-150] and/or ischemia [151-155] produce net loss of potassium from heart muscle. Progressive intracellular depletion of potassium results in shortening and increased slope of phase 2 of the action potential to decrease its duration, effects partial depolarization (decreasing $|\mathcal{E}_m|$), slows the upstroke (phase 0) of the action potential (dV/dt) and reduces the amplitude of the action potential. The effective refractory period, a function of the action potential duration, is also abbreviated. Ischemia and hypoxia, as discussed, also shorten action potential duration [112-114] and the refractory period,[155-157] increase the slope of the downstroke (phase 2) of the action potential, hypopolarize the heart cell membrane,[113] and decrease the rate of rise of phase 0 of the action potential.[157] It was therefore not unreasonable that these electrophysiologic changes associated with ischemia and hypoxia were postulated to result from net intracellular $K^+$-loss from the myocardium.[108, 110] Since glucose or glucose and insulin could reverse the electrophysiologic abnormalities of glucose-free nonoxygenated medium on papillary muscles,[107, 113, 123, 157] was this action mediated by an energy-dependent $K^+$-conserving mechanism by the myocyte? If so, what would be the effect and advantage of administering exogenous potassium?

Decreased efflux of potassium occurs in response to hyperglycemia under hypoxic conditions.[151] A monotone relationship exists between the extent of change in action potential duration, ATP content, lactate production, and severity and duration of anoxia (Figs. 17-19). Following anoxic incubation of heart muscles, intracellular potassium declined in proportion to the decline in ATP content, lactate produced, and abbreviation of action potential duration (Fig 20).[158] Moreover, this effect was more marked in ventricular muscle, probably because of relatively greater glycogen stores in atrial muscle, conferring greater

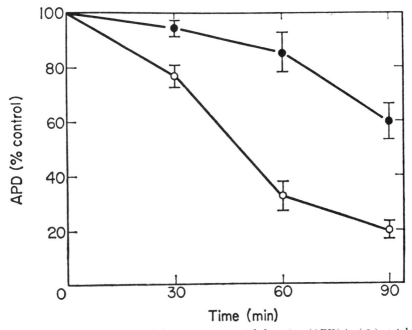

**Figure 17** The decline of the action potential duration (APD) in ( ● ) atrial muscle and ( ○ ) papillary muscle incubated under anoxic conditions in 5 mM glucose medium. Control action potential duration was recorded following a 1 hour aerobic incubation. Each point represents the mean value from 6 muscles. Vertical bars are S.E.M. Reproduced with permission.[158]

resistance to anoxia. Such net potassium loss occurred from a decrease in the rate of influx rather than an increased rate of efflux from the cell.[110, 129, 130, 149] Since potassium uptake was an energy-dependent process, the greater energy production of anoxic atrial muscle as compared with anoxic ventricular myocardium could account for its higher rate of potassium influx. A greater glucose concentration (50 mM) in the medium significantly slowed net myocardial $K^+$ loss (Fig. 20).[129, 158]

These data prove that intracellular potassium concentration is maintained by an energy-dependent process. The resting potential of anoxic ventricular muscle has been separated into two components, one dependent upon the equilibrium potential of potassium alone, $\mathcal{E}_{K^+}$, and the other upon active electrogenic sodium pumping.[159] Therefore, maintenance of intracellular potassium concentration is primarily dependent upon active ion transport.

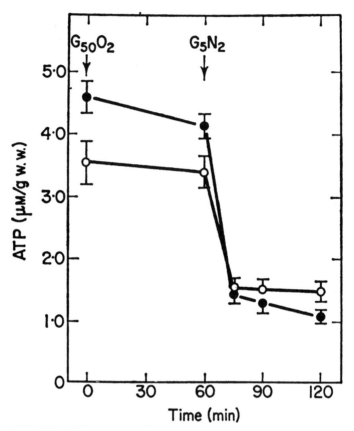

**Figure 18** The ATP content of guinea pig cardiac muscle during a 1 hour aerobic incubation $(G_{50}O_2)$ and subsequent 1 hour anoxic incubation in 5 mM glucose medium $(G_5N_2)$. Mean ± S.E., n=8-12. (○) from atrial muscle (●) from ventricular muscle. Reproduced with permission.[158]

The ability of ouabain, a potent inhibitor of cardiac $Na^+$, $K^+$-ATPase, to attenuate the ability of glucose to lengthen the abbreviated action potential of anoxic myocardium has been mentioned.[112] The need for energy within the myocyte for the expression of ouabain's positive inotropic action is well established.[142] Inhibition of sarcolemmal $Na^+$, $K^+$-ATPase increases the intracellular sodium pool and decreases net intracellular potassium content. Even in the presence of added sufficient substrate (glucose), chemical inhibition of this enzyme by ouabain precludes replenishment of intracellular $K^+$ and its electrophysiological correlate, restoration of the action potential duration. Similarly, the reduction in action potential duration and augmented contractility

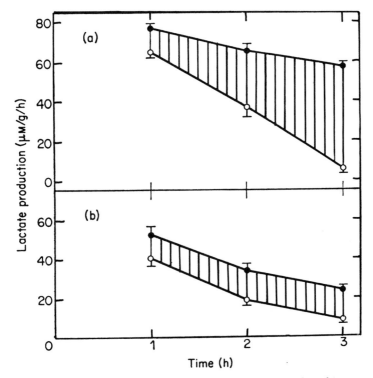

**Figure 19** The lactate production ($\mu$mol/g wet tissue/h) of guinea pig atrial (a) and ventricular (b) muscle incubated under anoxic conditions in either ($\bullet$) 5 mM glucose medium ($G_5N_2$) or ($\bigcirc$) glucose-free medium ($G_0N_2$). Mean $\pm$ S.E., n=8. Reproduced with permission.[158]

observed in human papillary muscle in KCl-free solution may be due to inhibition of membrane ATPase. Stimulation of $Na^+$, $K^+$-ATPase by rubidium chloride produces an increased duration of the cardiac action potential, conduction delay, and muscle inexcitability, in association with a decrease in the force of contraction.[114] The widened action potential is presumably caused by net accumulation of intracellular potassium. While the precise reasons for variation in contractility are beyond the scope of this review, inhibition of $Na^+$, $K^+$-ATPase probably leads to augmented exchange of intracellular sodium for extracellular calcium and hence provides a greater intracellular calcium concentration for the initiation of contraction and was further discussed in Chapter 3.[160]

The hypothesis that lack of high energy substrate for this ATPase and slowing of the $Na^+$, $K^+$ pump is responsible for ischemic intracellular $K^+$-loss and its electrophysiological consequences has been proposed

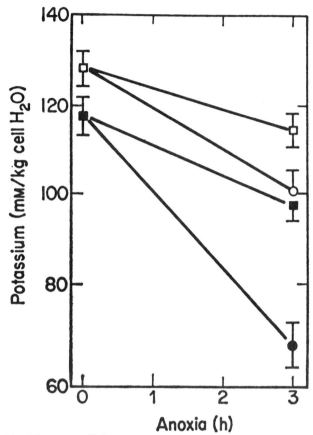

**Figure 20**   The intracellular potassium concentration of guinea pig cardiac muscle during anoxic incubation. Values at 0 hour were determined after an initial 1 hour aerobic incubation. Atrial muscle (open symbols) and ventricular muscle (filled symbols) were incubated for 3 hours under anoxic conditions in either (circles) 5 mM $(G_5N_2)$ or (squares) 50 mM $(G_{50}N_2)$ glucose medium. Mean ± S.E., n=9. Reproduced with permission.[158]

by several investigators.[161] Recently, however, Schwartz and colleagues [162] showed that the initial $K^+$-loss of ischemic myocardium was not accompanied by depressed $Na^+$, $K^+$-ATPase activity, whereas several days later, the function of this enzyme was impaired. These investigators concluded that diminution of $Na^+$, $K^+$-ATPase activity need not have been the cause of immediate potassium loss at a time when contractility was severely reduced, but that restoration of intracellular potassium levels during recovery from ischemia was indeed dependent upon adequate $Na^+$, $K^+$-ATPase function.

## E. Effect of KCl on the action potential of anoxic and ischemic heart muscle

The effect of adding potassium to papillary muscles in nonoxygenated Krebs-Ringer solutions was recently studied.[157] As before, anoxia and a low glucose concentration produced shortening of the action potential duration and effective refractory period (Fig. 21B). Potassium chloride 2 mM further shortened the action potential duration and effective refractory period, further decreased the resting transmembrane potential (decreasing $|\mathcal{E}_m|$) and further depressed the rate of rise in phase 0 of the action potential (Fig. 21C). While exposure of anoxic papillary muscles sequentially from glucose-free media to media containing 50 mM glucose or glucose and insulin restored the abbreviated action potential, the exposure of muscles to glucose (50 mM), insulin (40 mU/ml) and KCl (2 mM) produced a lengthening of action potential duration (Fig. 22). These changes were less than the changes produced by either glucose alone or glucose and insulin together. Rate of rise of phase 0 of the action potential, however, was further reduced by the combination glucose, insulin and potassium.

These data suggested that potassium hindered the actions of glucose and insulin on the abbreviated action potential in anoxic heart muscle. Accordingly, the elimination of potassium from the combination GIK was advised and it was further proposed that the ineffectiveness of polarizing solution might be related to an increase in incidence of arrhythmias due to the ill effects of potassium.[157] Such a view is to be contrasted with those of other workers who stress the antiarrhythmic actions of potassium, although in a completely different setting.[163-165]

Nonetheless the ability of KCl to shorten the action potential duration and refractory period, decrease the resting transmembrane potential and depress the rate of rise of phase 0 (dV/dt) of the action potential is well known.[166-169] Such experiments are similar to the study described above in that the extracellular potassium concentration is acutely raised. Under these circumstances the ratio $[K^+]_i/[K^+]_o$, upon which transmembrane potential depends, decreases due to an increase in the denominator. Surawicz[170] mentions "there is no evidence that loading with potassium and increasing the extracellular potassium concentration will appreciably alter the intracellular potassium of normal myocardium." During anaerobic metabolism this relationship changes, but perhaps as much as 45 percent of tissue intracellular potassium is nonexchangeable, and therefore may be independent of extracellular potassium levels.[171] Indeed, myocardial loss of $K^+$ during

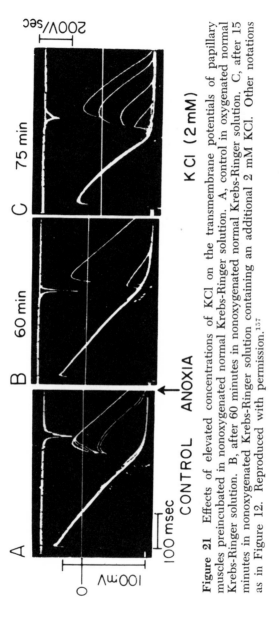

**Figure 21**  Effects of elevated concentrations of KCl on the transmembrane potentials of papillary muscles preincubated in nonoxygenated normal Krebs-Ringer solution. A, control in oxygenated normal Krebs-Ringer solution. B, after 60 minutes in nonoxygenated normal Krebs-Ringer solution. C, after 15 minutes in nonoxygenated Krebs-Ringer solution containing an additional 2 mM KCl. Other notations as in Figure 12. Reproduced with permission.[157]

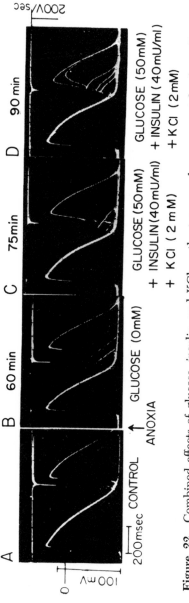

**Figure 22** Combined effects of glucose, insulin, and KCl on the transmembrane potentials of papillary muscles preincubated in nonoxygenated glucose-free Krebs-Ringer solution. A, control in oxygenated normal Krebs-Ringer solution. B, after 60 minutes in nonoxygenated glucose-free Krebs-Ringer solution. C and D, after 15 and 30 minutes, respectively in nonoxygenated Krebs-Ringer solution containing 50 mM glucose, 40 mU. per milliliter of insulin, and 6.5 mM KCl. Other notations as in Figure 12. Reproduced with permission.[157]

ischemia is simulated by regional hyperkalemia during which KCl [104, 105, 172] is infused into a given coronary artery.

These data are further underscored by the recent report by Gould and co-workers [301] who infused GIK in twenty-one patients with organic heart disease. Using His bundle electrograms, these investigators found that GIK produced a significant increase in the A-H interval with only minimal effects on the P-A, H-Q and H-S intervals, representing a conduction delay at the level of the atrioventricular node, most likely due to the potassium in the solution.

## F. Electrophysiological contrast between ischemia and hypoxia— relevance to GIK therapy

In Chapter 1, certain metabolic differences between hypoxia and ischemia were mentioned. Lactate accumulates rapidly in ischemic myocardium, an effect which would be accentuated when anaerobic glycolysis is accelerated during GIK treatment.

In Chapter 3, the association-induction hypothesis was discussed. In contrast with classical membrane theory, which regards the resting membrane potential as an oxidation-reduction potential, this hypothesis postulates an entirely different origin of the transmembrane potential.[173-189] In this theory, the resting and active potentials have no direct relation to ionic permeability, but are seen as phase-boundary potentials between the cell phase and the extracellular phase. Hence the resting potential is generated when some of the counter ions—$K^+$— diffuse away, leaving negatively charged sites open near the cell surface.

The interruption of high energy phosphate production with metabolic inhibitors brings about net $[K^+]_i$ loss and various electrophysiologic changes. This information has been considered evidence that $Na^+$, $K^+$-pumping needs metabolic energy. However, because of thermodynamic limitations,[189a, 189b] the association-induction hypothesis regards ATP as a key *adsorbent*. Adsorption of ATP on cardinal sites maintains gangs of protein sites such that $K^+$ is preferentially adsorbed in relation to $Na^+$, and water exists in a state of polarized multilayers capable of excluding $Na^+$ ions.[190] Edelman [190a] has recently shown that the relative effectiveness of $K^+$, $Rb^+$, and $Cs^+$ ions in lowering the transmembrane resting potential bears no relation to the membrane permeabilities of these ions in guinea pig heart muscle, but follows quantitatively after their measured adsorption constants.

With this background in mind, Wissner [190b] recently proposed that ischemia of the Purkinje fiber was characterized by depolarization, biphasic response to the duration of the plateau of the action potential, shortening of the plateau with a rebound prolongation upon return to normal Tyrode solution, and enhancement of phase 4 depolarization (Figs. 23-25). Wissner maintains that these effects are due to excess intracellular lactate and are to be contrasted with the electrophysiologic changes associated with $[K^+]_i$ loss from the ischemic cell discussed above. According to Wissner, the action potentials of ischemic—and hypokalemic—fibers are similar only in depolarization, but differ markedly in the changes of the plateau. Together with the relative resistance of Purkinje fibers to increases in extracellular $K^+$, and the low probability of local $K^+$ accumulation in a beating heart, Wissner concludes that excess lactate is an important determinant of electrophysiological changes associated with ischemia.

### G. Arrhythmias and glucose, insulin, potassium infusion

The increased vulnerability of the left ventricle to ventricular fibrillation soon after myocardial infarction is a well-recognized phenomenon.[9, 11, 191, 192] Although the mechanism for this remains unknown, such arrhythmias are believed to be due to enhanced automaticity or reentry, related to either the shortened refractory period of ischemic muscle, or to ischemia-induced injury currents.[193-195] In addition, substrate-free Tyrode solution may produce ventricular fibrillation which may be prevented by glucose administration,[196] but not by ATP presented extracellularly.[197]

Several early studies reported a reduction in the incidence of arrhythmias and electrocardiographic improvement using various proportions of glucose, insulin, and potassium in patients with myocardial infarction.[1-3, 14, 21, 196, 198] Mittra[199] reported on oral potassium and glucose supplements and subcutaneously injected insulin in 170 patients with acute myocardial infarction. The mortality rate was reduced from 28.2 percent in the control group to 11.7 percent in the treated groups, and was attributed to a decrease in arrhythmia deaths. Mittra,[199-207] a strong supporter of glucose-insulin-potassium therapy, noted that in his original series that the overall incidence of arrhythmias complicating myocardial infarction was similar in both treated and control groups (Fig. 26). However, the arrhythmias in the treated group were less "serious," of shorter duration, and not as lethal as those encountered in the control group (Fig. 27) (Table III). Interestingly, Mittra noted that the regimen was of little benefit in female patients, and explained this on the basis that "men were more liable to succumb to an arrhythmia."[201, 204] No deaths occurred in either

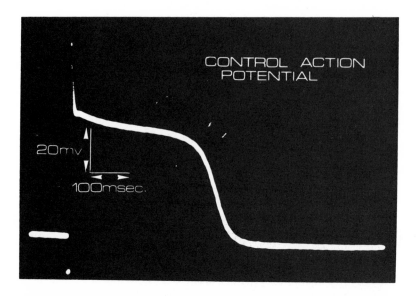

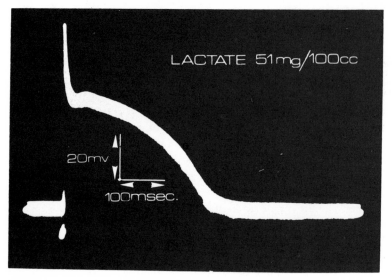

**Figure 23**   A. Control action potential.   B. Action potential after lactic acid introduction into the perfusate at a concentration of 51 mg/100cc.   C. Action potential after introduction of lactic acid into perfusate at 170 mg/100cc. D. Action potential after return to a normal Tyrode solution. Note prolongation of the duration of the plateau. Reproduced with permission.[190b]

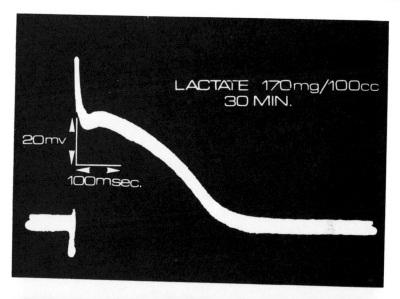

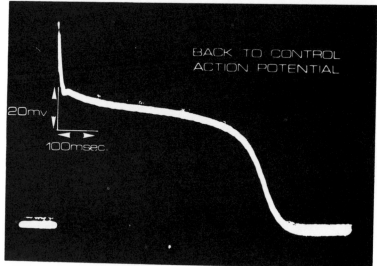

Figure 23—Continued

group—treated or control—in patients without arrhythmias, but the reported incidence of "sudden death" was decreased in controls. Mittra also observed earlier resolution of electrocardiographic signs of injury and ischemia in his treated patients (Fig. 28) in accord with earlier reports of other investigators.[18-30, 208] This phenomenon was interpreted as proof that the regimen did in fact restore intracellular

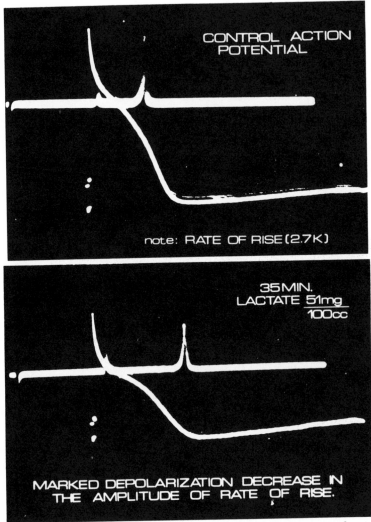

**Figure 24**    A. Control action potential with differentiated spike to the right. Note height of the differentiated spike. B. After the introduction of lactic acid and an interval of thirty-five minutes there is both a depolarization of the transmembrane potential and a decreased amplitude of the rate of rise of the action potential. C. With the return of a normal Tyrode solution there is a return of the action potential to normal. Note the differentiated spike again. Reproduced with permission.[190b]

potassium and resting membrane potential in those cells partially depolarized by ischemia and anoxia.

These studies of Mittra require special comment. The regimen used

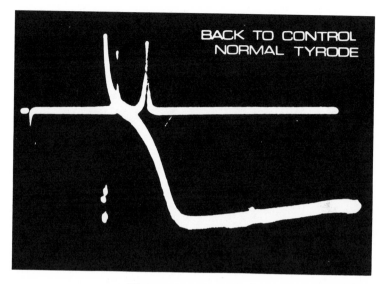

**Figure 24**—Continued

involved oral potassium ingestion rather than intravenously-administered KCl, as originally advocated by Sodi-Pallares and co-workers.[22-29] Oral potassium chiefly results in enhanced liver uptake of $K^+$ [22] and for this reason must be given intravenously. In fact, glucose and insulin were originally added by Sodi-Pallares to prevent systemic hyperkalemia. Using Mittra's regimen, other authors reported no improvement in patients (age less than 60) post myocardial infarction.[209] The natural history of Mittra's patients were also unique in the lack of any incidence of ventricular power failure and arrhythmias in women.

Many other investigators variously reported on the incidence of arrhythmias and mortality in patients treated with glucose-insulin-potassium, some supporting the beneficial results noted above,[20-30, 209-215] and others failing to confirm any benefits [15, 16, 216-218] (Tables IV and V). These clinical trials could not be compared because of variations in patient selection, the differing time intervals between the onset of the ischemic process and institution of therapy, wide differences in mode of administration and concentrations of ingredients used, variation in treatment, facilities and recording techniques and incomplete reporting of observations. A careful consideration of all the studies mentioned does not enable the reviewer to conclude that GIK—in any route—does or does not reduce the incidence of "serious" arrhythmias, nor render them less lethal when they do occur. It has been suggested that treatment of patients with acute myocardial infarction in a

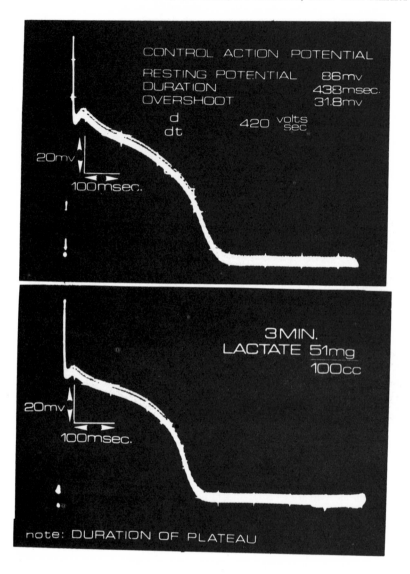

**Figure 25**   A. The classic parameters of the action potential are noted. B. Upon the introduction of lactic acid there is a biphasic response to the action potential. Note the slope of phase 2 of the action potential. C. Lactic acid at its maximum effect. The classic parameters are noted. Note that here there is a shortening of the duration of the plateau of the action potential. D. With the return of a normal Tyrode solution there is a rebound in the duration of the plateau of the action potential. Reproduced with permission.[190b]

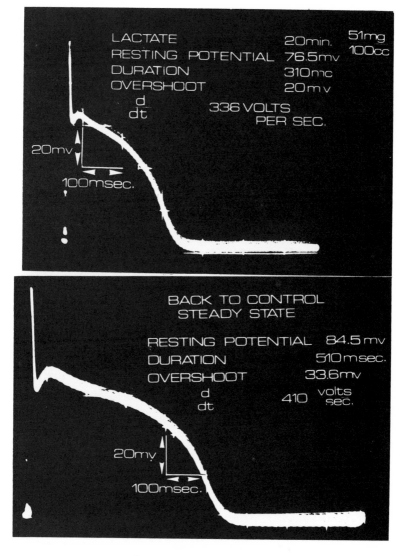

(**Figure 25**—continued)

coronary care unit may mask the antiarrhythmic actions of intravenous GIK, since reversal of electrical failure in this setting is greater than that achieved with GIK alone.[207, 215]

Recently, however, the results in several series of laboratory animals given GIK after experimental coronary occlusion tend to support a reduction in fatal arrhythmias as claimed, in association with dimin-

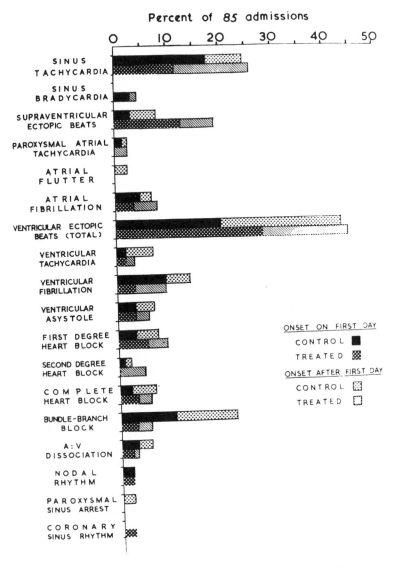

Figure 26   The regimen did not significantly reduce the incidence of various arrhythmias complicating myocardial infarction. Comparatively lower incidence of ventricular tachycardia, ventricular fibrillation and advanced heart block was observed in the treated group. Reproduced with permission from Mittra.[204]

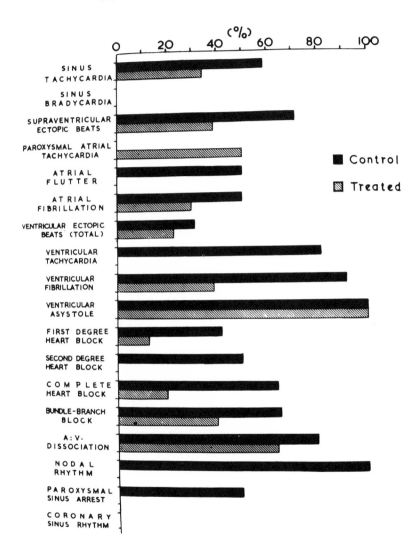

**Figure 27** Significant reduction in mortality was observed among treated patients with ventricular tachycardia and fibrillation and heart block when compared with controls. Although some reduction was observed among treated patients with other arrhythmias when compared with controls, the differences were not statistically significant. Reproduced with permission.[204]

**Table III**  Comparison of patients with and without arrhythmias in a control and treated group of a trial by Mittra.[204] Reproduced with permission.

Comparison of Patients With and Without Arrhythmias in the Control and Treated Groups of the Trial

| GROUP | Control | | | | Treated | | | |
|---|---|---|---|---|---|---|---|---|
| | Incidence | | Deaths | | Incidence | | Deaths | |
| | No. | % | No. | % | No. | % | No. | % |
| I. No arrhythmias | 23 | 27 | 0 | 0 | 18 | 21 | 0 | 0 |
| II. Arrhythmias present | 62 | 73 | 30 | 48.4 | 67 | 79 | 14 | 21 |
| (a) "Minor" forms of arrhythmias only | 11 | 13 | 1 | 9 | 23 | 27 | 1 | 4.3 |
| (b) "Serious"* arrhythmias | 51 | 60 | 29 | 57 | 44 | 52 | 13 | 29.5 |
| TOTAL NUMBER OF PATIENTS | 85 | 100 | 30 | 35.3 | 85 | 100 | 14 | 16.5 |

*"Serious" arrhythmias included frequent ventricular ectopic beats, atrial tachycardia, flutter and fibrillation, nodal rhythm, ventricular tachycardia and fibrillation and advanced heart block.

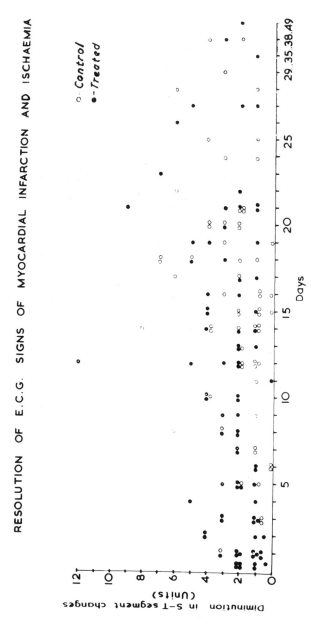

**Figure 28** Differences between maximum and minimum elevation of S-T segment or inversion of T-wave (measured in units) were plotted against time (in days) taken to achieve such a degree of improvement. Resolution of ECG signs of injury and ischemia was noted to be significantly (p < 0.01) rapid in the treated group when compared with the controls. Reproduced with permission.[204]

**Table IV** Trials of intravenous infusion of glucose, insulin and potassium (GIK) in myocardial infarction. Reproduced with permission.[207]

| Authors | Type of Ward | GIK no. of pts | GIK Length of treatment | Control (no. of pts) | Results |
|---|---|---|---|---|---|
| Lundman and Orinius (1965) | *GW | 26 | 3 days | Nil | Incidence of arrhythmias lower than expected |
| Day and Averill (1966) | **CCU | 141 | 3 days | 134 | Considerable reduction in the incidence of ventricular fibrillation (3.5% treated; 16.4% controls) in the first 3–5 days after admission |
| Autio et al. (1966) | GW | 91 | 3 days | Nil | 9.9% mortality. No reduction in incidence of arrhythmias |
| Kernohan (1967) | CCU | 118 | 5 days | 100 (retrospectively) | 17% mortality in treated group and 28% in controls |
| Malach (1967) | CCU | 47 | 3 days | 54 (received glucose and Heparin) | Incidence of 'serious' arrhythmias higher among treated group (45%) than controls (15%). However, mortality similar in two groups (treated 12.7%, control 14.8%) |
| Fletcher et al. (1968) | Mostly CCU | 16 | 3 days | 4 groups of 16 pts each a. Glucose b. Glucose + K c. Glucose + insulin d. Nil | Unsatisfactorily conducted trial. No difference in incidence of arrhythmias, ECG improvement or mortality (overall – 13.7%; 19% in patients treated with GIK) |
| Pentecost et al. (1968) | CCU | 100 | 2 days | 100 | Mortality (treated 15%; controls 16%) and incidence of arrhythmias similar in the two groups |
| Lal and Caroli (1968) | GW | 400 | 14 days (intermittent) | Nil | 7% mortality. Much higher mortality rates were recorded in the same hospital following treatment with anticoagulants or Lomodex infusion |
| Sodi-Pallares et al. (1969) | GW | 125 | ? 21 days | Nil | Mortality 4.8% 'low-risk' private patients |

*GW – General Ward; **CCU = Coronary care unit.

Table V  Mortality in patients with myocardial infarction treated with oral potassium and glucose, and subcutaneous insulin (PGI regimen after Mittra) compared with controls. Reproduced with permission.[207]

| Authors | PGI | | | Control | | | Interpretation of results |
|---|---|---|---|---|---|---|---|
| | No. of pts | No. of deaths | Mortality (%) | No. of pts | No. of deaths | Mortality (%) | |
| Mittra (1965) | 85 | 10 | 11.7 | 85 | 24 | 28.2 | Significant difference (P < 0.05) in favour of treatment |
| Pilcher et al. (1967) | 49 | 6 | 12.2 | 53 | 12 | 22.6 | Significant difference (P < 0.001) in favour of treatment (mainly in over-60 age group) |
| M.R.C. Working Party (1968) | 410 | 98 | 23.9 | 430 | 109 | 25.3 | No significant difference |
| Iisalo and Kallio (1969) | 124 | 16 | 12.9 | 132 | 24 | 18.2 | No significant difference in the total mortality (significant difference in favour of treatment at the end of first 48 hours) |
| Cotterill et al. (1970) | 112 | 22 | 19.5 | 174 | 81 | 46.5 | Significant difference (P<0.001) in favour of treatment |
| Total of all studies | 780 | 152 | 19.5 | 874 | 250 | 28.6 | Significant difference (P < 0.01) in favour of treatment |

ished myocardial potassium loss.[151, 219, 220] The incidence of ventricular fibrillation decreased when glucose and insulin were given intravenously, but hypertonic glucose, saline and sucrose were all equally efficacious in reducing ischemic arrhythmias and K⁺-efflux.[219, 220] Insulin was administered intravenously alone in large doses (8-25 units/ Kg) to dogs periodically after ligation of the circumflex branch of the left coronary artery.[221] All control animals, treated either with glucagon or saline, promptly showed electrocardiographic changes followed by progressively longer paroxysms of ventricular tachycardia, terminating in fatal ventricular fibrillation within 1 to 16 minutes. Although it was possible that glucagon contamination of insulin may have accounted for insulin's reputed positive effect,[222, 223] comparison of the insulin-treated and glucagon-treated groups revealed a significant difference. In treated dogs, insulin suppressed ventricular ectopic activity, and reduced paroxysms of ventricular fibrillation, early electrocardiographic changes of injury and considerably prolonged survival. Blood glucose was stabilized by varying the rate of exogenous glucose infusion. Insulin-induced blockage of the cardioaccelerator effect of the catecholamines was thought to contribute to the protection observed.[224, 225] The doses of insulin used in these laboratory animals were much higher than those usually recommended for glucose-insulin-potassium infusion in man. Using lower doses of insulin in dogs after experimental myocardial infarction, but still higher than those given clinically, Maroko and associates [100] observed no reduction in the incidence of arrhythmias.

## IV. CLINICAL TRIALS OF GIK: OVERALL ACTIONS

### A. Acute ischemic heart disease

As discussed, many of the early studies (Table III) using GIK in patients with heart disease were not comparable in that varying dose regimens were employed, the time intervals to the initiation of therapy after an acute insult varied, criteria for the selection of patients differed even within the same series, and choice of assessment variables was varied as well. The incidence of potentially lethal arrhythmias and mortality were chiefly used to judge the efficacy of treatment, each of which in turn is a complex and unknown function of many interrelated variables. Mittra [199-207] reported improved mortality in one of the largest series of 370 patient evaluations. The Medical Research Council of Great Britain [217] pooled data from 13 hospitals involving 986 patients and concluded that no significant difference existed between treated and untreated patients. Interestingly, there was a significant variation in mortality between hospitals, recording figures of 12.2 to 35.4 percent for their control patients and 9.7 to 33.7 percent for their treated patients. Mittra [207] recently compared his results with those of other investigators and defended the potential usefulness of GIK infusion in patients with acute myocardial infarctions treated in hospitals without coronary care units.

Sodi-Pallares and collaborators,[20-29] pioneers in the development and investigation of GIK therapy for heart disease, offered their latest program of treatment,[26, 27, 226] associated with a mortality of 4.8 percent in selected patients. These investigators stress the need for dietary control as an essential part of GIK treatment and appeal for standardization of regimens to their own.

### B. Combined effects of GIK on metabolism

The combined effects of GIK infusion on metabolism is of interest, considering the potentially varied and considerable actions of each of its components. The high plasma free fatty acid levels observed in subgroups of patients with ischemic heart disease [227] correlates with intense suppression of insulin secretion and the extent of hemodynamic insult produced.[228] Moffitt and co-workers [229, 230] studied thirty-three patients with low cardiac outputs following open-heart surgery treated with two liters of 10 percent dextrose in water with 80 units regular insulin and 160 mEq $K^+$, and two liters of the same solution without glucose or potassium and a control (5 percent glucose). During GIK infusion, mean arterial levels of osmolarity, glucose, lactate, free fatty acids and ketone bodies decreased, as compared with these parameters in control groups. Arterial pyruvate, oxygen content, growth hormone and insulin levels remained unchanged during GIK infusion. Therefore these investigators concluded that GIK promoted aerobic carbohydrate metabolism rather than lipid metabolism.

These data are somewhat supported by preliminary reports from Stanley and coauthors [231, 232] who studied eleven patients with coronary artery disease given GIK. Arterial and coronary sinus samples were collected thirty minutes before and after a bolus of glucose (ten grams) and insulin (5 units) followed by 1-2 ml/min of a solution composed of 300 g glucose, 50 units insulin and 80 mEq KCl per liter. At the conclusion of the thirty minute infusion period, arterial free fatty acid levels dropped 60 percent, arterial glucose levels rose 64 percent and arterial lactate levels doubled. The arterial-coronary sinus difference for free fatty acids fell 80 percent while the glucose difference increased 140 percent, and that for lactate increased 170 percent.

During the period when myocardial substrate extraction changed, myocardial oxygen extraction fell 8 percent. Thus, at least in fasting patients with coronary artery disease, GIK changes myocardial substrate utilization from fat to carbohydrate and is associated with a small drop in myocardial oxygen extraction.

This conclusion is consistent with the "glucose hypothesis" of Opie,[233] which predicts that increased glucose provided to the ischemic heart would promote anaerobic glycolysis, decrease potassium loss and maintain the action potential, and depress high circulating free fatty acid levels. The data of Maroko and co-workers,[100] previously considered, support the contention that GIK infusion does in fact activate anaerobic glycolysis in the ischemic heart. In contrast, however, are recent reports from Lochner, Opie and associates [234] that GIK therapy does not favorably affect myocardial energy metabolism after experimental myocardial infarction in the cape chacma baboon heart, as evidenced by failure to alter a defective mitochondrial P/O ratio, and restore tissue ATP, phosphocreatine, and tissue lactate levels.

### C. GIK effect in congestive heart failure

On theoretical grounds, the combination of GIK has been strongly advocated for congestive heart failure associated with ischemic heart disease.[235-237] In man, insulin secretion is severely suppressed when cardiac performance is poor and the syndrome of congestive failure is present.[238, 239] Accordingly, since a reduction in myocardial ischemia [240] and hypoxia [241] improves ventricular contractility, Majid and co-workers [242] evaluated the hemodynamic response to GIK in six patients with "ischemic heart failure." Subjects were given 1.5 g/Kg oral glucose followed in ten minutes by an intravenous infusion over five minutes of a 100 ml solution of 0.5 g/Kg glucose, 1.5 units/Kg insulin and 10 mEq potassium chloride. Hemodynamic studies were conducted before and five minutes after completion of the infusion through a pulmonary artery catheter, and results were compared with those recorded in normal controls. Except for a transient feeling of warmth during the infusion, no adverse symptoms or signs were reported; there were no dysrrhythmias nor any change in configuration of the electrocardiographic complexes resulting from the infusion. Intravenous glucose-insulin-potassium increased cardiac output and maximum rate of rise in left ventricular pressure (LV dp/dt), but decreased left ventricular end-diastolic pressure in both groups at rest (Fig. 29). The

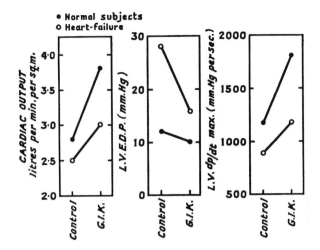

**Figure 29**  Hemodynamic changes at rest after GIK infusion in 6 patients in ischemic heart failure and in 6 normal subjects. Reproduced with permission from Majid et al.[212]

mean systemic arterial pressure was unchanged in both groups, whereas the heart rate was elevated in the normal subjects, but not in the patients with heart failure. During exercise, GIK infusion again changed cardiac output, LV(dp/dt)$_{max}$, and left ventricular end-diastolic pressure in similar directions, and reduced pulmonary artery pressure in both groups (Fig. 30). Heart rate and mean arterial pressure were unchanged.

During GIK infusion, total body oxygen consumption and minute ventilation rose in both groups of subjects, with no change in the pulmonary alveolar/arterial oxygen tension gradient in either group. The systemic arterial oxygen tension was significantly increased in the normal subjects but unchanged in patients with heart failure. Glucose infusion alone did not produce any signficant changes in the hemodynamic variables studied except for LV(dp/dt)$_{max}$ at rest (Fig. 31).

The blood glucose and plasma insulin levels were normal in all patients and levels of both increased in response to GIK in all subjects. Plasma potassium levels fell slightly after GIK was begun, but remained within the normal range.

Based upon the similarity in electrolyte profiles of burned patients and patients with congestive heart failure, and the effect of glucose and insulin infusion in burned patients,[331, 332] Allison and co-workers[333]

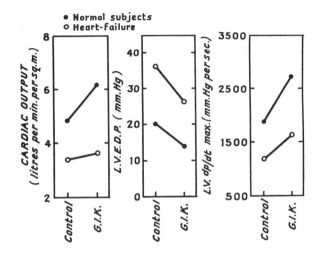

**Figure 30** Hemodynamic changes on exercise after GIK infusion in 6 patients in ischemic heart failure and in 6 normal subjects. Reproduced with permission from Majid et al.[242]

studied the actions of GIK infusion on six patients with congestive failure and hyponatremia, resistant to diuretic and digoxin therapy. A daily infusion of 500-1000 ml of 50 percent glucose containing 100-200 units of soluble insulin and 100-200 mEq of KCl per liter was given and the patients' clinical response was recorded. Four patients sustained a significant sodium and water diuresis and a rise in the serum sodium level, and two of these converted from atrial fibrillation to a sinus rhythm. Two patients showed no response to the GIK infusion.

These data may indicate that GIK infusion is positively inotropic in hearts failing from chronic ischemic heart disease. This situation should be distinguished from previously discussed work concerned with the incidence of arrhythmias, as judged by mortality, or the extent of ischemic injury in the context of acute myocardial infarction.

Even more recently, Espina and associates [243] recorded catheterization data in ten patients with heart disease immediately prior to and after a ten minute infusion of a mixture composed of 0.50 gm glucose, 10 mEq potassium and 20 units regular insulin. The cardiac index and stroke index rose significantly, but were associated with concommitant rises in left ventricular end-diastolic pressure and tension-time index. Therefore these authors concluded that overall left ventricular performance was not improved by GIK in the doses used.

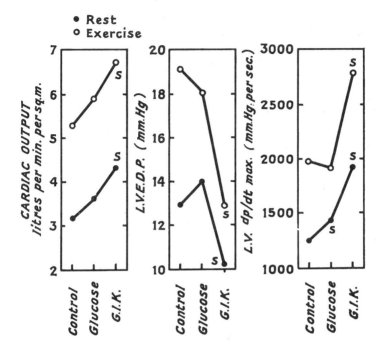

**Figure 31** Comparison of hemodynamic effects of glucose alone and GIK in 4 normal subjects. Reproduced with permission.[242]

Of interest in this regard is the report of Wildenthal and co-workers [244] who studied the hemodynamic effects of GIK on depressed canine myocardium during severe systemic hypoxia. GIK infusion alone did not improve the hemodynamic profile, but when given in conjunction with the beta-adrenergic blocking agent propranolol GIK was felt to be beneficial and increased survival.

### D. GIK effect after open-heart surgery

Moffitt and co-workers [229, 230, 245, 246] extensively studied the clinical course and metabolism of patients following cardiac surgery. They documented postoperative metabolic changes (hyperglycemia, increased blood lactate levels) consistent with anaerobic metabolism and

relative insulin-lack and consequently administered GIK to some patients postoperatively. After two liters containing 10 percent glucose,
80 units regular insulin and 160 mEq potassium given to patients with
(New York Heart Association) functional class III or IV disease, cardiac
output (left atrial-to-thoracic aorta dye curve) was significantly higher
than in controls given 5 percent glucose in water solutions.[229]

More detailed hemodynamic data were offered by Bradley and
Branthwaite[247] who administered 100 ml 50 percent glucose with 10
units insulin and 10 mEq potassium through a caval catheter over 30 to
45 minutes to ten patients postop valve replacement. A small increase
in cardiac index was recorded, but was accompanied by larger elevations in both right- and left-atrial pressures and pulmonary artery
pressure. Thus, GIK in this study was unable to produce any favorable
effect on stroke volume with respect to left ventricular filling pressure,
*i.e.*, increase the level of contractility and change the ventricular function curve.


### E. Potential modulation of GIK actions by other pharmacologic agents [43]

Not only may the effects of GIK on the heart be dependent upon
the history of the myocardium studied, etiology and extent of heart
disease present, arterial level of insulin, substrates and electrolytes
present, and dose and method of infusion of GIK, but other drugs
simultaneously being administered may influence any GIK effect.[248]
Although insulin secretion is suppressed by the high adrenergic drive
associated with the stress of heart disease, many cardioactive agents
affect insulin release as well.

Ouabain has been implicated as a direct insulin secretagogue from
work done in slices of rabbit pancreas and in the anesthetized dog.[249]
However, this has not been confirmed in more recent work studying
the effect of intravenous ouabain in normal man.[250] No data is available in patients with heart disease, but it is known that ouabain is
capable of inhibiting the metabolic actions of epinephrine [251, 252] and
may suppress norepinephrine production.[250] As a positive inotropic
agent, the expression of digitalis-related actions are energy-dependent
and are therefore a function of glucose availability [254-256] and the
presence of insulin [115, 257] when glucose serves as the principle substrate for the ischemic heart.

The thiazide diuretics may elevate blood glucose,[254-261] probably via
a direct suppression of insulin secretion,[262] although their diabetogenic
property is not reversed by tolbutamide [263] and histologic changes in

the pancreatic beta cell have not been associated with their use.[264] Benzothiadiazine, a nondiuretic antihypertensive, may release sympathomimetic amines in some species [265, 266] but not in man.[267] Yet this compound may produce hyperglycemia in man, and its insulin-suppressing action is potentiated by the catecholamines [268] and reduced by beta-blocking agents.[209]

The methylxanthines may stimulate insulin release,[270] a process which is glucose-dependent.[271] No data is presently available connecting the use of these compounds with clinically-manifest hyperglycemia in man.

Commercial insulin used for many GIK studies is contaminated with small amounts of glucagon. Pancreatic glucagon is released endogenously in response to stress [272] and acute myocardial infarction.[273] Glucagon has a significant positive inotropic action [223] and may in part account for some of the increases in myocardial contractility reported, although the doses involved are much lower than clinically used to demonstrate glucagon's positive inotropic property.

One group of investigators used glucagon in one of their control groups and showed the comparative beneficial action of GIK on survival after experimental myocardial infarction.[221] Recently the effects of intravenous glucagon infusion on insulin, free fatty acid and glucose response was studied in man after acute myocardial infarction.[316] During the first week after the insult a modest dose of 1 mg glucagon intravenously elicited significant rises in insulin, free fatty acid and glucose levels. Six weeks after the myocardial infarction, the mean fasting blood glucose fell and insulin levels rose to the normal range. Glucagon administration again caused a rise in glucose, free fatty acid and insulin levels. These data suggested that postmyocardial infarction insulin resistance is of greater significance than depression of insulin secretion. In addition, the theoretical prediction that the relatively large doses of glucagon used for treatment of acute myocardial infarction (up to 250 mg/24 hr) could elevate glucose and insulin levels sufficiently to be therapeutic remains open. The relative contribution of glucagon to the observed effects of GIK remains to be specifically evaluated.

### F. Objections to the use of GIK solution

Objections to the use of GIK infusions and its individual components, including side effects and contraindications, have been raised periodically. As with any agent or therapeutic maneuver, lack of efficacy or indication in itself constitutes a contraindication and this applies particularly to GIK, since each of the ingredients may have far-reaching metabolic effects. Lack of absolute proof of effectiveness was stressed by Surawicz [170] in a review of the early clinical experience with GIK, again noting the lack of comparable criteria for efficacy, doses, timing of treatment, delay before institution of same and so forth. He also underscored the paucity of direct evidence indicating that ischemic myocardial fibers, relatively potassium-deficient, may have their intracellular potassium restored by systemically-infused potassium, citing the potentially limited transport of $K^+$ to an infarcted area of heart muscle by severely compromised coronary blood flow. Surawicz also questioned why the intravenous infusion of glucose and potassium should be less or more effective than orally administered glucose and potassium.

Brachfeld [309] recently mentioned his doubt that systemically administered GIK reaches an ischemic zone of myocardium, since GIK solution is ineffective when given by direct intracoronary infusion. The rapid infusion of 10 to 20 percent glucose solutions depresses $[K^+]_o$ for up to six to nine hours and changes the electrocardiogram. An unusual complication of intravenous infusion of high glucose concentrations is the precipitation of angina. [310]

The changes in plasma $K^+$ concentration effected by GIK infusions are difficult to predict. Some evidence indicates that in patients with acute myocardial infarctions plasma $K^+$ may be elevated for several days. [253, 274] Patients with congestive heart failure may be prone to develop hyperkalemia sooner than anticipated. [275, 276] The hazards of hyperkalemia have been discussed elsewhere [163-165, 169] and are beyond the scope of this discussion. On the other hand, since serum potassium need not correlate with total body potassium nor total myocardial potassium content, hypokalemia may be produced in potassium-depleted and even otherwise normal subjects during GIK administration, as a function of both glucose and insulin concentration infused over a given period of time. [277] Hyperkalemia may also be produced during GIK infusions. [242]

Theoretically, if infused potassium is not in great part distributed intracellularly, under the influence of concommitantly administered glucose and insulin, then the rise in ratio of $[K^+]_o/[K^+]_i$ very well might precipitate arrhythmias. The regional hyperkalemic model has already been discussed, in which the importance of locally high values of $[K^+]_o/[K^+]_i$ in decreasing vulnerability threshold were demonstrated. [104, 105, 172] Of interest in this context are the studies of Prasad and Callaghan [157] who specifically showed that KCl added to glucose and insulin accentuated the shortening of the action potential duration and effective refractory period and further slowed the rate of rise of phase 0 (dV/dt) of the action potential associated with hypoxia of human papillary muscles. These actions were believed to be harmful and therefore these authors concluded that glucose and insulin alone would be preferable to glucose and insulin with potassium.

The adverse effects of too much or too little insulin in relation to the metabolic status of the patient and the concentrations of glucose infused are relatively better understood by clinicians. Sudden hypoglycemia in patients with heart disease may precipitate angina and even myocardial necrosis. However, hyperglycemia appears to be the more frequent occurrence during GIK infusion. The work of Burke and associates[278] showed that glucose is not a necessary ingredient to prevent myocellular potassium loss during ischemia, but rather the volume and osmolarity of the perfusate is of greater importance.

During the actual GIK infusion side effects are reported to be minimal. Mittra[204] mentions that "slight" azotemia and hyperkalemia were not considered absolute contraindications in his series. Oral intake of glucose prevented hypoglycemia according to Mittra, so that monitoring of plasma glucose was not essential. Majid and co-workers[242] remarked that a feeling of warmth was reported by their patients, but no other side effect was noted during GIK infusion. Serum glucose remained fairly constant in their subjects.

It is appropriate to mention that not all series reflect or confirm any beneficial hemodynamic action of GIK or improvement in overall myocardial energy balance. The early uncontrolled series which failed to confirm the beneficial actions of GIK in other series with unacceptable experimental design have already been mentioned.[15, 16, 216, 218] The Medical Research Council Working Party series,[217] perhaps the best available, did not find any significant difference in mortality or serious arrhythmias between treated and control patients.

Lochner and associates[234] failed to note any metabolic evidence of a more favorable myocardial energy balance induced by GIK. The work of Dixon and coauthors[311] refuted that GIK drove K⁺ into myocytes and reduced the incidence of fatal ventricular fibrillation after acute coronary artery ligation.

Bradley and Branthwaite[247] showed that GIK infusion was incapable of improving overall left ventricular function. However, they also noted that serum calcium and potassium levels and hematocrits fell during GIK therapy and attributed this to osmotic hemodilution following the infusion of hypertonic glucose. An associated osmotic diuresis was also observed.

In a recent study designed to test the effect of GIK on ischemic stress in humans with heart disease, Lesch and associates [312] administered GIK to eight patients with positive exercise electrocardiograms during rapid atrial pacing. These investigators reasoned that if the ability of patients to withstand such a stress were extended by GIK, this evidence would be manifest while the plasma concentrations of glucose and insulin were elevated, and in association with enhanced myocardial lactate production. Their patients were subjected to atrial pacing-induced tachycardia before and during GIK infusion. The GIK program consisted of a 50 ml bolus of 25 g glucose and 10 units CZI insulin into a central venous line over five minutes, followed by 150 ml of a solution containing 75 g glucose, 9 units CZI insulin, and 30 mEq KCl infused over one hour. Steady-state elevation of glucose and insulin was achieved prior to atrial pacing during GIK infusion. Five of eight patients developed diminished tolerance to pacing during the GIK-paced state (Fig. 32). Left ventricular end-diastolic pressure (LVEDP) was elevated in all patients at rest during GIK infusion as compared with the rest control state. During pacing, varying degrees of elevation in LVEDP were unaffected by GIK. The transmyocardial

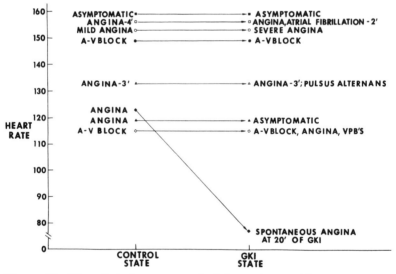

**Figure 32** The clinical response of eight patients with coronary artery disease to the stress of pacing-induced tachycardia in the control state (see text) is presented on the left. The clinical response to an identical pacing stress following infusion of glucose, potassium and insulin (GKI-state) is presented on the right. One patient (♦) developed spontaneous angina after 20 min. of GKI infusion. VPB = ventricular premature beat. Reproduced with permission.[312]

arterial-coronary sinus glucose difference rose significantly in the GIK paced state as compared with the control paced state. The transmyocardial arteriovenous potassium levels were unaltered by GIK. Lactate extraction was positive at rest in both control and GIK states, and was lower during pacing as compared to resting values in the control state in all eight patients. However, there was no stoichiometric relationship between enhanced glucose uptake and myocardial lactate production in this study. Of special interest were the large negative transmyocardial glucose differences reported. The lack of an expected relation between increased glucose uptake and myocardial lactate production has been variously explained.[309, 312, 313] Nonetheless, this report documents that GIK solution may adversely affect left ventricular function and under the experimental conditions used (rapid atrial pacing) suggests that GIK does not extend tolerance to ischemia during stress.

## V. POSSIBLE MECHANISMS OF ACTION OF GIK SOLUTION

After reviewing the experimental evidence affirming some beneficial actions of glucose-insulin-potassium solution, and considering the fundamental properties of each component, what conclusions may be reached concerning the possible mechanisms of GIK infusion when administered together? Unfortunately, not only are the clinical data conflicting regarding the efficacy of GIK, but the analysis of metabolic data leads to more questions than may be answered at present about the mechanism of action.[309]

### A. Mechanism of effect on arrhythmias

Potassium is lost from ischemic heart cells. The currently available evidence strongly suggests that arrhythmias may be initiated by the adverse effects of intracellular potassium loss on electrical properties of excitable membranes. Although it is said that convincing proof that GIK given intravenously significantly increases intracellular potassium is lacking, several studies suggest that net potassium movement into the myocyte is due to the combined metabolic action of glucose and insulin.[219, 278] At the same time, there is substantial evidence that the administered $K^+$ does not significantly enter the cell and may in fact be harmful.[157] While high concentrations of free fatty acids have been incriminated in the production of arrhythmias,[227] much evidence also argues against a major role of free fatty acidemia in the production of "ischemic arrhythmias".[279]

## B. Mechanism of effect on extent of ischemic necrosis

The ischemic myocardium is primarily dependent upon glucose for energy production. Hypoxia doubles the myocardial uptake of glucose, but with insulin the uptake is increased fivefold. Once membrane glucose transport is assured in the presence of insulin, only the activity of phosphofructokinase and hexokinase limits glucose metabolism. Glucose-insulin-potassium does in fact stimulate these phosphorylating enzymes.[30] When the myocardium is hypoxic, the stimulation of anaerobic pathways will improve the energy balance of the cell. Even optimal anaerobic metabolism cannot meet the energy requirements of normally contracting myocardium but is certainly capable of maintaining some electrical properties. However, augmented anaerobic activity also increases intracellular lactate levels, associated with a progressive decrease in intracellular pH. The work of Maroko and associates,[100] showing that GIK decreases the severity of myocardial ischemic injury, presumably reflects the improvement in myocellular energy balance affected by GIK infusion. Lochner and co-workers [234] have recently contested these data. A more favorable myocardial energy balance also predicts improvement in mechanical muscle performance.[240, 241] Recent studies [123] have clearly established that the nonmetabolizable sugars cannot reverse the electrical markers of hypoxia and hence support these notions.

During ischemia, inorganic phosphate is lost from the myocardial cell.[314] The infusion of glucose drives inorganic phosphate into cells. Experimentally, orthophosphate has been shown to stimulate glycolysis and glycogenolysis by activating phosphofructokinase and providing a substrate for glycogen phosphorylase and glyceraldehyde-3-phosphate dehydrogenase. Therefore the precise biochemical reason for activation of the phosphorylating enzymes associated with GIK remains undefined.

The possibility of an increase in myocardial perfusion from lactate-induced vasodilatation during GIK infusion must also be mentioned.[315]

Insulin-induced protein synthesis and restriction of protein degradation in the ischemic heart may provide still another mechanism by which insulin could protect against ischemic necrosis. Recently Rannels and co-workers [307] reported that provision of insulin to perfused rat hearts could prevent or reverse the protein degradation that was usually observed in this preparation. Even more significant was the associated lowered free activity of the two lysosomal enzymes, $\beta$-acetylglucosaminidase and cathepsin-D, suggesting that insulin altered the autolytic process.

## C. Osmotic effect of GIK

The relationship between left ventricular pressure and volume, or myocardial compliance, is an important determinant of left ventricular performance.[280-282] The compliance of ischemic and/or infarcted heart muscle may initially increase,[283] then may decrease as the ventricular wall becomes stiff.[284] As recovery progresses, left ventricular compliance may return to approach preischemic values. The details of the viscoelastic properties of the myocardium and stress-strain relationships are beyond the scope of this discussion and are reviewed elsewhere.[285]

While the molecular and structural reasons for the effect of heart disease on ventricular compliance are unknown, a defect in relaxation, possibly mediated by impaired sequestration of calcium by the sarcoplasmic reticulum [286] and/or by physical swelling of ischemic myocytes, may provide an explanation with experimental support.

When the aerobic metabolism of heart muscle is impaired during hypoxia and ischemia, the $Na^+$, $K^+$-pump is unable to keep pace with the intracellular sodium entering the cell. Net intracellular sodium accumulates, thereby in part dissipating the resting transmembrane potential (Fig. 33). Partial depolarization of the cell may be accompanied by chloride diffusion into the cell. Although potassium simultaneously leaks out of the cell, it does not equal the sodium and chloride gained.[287] A net gain of intracellular osmotically-active particles is followed by water diffusion into the cell. Dilution of cellular constituents, including calcium available for myofilament sliding, may further impair contractility. This process becomes accentuated if ischemia is of sufficient intensity to destroy membrane integrity and thus allow larger molecules to enter the cell, or permit large molecules within the cell to lyse into smaller ones with greater osmotic activity.

Cell swelling during a transient ischemic episode may increase interstitial pressure and may block blood flow within a tissue.[288-290] Experimentally, edema and the associated elevation in interstitial pressure is capable of restricting arteriolar dilation.[328] Thus not only is cell swelling a result of ischemia, but it is also a cause of ischemia and tends to create a positive feedback perpetuation of the problem. After clamping a renal artery, release of the clamp is not accompanied by a full restoration of blood flow—the so-called "no-reflow" phenomenon.[291] Willerson and co-workers [292, 293] demonstrated that infusion of hypertonic mannitol during or before occlusion of the left anterior descending coronary artery lowered the S-T segment elevation over the affected muscle, augmented its contractility, and was accompanied by an increase in collateral blood flow into the area. These data have been

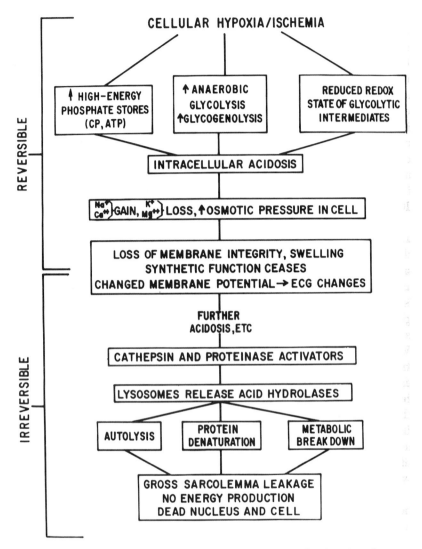

**Figure 33**  Postulated events leading to myocyte death after hypoxia and/or ischemia. Lines connecting processes do not necessarily imply an exact temporal sequence, nor a cause and effect relation.

confirmed by Powell and associates,[294] underscoring the contribution of cell swelling to the pathogenesis of myocardial ischemia. Hyperosmolar agents also improve the function of hypoxic papillary muscles.[302]

A moderate sudden increase in serum osmolarity may produce a positive inotropic action [258, 296] independent of the osmotic agent used.[297] This action, not dependent upon changes in sympathetic nervous activity nor on the Frank-Starling mechanism, results in enhanced stroke volume and left ventricular $(dp/dt)_{max}$ in the resting intact dog[298] and in the anoxic perfused rat heart in the absence of any change in myocardial energy metabolism.[299] The preliminary data of Willerson and co-authors[300] support the hypothesis that the positive inotropic action of myocardial perfusion with hyperosmolar solutions results from a decrease in cell size, thereby effectively increasing the concentration of intracellular calcium. The ability of hypertonic mannitol to improve myocardial contractility and coronary blood flow in patients with heart disease when serum osmolarity is increased only 10 mOsm has also been reported.[295]

In the studies of Regan and associates,[220, 278] the antiarrhythmic actions of GIK were evident during intravenous administration, and the constituents of the solution were less critical than the rate of infusion and its osmolarity. Hence hypertonic solutions without glucose, as well as isotonic saline, spared myocardial potassium loss during ischemia and manifested an antiarrhythmic effect without enhancing glucose uptake.[278] Moreover, the greater the osmolarity of the GIK solution chosen, the greater the antiarrhythmic action.[220] However, Wildenthal and co-workers[244] were also able to demonstrate a protective effect of GIK when administered in an isotonic solution, although pretreatment with propranolol was necessary to "unmask" the beneficial action in their studies. If true, it is necessary to explain the data of MacLeod and Prasad,[123] who clearly showed that nonmetabolizable sugars could not produce glucose-like effects on the abbreviated action potential duration associated with papillary muscle anoxia, affirming that the ability of glucose to reverse such electrical changes was dependent upon the metabolism of glucose.

Extrapolation of these data to the clinical situation is fraught with hazard, since there is no evidence that the osmolality of coronary arterial blood is raised during GIK infusions.

## VI. CONCLUSION

### A. Unanswered questions about cardiac metabolism

There is little question that a better understanding of cardiac metabolism may enable a systematic experimental approach to the prevention of heart cell death, and improve performance of poorly functioning myocardial tissue. However, there remain a significant number of unanswered questions concerning cardiac metabolism during ischemia and anoxia: *

1. Can absolute blood flow be enhanced to a jeopardized or blighted zone?
2. What are the details of *in vivo* control of coronary vascular resistance and specifically the actions of adenosine and tissue $pO_2$?
3. What is the role of the microvasculature in the progression of myocardial necrosis, and the action of the many cardioactive agents used daily in the treatment of heart disease upon the microvasculature?
4. Will it be possible to protect the myocardium easily by increasing glycogen stores before an ischemic episode occurs, and how?
5. What limits glycolytic energy production in the mammalian heart as compared with the turtle heart, and can this be partially overcome?
6. What is the optimum substrate mixture for the ischemic myocyte?
7. Are free fatty acids or their release "harmful" to the ischemic heart?
8. What are the precise differences between ischemia and anoxia on the mammalian heart? Does acidosis and suppression of glycolysis account for the greater severity of damage observed during ischemia?
9. What is (are) the precise biochemical step(s) that account for the transition from jeopardized to blighted, and from blighted to necrotic zones?
10. Will conventional therapeutic maneuvers which increase myocardial contractility irreversibly cause transitions from jeopardized to blighted zones, and if so, can this be monitored, modified, or prevented?
11. Are the biochemical correlates of ischemia associated with angina identical with those in the jeopardized zone surrounding a necrotic one in the center of a myocardial infarction? If so, then what accounts for the difference in S-T segment changes? How can the S-T segment changes of Prinzmetal's angina be explained in this context?
12. Do lysosomal hydrolases initiate the terminal processes of myo-

---

* Modified after Brachfeld.[309]

cyte death? Is this the mechanism of action of corticosteroids in reducing myocardial infarct size?

## B. Unanswered questions about GIK

Since the suggestion by Sodi-Pallares in 1960 that GIK would benefit patients with heart disease by replacing myocardial intracellular potassium, it is still unknown whether in fact administered GIK does replace intracellular stores of potassium. Despite the voluminous reports on GIK that followed, the role of reduced intracellular potassium in the production of "ischemic arrhythmias," question of compartmentalization of $K^+$ within the myocyte and possible effects of "replacement" of intracellular $K^+$ are unresolved. Potassium is lost from ischemic cells, and serious arrhythmias may be caused both by acute changes in $K^+$ pools and by ischemia. $K^+$-loss may mimic some of the electrophysiological changes accompanying ischemia and/or anoxia. Yet there are significant metabolic and electrophysiological differences between ischemia and anoxia. Exactly which electrophysiologic parameter is altered by $K^+$-loss in each instance is yet to be determined. Perhaps one of the most difficult problems is the relationship of $K^+$ lost from a cell and blood flow in the same ischemic area. Specifically, to what extent is extracellular $K^+$ washed away from the ischemic zone?

A great deal of experimental basic work has shown that glucose and/or GIK solutions are capable of improving certain aspects of cardiac function and metabolism during hypoxia and ischemia. While Maroko's series suggested that the administration of GIK solutions protected against myocardial ischemic necrosis, the concentrations of glucose used were several-fold higher than usually administered. There was no significant difference between the use of GIK and glucose. Other work in laboratory animals does not support the view that GIK reduces myocardial infarct size by improving overall myocardial energy balance through an acceleration of anaerobic glycolysis.

The ability of glucose to reverse the deleterious effects of anoxia on the cardiac action potential is well documented. Again, however, a high concentration of glucose (50mM as opposed to normal, or 5mM glucose) is necessary to do so in the bathed isolated tissue. For this and other reasons, extrapolation of the data of Maroko and the electrophysiologic data to the clinical situation is hazardous.

The initial studies evaluating GIK in man attempted to demonstrate that GIK could prevent ventricular arrhythmias and deaths after acute myocardial infarction. In perhaps the best of a number of early uncontrolled studies, the Medical Research Council Working Party found no significant difference in mortality or incidence of ventricular arrhythmias between nontreated and GIK-treated patients with acute myocardial infarction.

Since this work, and especially in view of the demonstration that insulin secretion is suppressed in proportion to the decrease in cardiac index in congestive heart failure or after acute myocardial infarction, other investigators have found GIK a useful adjunct in the management of their patients with different types of heart disease. Data recently available suggest that the significant part of any GIK effect rests with the accompanying hyperosmolarity and consequent reduction in tissue pressure, thereby allowing a greater perfusion of the ischemic myocardium. Further work is, of course, necessary to clearly define this phenomenon.

Despite the plethora of data and great interest in GIK infusions for heart disease, and even though the metabolic actions of each ingredient of GIK solutions are better understood, there is much more yet to learn. Serious theoretical questions exist concerning the effects of each component and of GIK together. Unequivocal proof of a clear benefit of intravenous GIK in patients with heart disease is yet to be demonstrated. Nevertheless, there is sufficient evidence showing GIK benefits ischemic heart muscle and myocardial performance to warrant additional clinical research to clarify the role of GIK in cardiovascular therapy.

## References

1. Laborit, H.: The treatment of cardiovascular insufficiency and myocardial infarct with the combination of insulin, hypertonic glucose, and potassium salts. *Presse Med* **71**:1-3, 1963.
2. Kunlin, J., Laborit, H.: Experimental cardiac resuscitation: Importance of cardiac massage with clamping of the thoracic aorta, of insulinated hypertonic glucose and of potassium chloride. *Bull Soc Int Clin* **19**:96-98, 1960.
3. Weber, B., Laborit, H., Jouany, J., et al.: Modificationes des signes electrocardiographiques de l'infarctus du myocarde experimental chez le lapin par l'injection de sels de l'acide aspartique. *Compt Rend Soc Biol* **152**:431-436, 1958.
4. Harris, A. S.: Potassium and experimental coronary occlusion. *Amer Heart J* **71**:797-802, 1966.
5. Blumgart, H. L., Gilligan, D. R., Schlesinger, M. J.: Experimental studies on effect of temporary occlusion of coronary arteries: production of myocardial infarction. *Amer Heart J* **22**:374-389, 1941.
6. Sewell, W. M., Koth, D. R., Huggins, C. E.: Ventricular fibrillation in dogs after sudden return of flow to the coronary artery. *Surgery* **38**:1050-1053, 1955.
7. Danese, C.: Pathogenesis of ventricular fibrillation in coronary occlusion. *J Amer Med Assn* **179**:52-53, 1962.

8. Petropoulos, P. C., Meijne, N. G.: Cardiac function during perfusion of the circumflex coronary artery with venous blood, low-molecular dextran, or tyrode solution. *Amer Heart J* **68**:370-382, 1964.
9. Harris, A. S., Bisteni, A., Russell, R. A., et al.: Excitatory factors in ventricular tachycardia resulting from myocardial ischemia. Potassium major excitant. *Science* **119**:200-203, 1960.
10. Cummings, J. R.: Electrolyte changes in cardiac tissue and coronary arterial and venous plasma after coronary occlusion. *Circ Res* **8**:865-870, 1960.
11. Cherbakoff, A., Toyama, S., Hamilton, W. F.: Relation between coronary sinus potassium and cardiac arrhythmias. *Circ Res* **5**:517-521, 1957.
12. Garcia-Ramos, J.: Los mecanismos electrofisiologicas de la produción de extrasistoles y fibrilación. *Acta Physiol Lat Amer* **12**:36-43, 1962.
13. Hoffman, B. F., Cranefield, P. F.: *Electrophysiology of the Heart*, McGraw-Hill Book Co., New York, 1960, p. 245.
14. Ratti, G., Sanna, G. P.: L'infarcto del miocardo dal punto di vista elettrico e ionico-mecanismo d'azione ed effetti delle soluzioni polarizzanti. *Recent Progr Med (Rome)* **35**:345-369, 1963.
15. Autio, L., Hakkila, J., Härtel, G., et al.: Anticoagulants and Sodi-Pallares infusion in acute myocardial infarction. *Acta Med Scand* **179**:355-360, 1966.
16. Fletcher, G. F., Hurst, J. W., Schlant, R. C.: Preliminary report of a double-blind controlled study of the use of "polarizing" solutions in acute myocardial infarctions. *Circulation* **34**:102, 1966.
17. Selye, H., Mishra, R. K.: Prevention of the "phosphate-steroid-cardiopathy" by various electrolytes. *Amer Heart J* **55**:163-173, 1958.
18. Larcan, A.: Pathophysiological basis and practical application of a "metabolic" therapy of myocardial infarction, in *Electrolytes and Cardiovascular Diseases*, edited by Bajusz, E., Vol. 2, Basel, S. Karger, 1966, pp. 277-301.
19. Sodi-Pallares, D., Polansky, B. J.: On the neglected role of water and potassium in cardiovascular therapy. *Amer Heart J* **61**:568-569, 1961.
20. Sodi-Pallares, D., Bisteni, A., Medrano, G. A., et al.: Effects of a low sodium, high potassium and high water diet on the clinical and electrocardiographic development of various cardiomyopathies. *Acta Cardiol* **16**:166-200, 1961.
21. Ponce de Leon, J., Oriol, A., Sodi-Pallares, D.: Clinical course of acute myocardial infarction treated with polarizing solution of glucose, insulin and potassium. *Abstr Int Congr Cardiol (Cardiovasc Res Suppl)*: 45, 1962.
22. Sodi-Pallares, D., Testelli, M. R., Fishlender, B. L., et al.: Effects of an intravenous infusion of a potassium glucose-insulin solution on the electrocardiographic signs of myocardial infarction. A preliminary clinical report. *Amer J Cardiol* **9**:166-181, 1962.
23. Sodi-Pallares, D., De Micheli, A., Medrano, G., et al.: Effect of glucose-insulin-potassium solutions on the electrocardiogram in acute and chronic coronary insufficiency. *Mal Cardiovasc* **3**:41-79, 1962.
24. Sodi-Pallares, D., Bisteni, A., Medrano, G. A., et al.: The polarizing treatment of acute myocardial infarction. Possibility of its use in other cardiovascular conditions. *Dis Chest* **43**:424-432, 1963.
25. Sodi-Pallares, D., Bisteni, A., Ponce de Leon, J., et al.: The "polarizing" treatment of myocardial infarction, in *Sudden Death*, edited by Surawicz, B., Pelegrino, E. D., Grune & Stratton, New York, 1964, pp. 171-179.
26. Sodi-Pallares, D., Bisteni, A., Medrano, G. A., et al.: The polarizing treatment for myocardial infarction. *Amer J Cardiol* **24**:607-608, 1969.
27. Sodi-Pallares, D., Bisteni, A., Medrano, G. A., et al.: Polarizing treatment for myocardial infarction. *Circulation* **40**:607-608, 1969.
28. Sodi-Pallares, D., Bisteni, A., Medrano, G. A., et al.: The polarizing treatment in cardiovascular conditions. Experimental basis and clinical applica-

tion, in *Electrolytes and Cardiovascular Diseases*, edited by Bajusz, E., Vol. 2, Basel, S. Karger, 1966, pp. 198-238.

29. Sodi-Pallares, D., Medrano, G. A., Bisteni, A., Ponce de Leon, J.: *Deductive and Polyparametric Electrocardiography*, Mexico, D.F. Published privately by D. Sodi-Pallares, Instituto Nacional de Cardiologia, Ave. Cuauhtemoc 300, 1970, pp. 398-459.

30. Calva, E., Majica, A., Bisteni, A., et al.: Oxidative phosphorylation in cardiac infarct. Effect of glucose-KCl-insulin solution. *Amer J Physiol* **209**:371-375, 1965.

31. Scheit, S., Ascheim, R., Killip, T., III: Shock after acute myocarial infarction. A clinical and hemodynamic profile. *Amer J Cardiol* **26**:556-564, 1970.

32. Scheidt, S., Alonso, D., Post, M., et al.: Pathophysiology of cardiogenic shock: quantification of myocardial necrosis. *Int J Clin Pharmacol* **7**:150-155, 1973.

33. Kones, R. J.: Recent advances in the pathophysiology of cardiogenic shock. *N Y State J Med* **73**:1662-1670, 1793-1804, 1973.

34. Page, D. L., Caulfield, J. B., Kastor, J. A., et al.: Myocardial changes associated with cardiogenic shock. *New Eng J Med* **285**:133-137, 1971.

35. Alonso, D. R., Scheidt, S., Post, M., et al.: Pathophysiology of cardiogenic shock. Quantification of myocarial necrosis, clinical, pathologic and electrocardiographic correlations. *Circulation* **48**:588-596, 1973.

36. Jennings, R. B., Sommers, H. M., Herdson, P. B., et al.: Ischemic injury of myocardium. *Ann N Y Acad Sci* **156**:61-78, 1969.

37. Cox, J. L., McLaughlin, V. W., Flowers, N. C., et al.: The ischemic zone surrounding acute myocardial infarction: its morphology as detected by dehydrogenase staining. *Amer Heart J* **76**:650-659, 1968.

38. Lushnikov, E. F.: Histochemical study of experimentally produced myocardial infarction. *Fed Proc* **22**:906, 1963.

39. Kushner, I., Rakita, L., Kaplan, M. H.: Studies of acute phase protein. II. Localization of co-reactive protein in heart in induced myocardial infarction in rabbits. *J Clin Invest* **42**:286-292, 1963.

40. Hüttner, I., Rona, G., More, R. H.: Fibrin deposition within cardiac muscle cells in malignant hypertension. An electron microscopic study. *Arch Path* **91**:19-28, 1971.

41. Lie, J. T., Holley, K. E., Kampa, W. R., et al.: New histochemical method for morphologic diagnosis of early stages of myocardial ischemia. *Mayo Clin Proc* **46**:319-327, 1971.

42. Sobel, B. E., Shell, W. E.: Jeopardized, blighted, and necrotic myocardium. *Circulation* **47**:215-216, 1973.

43. Shell, W. E., Lavelle, J. F., Covell, J. W., et al.: Early estimation of myocardial damage in conscious dogs and patients with evolving acute myocardial infarction. *J Clin Invest* **52**:2579-2590, 1973.

44. Klein, M. S., Shell, W. E., Sobel, B. E.: Serum creatine phosphokinase (CPK) isoenzymes after intramuscular injections, surgery, and myocardial infarction. *Cardiovasc Res* **7**:412-418, 1973.

45. Sarnoff, S. J., Braunwald, E., Welch, G. H., Jr., et al.: Hemodynamic determinants of oxygen consumption of the heart with special reference to the time-tension index. *Amer J Physiol* **192**:148-156, 1958.

46. Sonnenblick, E. H., Ross, J., Jr., Braunwald, E.: Oxygen consumption of the heart: newer concepts of its multifactorial determination. *Amer J Cardiol* **22**:328-336, 1968.

47. Braunwald, E.: Control of myocardiol oxygen consumption. *Amer J Cardiol* **27**:416-432, 1971.

48. Kones, R. J.: *Cardiogenic Shock*, Futura Publishing Co., Mt. Kisco, N.Y. 1974.

49. Henry, P. D., Eckberg, D., Gault, J. H., et al.: Depressed inotropic state and reduced myocardial oxygen consumption in the human heart. *Amer J Cardiol* 31:300-306, 1973.
50. Moss, A. J., Johnson, J., Sentman, J.: Increase in myocardial oxygenation with propranolol. *Cardiovasc Res* 4:441-442, 1970.
51. Lekven, J., Mjos, O. D., Kjekshus, J. K.: Compensatory mechanisms during graded myocardial ischemia. *Amer J Cardiol* 31:467-473, 1973.
52. Katz, A. M.: Biochemic "defect" in the hypertrophied and failing heart. Deleterious or compensatory? *Circulation* 47:1076-1079, 1973.
53. Shell, W. E., Sobel, B. E.: Deleterious effects of increased heart rate on infarct size in the conscious dog. *Amer J Cardiol* 31:474-479, 1973.
54. Smith, E. R., Redwood, D. R., McCarron, W. E., et al.: Coronary artery occlusion in the conscious dog. Effects of alterations in arterial pressure produced by nitroglycerin, hemorrhage, and alpha-adrenergic agonists on the degree of myocardial ischemia. *Circulation* 47:51-57, 1973.
55. Epstein, S. E.: Hypotension, nitroglycerin, an acute myocardial infarction. *Circulation* 47:217-219, 1973.
56. Wolferth, C. C., Wood, F. C.: The electrocardiographic diagnosis of coronary occlusion by the use of chest leads. *Amer J Med Sci* 183:30-35, 1932.
57. Wood, F. C., Wolferth, C. C., Bellet, S.: Infarction of the lateral wall of the left ventricle: electrocardiographic characteristics. *Amer Heart J* 16:387-410, 1938.
58. Myers, G. B., Klein, H. A., Stofer, B. E.: 1. Correlation of electrocardiographic and pathologic findings in anteroseptal infarction. *Amer Heart J* 36:535-575, 1948.
59. Myers, G. B., Klein, H. A., Hiratzka, T.: 2. Correlation of electrocardiographic and pathologic findings in large anterolateral infarcts. *Amer Heart J* 36:838-881, 1948.
60. Myers, G. B., Klein, H. A., Hirotzka, T.: 3. Correlation of electrocardiographic and pathologic findings in anteroposterior infarction. *Amer Heart J* 37:205-236, 1949.
61. Myers, G. B., Klein, H. A., Hirotzka, T.: 4. Correlation of electrocardiogram and pathologic findings in infarction of the interventricular septum and right ventricle. *Amer Heart J* 37:720-770, 1949.
62. Myers, G. B., Klein, H. A., Stofer, B. E.: Correlation of electrocardiogram and pathologic findings in lateral infarction. *Amer Heart J* 37:374-417, 1949.
63. Wilson, F. N., Macloed, A. G., Baker, P. S., et al.: The electrocardiogram in myocardial infarction with particular reference to the initial deflections of the ventricular complex. *Heart* 16:155-199, 1933.
64. Wilson, F. N., Johnston, F. D., Rosenbaum, F. F., et al.: The precordial electrocardiogram. *Amer Heart J* 27:19-85, 1944.
65. Wegria, R., Segers, M., Keating, R. P., et al.: Relationship between the reduction in coronary flow and the appearance of electrocardiographic changes. *Amer Heart J* 38:90-96, 1949.
66. Brachfeld, N., Scheuer, J.: Metabolism of glucose by the ischemic dog heart. *Amer J Physiol* 212:603-606, 1967.
67. Prinzmetal, M., Toyoshima, H., Ekmekci, A., et al.: Myocardial ischemia. Nature of ischemic electrocardiographic patterns in the mammalian ventricles as determined by intracellular electrocardiographic and metabolic changes. *Amer J Cardiol* 8:493-503, 1961.
68. Toyoshima, H., Prinzmetal, M., Horiba, M., et al.: The nature of normal and abnormal electrocardiograms. *Arch Int Med* 115:4-16, 1965.
69. Case, R. B., Nasser, M. G., Crampton, R. S.: Biochemical aspects of early myocardial ischemia. *Amer J Cardiol* 24:766-775, 1969.
70. Maroko, P. R., Kjekshus, J. K., Sobel, B. E., et al.: Factors influencing

infarct size following experimental coronary artery occlusions. *Circulation* **43**:67-82, 1971.

71. Maroko, P. R., Libby, P., Covell, J. W., et al.: Precordial ST segment elevation mapping: an atraumatic method for assessing alterations in the extent of myocardial ischemic injury. The effects of pharmacologic and hemodynamic interventions. *Amer J Cardiol* **29**:223-230, 1972.

72. Scheuer, J., Brachfeld, N.: Coronary insufficiency: Relations between hemodynamic, electrical and biochemical parameters. *Circ Res* **18**:178-189, 1966.

73. Shell, W. E., Sobel, B. E.: Infarct size index: an effective predictor of prognosis after myocardial infarction. *Circulation* **48**:IV-39, 1973.

74. Maroko, P. R., Kjekshus, J., Sobel, B., et al.: The correlation between myocardial creatine phosphokinase activity and epicardial changes following experimental myocardial infarction. *Clin Res* **18**:116, 1970.

75. Maroko, P. R., Libby, P., Kjekshus, J. K., et al.: Decrease in the size of experimental myocardial infarct following acute coronary occlusion by glucose- insulin-potassium infusion (GIP). *Clin Res* **19**:167, 1971.

76. Kjekshus, J. K., Sobel, B. E.: Depressed myocardial creatine phosphokinase activity following experimental myocardial infarction. *Circ Res* **27**:403-414, 1970.

77. Watanabe, T., Covell, J. W., Maroko, P. R., et al.: Effects of increased arterial pressure and positive inotropic agents on the severity of myocardial ischemia in the acutely depressed heart. *Amer J Cardiol* **30**:371-377, 1972.

78. Pelides, L. J., Reid, D. S., Thomas, M., et al.: Inhibition by β-blockade of the ST-segment elevation after acute myocardial infarction in man. *Cardiovasc Res* **6**:295-301, 1972.

79. Becker, L. C., Ferreira, R., Thomas, M.: Effect of propranolol and isoproterenol on regional left ventricular blood flow and epicardial ST segment height in experimental myocardial ischemia. *Amer J Cardiol* **31**:119, 1973.

80. Peterson, D. F., Kaspar, R. L., Bishop, V. S.: Reflex tachycardia due to temporary coronary occlusion in the conscious dog. *Circ Res* **32**:652-659, 1973.

81. Swank, R. L., Edwards, M. J.: Microvascular occlusion by platelet emboli after transfusion and shock. *Microvasc Res* **1**:15-22, 1968.

82. Shell, W. E., Sobel, B. E.: Changes in infarct size following administration of propranolol in the conscious dog. *Amer J Cardiol* **31**:157, 1973.

83. Scheidt, S.: Personal communication, 1974.

84. Maroko, P. R., Bernstein, E. F., Libby, P., et al.: Effects of intraaortic balloon counterpulsation on the severity of myocardial ischemic injury following acute coronary occlusion. Counterpulsation and myocardial injury. *Circulation* **45**:1150-1159, 1972.

85. Maroko, P. R., Libby, P., Ginks, W. R., et al.: Coronary artery reperfusion. I. Early effects on local myocardial function and the extent of myocardial necrosis. *J Clin Invest* **51**:2710-2716, 1972.

86. Ginks, W. R., Sybers, H. D., Maroko, P. R., et al.: Coronary artery reperfusion. II. Reduction of myocardial infarct size at one week after coronary occlusion. *J Clin Invest* **51**:2717-2723, 1972.

87. Libby, P., Maroko, P. R., Bloor, C. M.: Reduction of experimental myocardial infarct size by corticosteroid administration. *J Clin Invest* **52**:599-607, 1973.

88. Kones, R. J.: Are corticosteroids in large doses beneficial in cardiogenic shock? *Jap Heart J* **14**:281-285, 1973.

89. Mjøs, O. D.: Effect of free fatty acids on myocardial function and oxygen consumption in intact dogs. *J Clin Invest* **50**:1386-1389, 1971.

90. Mjøs, O. D.: Effect of inhibition of lipolysis on myocardial oxygen consumption in the presence of isoproterenol. *J Clin Invest* **50**:1869-1873, 1971.

91. Henderson, A. H., Most, A. S., Parmley, W. W., et al.: Depression of myocardial contractility in rats by free fatty acids during hypoxia. *Circ Res* **26**:439-449, 1970.

92. Kjekshus, J. K., Mjøs, O. D.: Effect of free fatty acids on myocardial function and metabolism in the ischemic dog heart. *J Clin Invest* **51**:1767-1776, 1972.

93. Kjekshus, J. K., Sobel, B. E.: Depressed myocardial creatine phosphoskinase activity following experimental myocardial infarction in rabbit. *Circ Res* **27**:403-414, 1970.

94. Kjekshus, J. K., Mjøs, O. D.: Effect of inhibition of lipolysis on infarct size after experimental coronary artery occlusion. *J Clin Invest* **52**:1770-1778, 1973.

95. Maroko, P. R., Libby, P., Bloor, C. M., et al.: Reduction by hyaluronidase of myocardial necrosis following coronary artery occlusion. *Circulation* **46**: 430-437, 1972.

96. Reese, L., Scheidt, S., Killip, T.: Variability of precordial ST segment maps after acute myocardial infarction in man. *Circulation* **48** (suppl IV): IV-38, 1973.

97. Neil, W. A., Krasnow, N., Levine, H. J., et al.: Myocardial anaerobic metabolism in intact dogs. *Amer J Physiol* **204**:427-432, 1963.

98. Ballinger, W. F., II, Vollenweider, H.: Anaerobic metabolism of the heart. *Circ Res* **2**:681-685, 1962.

99. Jennings, R. B.: Myocardial ischemia-observations, definitions and speculations. *J Mol Cell Cardiol* **1**:345-349, 1970.

100. Maroko, P. R., Libby, P., Sobel, B. E., et al.: Effect of glucose-insulin-potassium infusion on myocardial infarction following experimental coronary artery occlusion. *Circulation* **45**:1160-1175, 1972.

101. In reference 29, pp. 172, 365-367, 477, 486.

102. Gunning, J. F., Harrison, E. C., Jr., Coleman, H. N., III: The effects of chronic potassium deficiency on myocardial contractility and oxygen consumption. *J Mol Cell Cardiol* **4**:139-153, 1972.

103. Harrison, E. C., Jr., Cooper, G., IV, Zujko, K. J., et al.: Myocardial and mitochondrial function in potassium depletion cardiomyopathy. *J Mol Cell Cardiol* **4**:633-649, 1972.

104. Logic, J. R.: Electrophysiologic effects of regional hyperkalemia in the canine heart. *Proc Soc Exp Biol Med* **141**:725-730, 1972.

105. Logic, J. R.: Enhancement of the vulnerability of the ventricle to fibrillation (VF) by regional hyperkalemia. *Cardiovasc Res* **7**:501-507, 1973.

106. Antoni, H.: Disturbances of transmembrane $Na^+$ and $K^+$ fluxes and their role in the pathogenesis of cardiac dysrhythmias. Proc VI Annual Meeting International Study Group for Research in Cardiac Metabolism; Freiburg, Germany, 25-28 Sept. 1973.

107. MacLeod, D. P., Daniel, E. E.: Influence of glucose on the transmembrane action potential of anoxic papillary muscle. *J Gen Physiol* **48**:887-889, 1965.

108. Prasad, K.: Glucose metabolism and transmembrane electrical activity of cardiac ventricular muscle. Univ. of Alberta, Ph.D. Thesis, 1967.

109. Prasad, K., MacLeod, D. P.: Agents affecting the action of glucose on the electrical activity of anoxic papillary muscle. *Proc Canad Fed Biol Soc* **9**:44-49, 1966.

110. Trautwein, W., Dudel, J.: Aktionpotential und Kontraktion des Herzmuskels im Sauerstoffmangel. *Pflueger Arch Ges Physiol* **263**:23-32, 1956.

111. Yang, W. C.: Anaerobic functional activity of isolated rabbit atria. *Amer J Physiol* **205**:781-784, 1963.

112. Prasad, K.: Substrate-dependent effects of ouabain on the transmembrane

action potentials and contractions of human heart *in vitro*. *Pharmacologist* **10**:186, 1968.

113. Prasad, K., Callaghan, J. C.: Effects of glucose metabolism on the trans-
     membrane action potential and contraction of human papillary muscle dur-
     ing surgical anoxia. *Ann Thoracic Surg* **7**:571-581, 1969.
114. Prasad, K., Callaghan, J. C.: Effect of replacement of potassium by rubidium
     on the transmembrane action potential and contractility of human papillary
     muscle. *Circ Res* **24**:157-166, 1969.
115. Morgan, H. E., Henderson, M. J., Regen, D. M., et al.: Regulation of glucose
     uptake in muscle. I. The effects of insulin and anoxia on glucose transport
     and phosphorylation in the isolated perfused rat heart of normal rats. *J Biol
     Chem* **236**:253-261, 1961.
116. Morgan, H. E., Neely, J. R., Wood, R. E., et al.: Factors affecting glucose
     transport in heart muscle and erythrocytes. *Fed Proc* **24**:1040-1045, 1965.
117. Morgan, H. E.: Regulation of metabolism in normal and ischemic heart
     muscle, Lecture, American College Cardiology 23rd Annual Session, New
     York City, Feb. 11, 1974.
118. Morgan, H. E., Randle, P. J.: Regulation of glucose uptake by muscle. III.
     Effects of insulin, anoxia, salicylate, 2′,4′-dinitrophenol on membrane trans-
     port and intracellular phosphorylation of glucose in the isolated rat heart.
     *Biochem J* **73**:573-579, 1959.
119. Weissler, A. M., Kruger, F. A., Baba, N., et al.: Role of anaerobic metab-
     olism in the preservation of functional capacity and structure of anoxic
     myocardium. *J Clin Invest* **47**:403-416, 1968.
120. Scheuer, J., Stezoski, S. W.: Protective role of increased myocardial glycogen
     stores in cardiac anoxia in the rat. *Circ Res* **27**:835-849, 1970.
121. Evans, C.: The glycogen content of the rat heart. *J Physiol* **82**:468-480,
     1934.
122. Daw, J. C., Wenger, D. P., Berne R. M.: Relationship between cardiac
     glycogen and tolerance to anoxia in the western painted turtle, *Chrysemys
     picta bellii*. *Comp Biochem Physiol* **22**:69-73, 1967.
123. MacLeod, D. P., Prasad, K.: Influence of glucose on the transmembrane
     action potential of papillary muscle. Effects of concentration phlorizin and
     insulin, nonmetabolizable sugars, and stimulators of glycolysis. *J Gen Physiol*
     **53**:792-815, 1969.
124. Nakamura, K., Saunders, P. R., Webb, J. L., et al.: Metabolism of the heart
     in relation to drug action. IV. Effects of various substrates upon the isolated
     perfused rat heart. *Amer J Physiol* **158**:269-278, 1949.
125. Opie, L. H., Shipp, J. C., Evans, J. R., et al.: Metabolism of glucose-U-C[14]
     in perfused rat heart. *Amer J Physiol* **203**:839-843, 1962.
126. Winburz, M. M.: Influence of glucose on contractile activity of papillary
     muscle during and after anoxia. *Amer J Physiol* **187**:135-138, 1956.
127. Kipnis, D. M., Cori, C. F.: Studies on tissue permeability. V. The penetra-
     tion and phosphorylation of 2-deoxyglucose in the rat diaphragm. *J Biol
     Chem* **234**:171-177, 1959.
128. Fisher, R. B., Zachariah, P.: The mechanism of the uptake of sugars by the
     rat heart and the action of insulin on this mechanism. *J Physiol* **158**:73-85,
     1961.
129. Hunter, E. G., McDonald, T. F., MacLeod, D. P.: Metabolic depression
     and myocardial potassium. *Pfluegers Arch Ges Physiol* **335**:266-278, 1972.
130. Webb, J. L., Hollander, P. B.: Metabolic aspects of the relationship between
     the contractility and membrane potentials of the rat atrium. *Circ Res* **4**:618-
     626, 1956.
131. Kipnis, D. M., Helmreich, E., Cori, C. F.: Studies on tissue permeability.

IV. Distribution of glucose between plasma and muscle. *J Biol Chem* **234**: 165-170, 1959.

132. Lotspeich, W. D.: Phlorizin and the cellular transport of glucose. *Harvey Lectures* **56**:63-91, 1960-1961.

133. Diedrich, D. F.: Competitive inhibition of intestinal glucose transport by phlorizin analogs. *Arch Biochem Biophys* **117**:248-256, 1966.

134. Kones, R. J.: The catecholamines: reappraisal of their use for acute myocardial infarction and the low cardiac output syndromes. *Crit Care Med* **1**:203-220, 1973.

135. Katz, A. M., Repke, D. I.: Calcium-membrane interactions in the myocardium: effects of ouabain, epinephrine, and 3′,5′-cyclic adenosine monophosphate. *Amer J Cardiol* **31**:193-201, 1973.

136. Kones, R. J.: The equivalent electric circuit for the heart cell membrane. *Medikon* (Belgium): in press.

137. Brooker, G.: Oscillation of cyclic adenosine monophosphate concentration during the myocardial contraction cycle. *Science* **182**:933-934, 1973.

138. Kones, R. J.: The molecular and ionic basis for altered myocardial contractility. *Res Commun Chem Pathol Pharmacol* **5** (suppl 1): 1-84, 1973.

139. Villar-Palasi, C., Larner, J.: A uridine co-enzyme linked pathway of glycogen synthesis in muscle. *Biochem Biophys Acta* **30**:449, 1958.

140. Villar-Palasi, C., Larner, J.: Insulin treatment and increased UDPG-glycogen transglucosylase activity in muscle. *Arch Biochem Biophys* **94**:436-442, 1961.

141. Williams, B. J., Mayer, S. E.: Hormonal effects on glycogen metabolism in the rat heart *in situ*. *Molec Pharmacol* **2**:454-464, 1966.

142. Prasad, K., Callaghan, J. C.: Influence of glucose metabolism on ouabain-induced changes in the transmembrane potential and contraction of human heart in vitro. *Canad J Physiol Pharmacol* **48**:801-812, 1970.

143. Prasad, K.: Influence of energy supply and calcium on the low sodium induced changes in the transmembrane potential and contraction of guinea pig papillary muscle. *Canad J Physiol Pharmacol* **48**:241-253, 1970.

144. Kones, R. J.: Digitalis-reappraisal of its use after myocardial infarction. *Cardiology* **59**:1-18, 1974.

145. Schwartz, A., Matsui, H., Laughter, A. H.: Tritiated digoxin binding to $(Na^+ + K^+)$-activated adenosine triphosphatase: possible allosteric site. *Science* **160**:323-325, 1968.

146. Prindle, K. H., Jr., Skelton, C. L., Epstein, S. E., et al.: Influence of extracellular potassium concentration on myocardial uptake and inotropic effect of tritiated digoxin. *Circ Res* **28**:337-345, 1971.

147. Goldman, R. H., Coltart, D. J., Friedman, J. P., et al.: The inotropic effects of digoxin in hyperkalemia. Relation to $(Na^+,K^+)$-ATPase inhibition in the intact animal. *Circulation* **48**:830-838, 1973.

148. Coren, H. L., Jr.: Effects of digitalis and hypoxia on potassium transfer and distribution in the dog heart. *Amer J Physiol* **184**:548-552, 1956.

149. McDonald, T. F., MacLeod, D. P.: The effect of 2′,4′-dinitrophenol on the electrical and mechanical activity metabolism and ion movements in guinea-pig ventricular muscle. *Brit J Pharmacol* **44**:711-722, 1972.

150. Gerlings, E. D., Miller, D. T., Gilmore, J. P.: Oxygen availability: a determinant of myocardial potassium balance. *Amer J Physiol* **216**:559-562, 1969.

151. Regan, T. J., Harman, M. A., Lehan, P. H., et al.: Ventricular arrhythmias and $K^+$ transfer during myocardial ischemia and intervention with procaine amide, insulin, or glucose solution. *J Clin Invest* **46**:1657-1668, 1967.

152. Case, R. B., Roselli, M. A., Crampton, R. S.: Relation of ST depression to metabolic and hemodynamic events. *Cardiologia* **48**:32-41, 1966.

153. Case, R. B., Nasser, M. G., Crampton, R.: Biochemical aspects of early myocardial ischemia. *Amer J Cardiol* **24**:766-774, 1969.

154. Jennings, R. B., Crout, J. R., Smitters, G. W.: Studies on distribution and localization of potassium in early myocardial ischemic injury. *Arch Path* **63**: 586-592, 1957.

155. Tsuchida, T.: Experimental studies of the excitability of ventricular musculature in infarcted region. *Jap Heart J* **6**:152-164, 1965.

156. Mandel, W. J., Burgess, M. J., Neville, J., Jr., et al.: Analysis of T-wave abnormalities associated with myocardial infarction using a theoretic model. *Circulation* **38**:178-188, 1968.

157. Prasad, K., Callaghan, J. C.: Electrophysiologic basis of use of a polarizing solution in the treatment of myocardial infarction. *Clin Pharm Therap* **12**: 666-675, 1971.

158. McDonald, T. F., MacLeod, D. P.: Anoxic atrial and ventricular muscle electrical activity, cell potassium, and metabolism: a comparative study. *J Mol Cell Cardiol* **5**:149-159, 1973.

159. McDonald, T. F., MacLeod, D. P.: Maintenance of resting potential in anoxic guinea pig ventricular muscle: electrogenic sodium pumping. *Science* **172**:570-572, 1971.

160. Kones, R. J., Benninger, G. W.: Digitalis in ischemic heart disease. *Heart and Lungs* **4**:99-103, 1975.

161. Obeid, A., Smulyan, H., Gilbert, R., et al.: Regional metabolic changes in the myocardium following coronary artery ligation in dogs. *Amer Heart J* **83**:189-196, 1972.

162. Schwartz, A., Wood, J. M., Allen, J. C., et al.: Biochemical and morphologic correlates of cardiac ischemia. I. Membrane systems. *Amer J Cardiol* **32**:46-61, 1973.

163. Zipes, D. P.: Electrolyte derangements in the genesis of arrhythmias, in *Cardiac Arrhythmias*, edited by Dreifus, L. S., Likoff, W., Grune and Stratton, New York, 1973, pp. 35-54.

164. Fisch, C.: Relation of electrolyte disturbances to cardiac arrhythmias. *Circulation* **47**:408-419, 1973.

165. Zipes, D. P., Fisch, C.: Potassium et troubles du rythme. *Coeur Med Intern* **11**:277-291, 1972.

166. Brandy, A. J., Woodbury, J. W.: Effects of sodium and potassium on repolarization in frog ventricular fibers, in *The Electrophysiology of the Heart*, edited by Hecht, H., *Ann N Y Acad Sci* **65**:687-692, 1957.

167. Coraboeuf, E., Otsuka, M.: L'action des solutions hyposodiques sur les potentiels cellulaires de tissu cardiaque de mammiferes. *C R Acad Sci D* **243**:441-444, 1956.

168. Délèze, J.: Perfusion of a strip of mammalian ventricle: Effects of K-rich and Na-deficient solutions on the transmembrane potentials. *Circ Res* **7**:461-465, 1959.

169. Fisch, C., Knoebel, S. B., Feigenbaum, H., et al.: Potassium and the monophasic action potential, electrocardiogram, conduction and arrhythmias. *Progr Cardiovasc Dis* **8**:387-418, 1966.

170. Surawicz, B.: Evaluation of treatment of acute myocardial infarction with potassium, glucose and insulin. *Progr Cardiovasc Dis* **10**:545-560, 1968.

171. Mudge, G. H.: Cellular mechanisms of potassium metabolism. *Lancet* **73**: 166-168, 1953.

172. Ettinger, P. O., Regan, T. J., Oldewurtel H. A., et al.: Ventricular conduction delay and arrhythmias during regional hyperkalemia in the dog. *Circ Res* **33**:521-531, 1973.

173. Ling, G. N.: *A Physical Theory of the Living State: The Association-Induction Hypothesis*, New York, Blaisdell, 1962.

174. Ling, G. N.: Physiology and anatomy of the cell membrane: The physical state of water in the living cell. *Fed Proc* **23**:103-112, 1965.
175. Ling, G. N.: Studies on ion permeability. I. What determines the rate of Na⁺ ion efflux from frog muscle cells? *Physiol Chem Phys* **2**:242-248, 1970.
176. Ling, G. N., Miller, C., Ochsenfeld, M. M.: The physical state of solutes and water in living cells according to the Association-Induction Hypothesis. *Ann N Y Acad Sci* **204**:6-50, 1973.
177. Ling, G. N., Bohr, G.: Studies on ion distribution in living cells. II. Cooperative interaction between intracellular potassium and sodium ions. *Biophys J* **10**:519-538, 1970.
178. Ling, G. N., Cope, F. W.: Potassium ion: Is the bulk of intracellular K⁺ adsorbed? *Science* **163**:1335-1336, 1969.
179. Ling, G. N., Gerard, R. W.: External potassium and the membrane potential of single muscle fibers. *Nature* **165**:113-114, 1950.
180. Ling, G. N.: Muscle electrolytes. *J Phys Med* **34**:89-101, 1955.
181. Ling, G. N., Gerguson, E.: Studies on ion permeability. 2. Does exchange diffusion make a significant contribution to the Na⁺ ion efflux in frog muscles? *Physiol Chem Phys* **2**:216, 1970.
182. Ling, G. N.: Tentative hypothesis for selective ionic accumulation in muscle cells. *Amer J Physiol* **167**:806-807, 1951.
183. Ling, G. N.: The role of phosphate in the maintenance of the resting potential and selective ionic accumulation in frog muscle cells in *Phosphorus Metabolism*, edited by McElroy, Glass, B., The Johns Hopkins Press, Baltimore, Vol. 2, 1952, pp. 748-797.
184. Ling, G. N.: The physical state of water in living cell and model systems. *Ann N Y Acad Sci* **125**:401-417, 1965.
185. Ling, G. N.: The membrane theory and other views for solute permeability, distribution and transport in living cells. *Persp Biol Med* **9**:87-106, 1965.
186. Ling, G. N.: All-or-none absorption by living cells and model protein-water systems: Discussion of the problem of "permease induction" and determination of secondary and tertiary structure of protein. *Fed Proc Symp* **25**:958-970, 1966.
187. Ling, G. N., Ochsenfeld, M. M.: Studies in ion accumulation in muscle cells. *J Gen Physiol* **49**:819-843, 1966.
188. Ling, G. N.: A new model for the living cell: a summary of the theory and recent experimental evidence in its support. *Intern Rev Cytol* **26**:1-61, 1969.
189. Ling, G. N.: Measurement of potassium ion activity in the cytoplasm of living cells. *Nature* **221**:386-387, 1969.
189a. Minkoff, L., Damodian, R.: Caloric catastrophe. *Biophys J* **13**:167-178, 1973.
189b. Minkoff, L., Damadian, R.: Reply to letters on "Caloric catastrophe." *Biophys J* **14**:69-72, 1974.
190. Ling, G. N., Ochsenfeld, M. M.: Control of cooperative adsorption of solutes and water in living cells by hormones, drugs and metabolic products. *Ann N Y Acad Sci* **204**:325-336, 1973.
190a. Edelmann, L.: The influence of rubidium and cesium ions on the resting potential of guinea-pig heart muscle cells as predicted by the association-induction hypothesis. *Ann N Y Acad Sci* **204**:534-537, 1973.
190b. Wissner, S. B.: The effect of excess lactate upon the excitability of the sheep Purkinje fiber. *J Electrocardiol* **7**:17-26, 1974.
191. Han, J.: Ventricular vulnerability during acute coronary occlusion. *Amer J Cardiol* **24**:857-864, 1969.
192. Burgess, M. J., Abildskov, J. A., Millar, K., et al.: Time course of vulner-

ability to fibrillation after experimental coronary occlusion. *Amer J Cardiol* **27**:617-621, 1971.

193. Tsuchida, T.: Experimental studies of the excitability of ventricular musculature in infarcted region. *Jap Heart J* **6**:152-164, 1965.

194. Mandel, W. J., Burgess, M. J., Neville, J., Jr., et al.: Analysis of T-wave abnormalities associated with myocardial infarction using a theoretic model. *Circulation* **38**:178-188, 1968.

195. Wolff, C. A., Veith, F., Lown, B.: A vulnerable period for ventricular tachycardia following myocardial infarction. *Cardiovasc Res* **2**:111-121, 1968.

196. Penna, M., Illanes, A., Rivera, J., et al.: Electrogram changes induced by lack of metabolites on isolated guinea pig heart. *Acta Physiol Lat Amer* **7**:110-116, 1957.

197. Penna, M., Illanes, A., Pupkin, M.: Effects of adenosinetriphosphate and potassium chloride on ventricular fibrillation induced by lack of substrates. *Circ Res* **10**:642-646, 1962.

198. Maciel, J. P., Mancini, D., Girnenez, H., et al.: Tratamients de algunas cardiopatias con la terpeutica polarizante. *Pren Méd Argent* **50**:2995-3005, 1963.

199. Mittra, B.: Potassium, glucose and insulin in treatment of myocardial infarction. *Lancet* **2**:607-609, 1965.

200. Mittra, B.: Potassium, glucose and insulin in treatment of heart block after myocardial infarction. *Lancet* **2**:1438-1441, 1966.

201. Mittra, B.: Potassium, glucose and insulin in the treatment of myocardial infarction. *Brit Heart J* **29**:616-620, 1967.

202. Mittra, B.: Resolution of ECG changes in myocardial infarction after potassium, glucose, and insulin therapy. *Postgrad Med J* **43**:701-705, 1967.

203. Mittra, B.: Effects of potassium, glucose and insulin therapy on cardiac arrest after myocardial infarction. *Irish J Med Sci* **1**:373-385, 1968.

204. Mittra, B.: Use of potassium, glucose and insulin in the treatment of myocardial infarction. *Progr Cardiovasc Dis* **10**:529-544, 1968.

205. Mittra, B.: Arrhythmias in myocardial infarction. *Geriatrics* **24/2**:155-168, 1969.

206. Mittra, B.: Potassium, glucose and insulin for arrhythmias in myocardial infarction. *Geriatrics* **24/3**:125-143, 1969.

207. Mittra, B.: Polarizing treatment in acute myocardial infarction in *Textbook of Coronary Care*, edited by Meltzer, L. E., Dunning, A. J., The Charles Press, Philadelphia, 1972, pp. 316-327.

208. Fritz, E.: Untersuchungen zur behandlung des myokardinfarktes mit insulin-glukose-infusionen. *Z Kreislaufforsch* **54**:274-287, 1965.

209. Pilcher, J., Etishamudin, M., Exon, P., et al.: Potassium, glucose and insulin in myocardial infarction. *Lancet* **1**:1109-1110, 1967.

210. Lundman, T., Orinius, E.: Insulin-glucose-potassium infusion in acute myocardial infarction. *Acta Med Scand* **178**:525-528, 1965.

211. Day, H. W., Averill, K.: Recorded arrhythmias in an acute coronary care area. *Dis Chest* **49**:113-118, 1966.

212. Kernohan, R. J.: Potassium, glucose and insulin in acute myocardial infarction. *Lancet* **1**:620, 1967.

213. Iisalo, E., Kallio, V.: Potassium, glucose and insulin in the treatment of acute myocardial infarction. *Curr Ther Res* **11**:209-215, 1969.

214. Lal, H. B., Caroli, R. K.: Observations on 400 cases of acute myocardial infarction treated with insulin, potassium and dextrose infusions. *Indian J Med Res* **56**:1120-1136, 1968.

215. Cotterill, J. A., Hughes, J. P., Jones, R., et al.: G.I.K. for myocardial infarction. *Lancet* **1**:1176-1177, 1970.

216. Malach, M.: Polarizing solution in acute myocardial infarction. *Amer J Cardiol* **19**:141, 1967.
217. Medical Research Council Working Party: Report on the treatment of myocardial infarction. Potassium, glucose and insulin treatment for acute myocardial infarction. *Lancet* **2**:1355-1360, 1968.
218. Pentecost, B. L., Mayne, N. M. C., Lamb, P.: Controlled trial of intravenous glucose, potassium and insulin in acute myocardial infarction. *Lancet* **1**:946-948, 1968.
219. Regan, T. J., Frank, M. J., Lehan, P. H., et al.: Relationship of insulin and strophanthidin in myocardial metabolism and function. *Amer J Physiol* **205**: 790-794, 1963.
220. Levinson, R. S., McIlduff, J. B., Regan, T. J.: Comparison of polarizing solution and isovolumic KCl in digitalis-induced ventricular tachycardia. *Amer Heart J* **80**:70-79, 1970.
221. Hiatt, N., Sheinkopf, J. A., Warner, N. E.: Prolongation of survival after circumflex artery ligation by treatment with massive doses of insulin. *Cardiovasc Res* **5**:48-53, 1971.
222. Visscher, M. B., Muller, E. A.: The influence of insulin on the mammalian heart. *J Physiol* **62**:341-348, 1926.
223. Kones, R. J., Phillips, J. H.: Glucagon-present status in cardiovascular disease. *Clin Pharm Therap* **12**:427-444, 1971.
224. Hiatt, N., Katz, J.: Modification of cardiac and hyperglycemic effects of epinephrine by insulin. *Life Sci* **8** (part 1): 551-558, 1969.
225. Hiatt, N., Sheinkopf, J. A., Katz, J.: Insulin blockade of epinephrine. *Endocrinology* **87**:186-191, 1970.
226. Sodi-Pallares, D., Ponce de Leon, J., Bisteni, A., et al.: Potassium, glucose and insulin in myocardial infarction. *Lancet* **1**:1315-1316, 1969.
227. Oliver, M. F., Kurien, V. A., Greenwood, T. W.: Relation between serum-free-fatty-acids and arrhythmias and death after acute myocardial infarction. *Lancet* **1**:710-714, 1968.
228. Dykes, J. R. W., Saxton, C., Taylor, S. H.: Insulin secretion in cardiogenic shock. *Brit Med J* **2**:490, 1969.
229. Moffitt, E. A., Molnar, G. D., Plath, J. R., et al.: Effects on metabolism and cardiac output of glucose-potassium solution, with and without insulin. *Ann Thoracic Surg* **15**:1-15, 1973.
230. Moffitt, E. A., Rosevear, J. W., Molnar, G. D., et al.: The effect of glucose-insulin-potassium solution on ketosis following cardiac surgery. *Anesthesia Analgesia* **50**:291-297, 1971.
231. Stanley, A. W., Moraski, R. E., Russell, R. O., et al.: Effects of glucose-insulin-potassium on myocardial fuel consumption. *Circulation* **48** (suppl IV): IV-221, 1973.
232. Stanley, A. W., Jr., Moraski, R. E., Russell, R. D., Jr., et al.: Alteration of myocardial fuel and oxygen extraction by glucose-insulin-potassium. *Clin Res* **22**:13A, 1974.
233. Opie, L. H.: The glucose hypothesis: relation to acute myocardial ischemia. *J Mol Cell Cardiol* **1**:107-115, 1970.
234. Lochner, A., Opie, L. H., Gray, A., et al.: Coronary artery ligation in the baboon as a model of acute myocardial infarction: failure of glucose, potassium, and insulin treatment to influence mitochondrial metabolism and energetics, in *Myocardial Metabolism: Recent Advances in Studies on Cardiac Structure and Metabolism*, edited by Dhalla, N. S., Rona, G., University Park Press, Baltimore, 1973, Vol. 3, pp. 685-690.
235. Taylor, S. H., Majid, P. A.: Insulin and the heart. *J Mol Cell Cardiol* **2**:293-317, 1971.
236. Majid, P. A., Ghosh, P., Pakrashi, B. C., et al.: Insulin secretion after open

heart surgery with particular respect to the pathogenesis of low cardiac output state. *Brit Heart J* **33**:6-11, 1971.

237. Taylor, S. H.: Insulin and heart failure. *Brit Heart J* **33**:329-333, 1971.
238. Sharma, B., Majid, P. A., Pakrashi, B. C., et al.: Insulin secretion in heart failure. *Brit Med J* **2**:396-398, 1970.
239. Majid, P. A., Saxton, C., Dykes, J. R. W., et al.: Autonomic control of insulin secretion and the treatment of heart failure. *Brit Med J* **2**:328-334, 1970.
240. Schelbert, H. R., Covell, J. W., Burns, J. W., et al.: Observations on factors affecting local forces in the left ventricular wall during acute myocardial ischemia. *Circ Res* **29**:306-316, 1971.
241. Henderson, A. H.: Heart muscle mechanics and hypoxia. *J Mol Cell Cardiol* **5**:121-124, 1973.
242. Majid, P. A., Sharma, B., Meeran, M. K. M., et al.: Insulin and glucose in the treatment of heart failure. *Lancet* **2**:937-941, 1972.
243. Espina, L., Gould, L., Reddy, C. V. R., et al.: Hemodynamic evaluation of glucose-insulin-potassium infusions. *Circulation* **48**:IV-161, 1973.
244. Wildenthal, K., Crie, J. S., Vastagh, G. F.: Cardiovascular function and survival during severe systemic hypoxemia: Influence of glucose-potassium-insulin solution and of beta-blockade. *Cardiovasc Res* **7**:174-180, 1973.
245. Moffitt, E. A., Rosevear, J. W., Molnar, G. D., et al.: Myocardial metabolism in open-heart surgery. *J Thoracic Cardiovasc Surg* **59**:691-706, 1969.
246. Moffitt, E. A., Molnar, G. D., McGoon, D. C.: Myocardial and body metabolism in fatal cardiogenic shock after valvular replacement. *Circulation* **44**:237-244, 1971.
247. Bradley, R. D., Branthwaite, M. A.: Circulatory effects of potassium, glucose and insulin following open-heart surgery. *Thorax* **25**:716-719, 1970.
248. Hales, C. N., Milner, R. D. G.: The role of sodium and potassium in insulin secretion from rabbit pancreas. *J Physiol* **194**:725-743, 1968.
249. Triner, L., Papayoanou, J., Killian, P., et al.: Effects of ouabain on insulin secretion in the dog. *Circ Res* **25**:119-127, 1969.
250. Saxton, C., Majid, P. A., Clough, G., et al.: Effect of ouabain on insulin secretion in man. *Clin Sci* **42**:57-62, 1972.
251. Kypson, J., Triner, L., Nahas, G. G.: Effects of ouabain and K⁺ free medium on activate lipolysis and epinephrine stimulated glycogenolysis. *J Pharmacol Exper Ther* **159**:8-17, 1968.
252. Triner, L., Kypson, J., Nahas, G. G.: Interaction of ouabain with the metabolic effects of epinephrine. *Pharmacologist* **9**:236-239, 1967.
253. Wilhelm, S. K.: Alterations in serum potassium and sodium in acute myocardial infarction. *Amer J Clin Path* **21**:146-148, 1957.
254. Berman, D. A., Masnoka, D. T., Saunders, P. R.: Potentiation by ouabain of contractile response of myocardium to glucose. *Science* **126**:746-747, 1957.
255. Kien, G. A., Sherrod, T. R.: The effect of digoxin on the intermediary metabolism of the heart as measured by glucose-C¹⁴ utilization in the intact dog. *Circ Res* **8**:188-198, 1960.
256. Lorber, V.: Energy Metabolism of the completely isolated mammalian heart in failure. *Circ Res* **1**:298-311, 1953.
257. Darforth, W. H., McKinsey, J. J., Stewart, J. T.: Transport and phosphorylation of glucose in the dog heart. *J Physiol* **162**:367-384, 1962.
258. Wildenthal, K., Skelton, C. L., Coleman, H. N.: Cardiac muscle mechanics in hyperosmotic solutions. *Amer J Physiol* **217**:302-306, 1969.
259. Goldner, M. G., Zarowitz, H., Akun, S.: Hyperglycemia and glycosuria due to thiazide derivatives administered in diabetes mellitus. *New Eng J Med* **262**:403-405, 1960.

260. Corin, J. W.: Hypertension. The potassium ion and impaired carbohydrate tolerance. *New Eng J Med* **273**:1135-1143, 1965.
261. Ferguson, M. J.: Saluretic drugs and diabetes mellitus. *Amer J Cardiol* **7**:568-569, 1961.
262. Howell, S. L., Taylor, K. W.: Effects of diazoxide on insulin secretion *in vitro*. *Lancet* **1**:128-129, 1966.
263. Wolff, F. W., Parmley, W. W.: Etiological factors in benzothiadiazine hyperglycemia. *Lancet* **2**:697, 1963.
264. Wolff, F. W., Langdon, R. G., Ruebner, B. H., et al.: A new form of experimental diabetes. *Diabetes* **12**:335-338, 1963.
265. Loubatieres, A., Mariani, M. M., Alric, R.: Demonstration of the actions of diazoxide on insulin secretion medullo-adrenal secretion and the liberation of catecholamines. *Ann N Y Acad Sci* **150**:226-241, 1968.
266. Staquet, M., Nabwangu, J., Wolff, F.: The effect of thiazide on the blood sugar of alloxanized and suballoxanized rats. *Metabolism* **14**:1307-1320, 1965.
267. Wales, J. K., Spechtmeyer, H., Viktora, J. K., et al.: Clinical studies in the use of vial diazoxide in postsurgical and functional hypoglycemia. *Med Ann* (D.C.) **37**:460-468, 1968.
268. Porte, D.: Inhibition of insulin release by diazoxide and its relation to catecholamine effects in man. *Ann N Y Acad Sci* **150**:281-291, 1968.
269. Tabachnik, I., Gulbenkian, A.: Mechanism studies with diazoxide. *Ann N Y Acad Sci* **150**:204-218, 1968.
270. Lambert, A. E., Jeanrenand, B., Renold, A. E.: Enhancement of caffeine of glucagon-induced and tolbutamide-induced insulin release from isolated foetal pancreatic tissue. *Lancet* **1**:820, 1967.
271. Malaisse, W. J., Malaisse-Lägae, F., Mayhew, D. A.: A possible role for the adenyl-cyclase system in insulin secretion. *J Clin Invest* **46**:1724-1734, 1967.
272. Bloom, S. R., Daniel, P. M., Johnston, D. I., et al.: Release of glucagon, induced by stress. *Quart J Exp Physiol* **58**:99-108, 1973.
273. Lanaido, S., Segal, P., Esrig, B.: The role of glucagon hypersecretion in the pathogenesis of hyperglycemia following acute myocardial infarction. *Circulation* **48**:797-800, 1973.
274. Gerchikova, T. N.: Changes in sodium and potassium content of plasma and erythrocytes in patients with myocardial infarction. *Fed Proc* **22**:893-896, 1963.
275. Brown, H., Tanner, G. L., Hecht, H. H.: The effects of potassium salts in subjects with heart disease. *J Lab Clin Med* **37**:506-514, 1951.
276. Soffer, A. (ed): *Potassium Therapy: A Seminar*, Charles C Thomas, Springfield, Illinois, 1968.
277. Kunin, A. S., Surawicz, B., Sims, E. A. H.: Decrease in serum potassium concentrations and appearance of cardiac arrhythmias during infusion of potassium with glucose in potassium-depleted patients. *New Eng J Med* **266**:228-233, 1962.
278. Burke, W. M., Asokan, S. K., Moschos, C. B., et al.: Effects of glucose and nonglucose infusions on myocardial potassium ion transfers and arrhythmias during ischemia. *Amer J Cardiol* **24**:713-722, 1969.
279. Kostis, J. B., Mavrogeorgis, E. A., Horstmann, E., et al.: Effect of high concentrations of free fatty acids on the ventricular fibrillation threshold of normal dogs and dogs with acute myocardial infarction. *Cardiology* **58**:89-98, 1973.
280. Dodge, H. T., Hay, R. E., Sandler, H.: Pressure-volume characteristics of the diastolic left ventricle of man with heart disease. *Amer Heart J* **64**:503-511, 1962.

281. McLaurin, L. P., Grossman, W., Stefadouros, M. A., et al.: A new technique for the study of left ventricular pressure volume relations in man. *Circulation* 48:56-64, 1973.

282. Diamond, G., Forrester, J. S., Hargis, J., et al.: The diastolic pressure-volume relationship of the canine left ventricle. *Circ Res* 29:267-275, 1971.

283. Forrester, J. S., Diamond, G., Parmley, W. W., et al.: Early increase in left ventricular compliance after myocardial infarction. *J Clin Invest* 51: 598-603, 1972.

284. Diamond, G., Forrester, J. S.: Effect of coronary artery disease and acute myocardial infarction on left ventricular compliance in man. *Circulation* 45:11-19, 1972.

285. Covell, J. W., Ross, J. W., Jr.: Nature and significance of alterations in myocardial compliance. *Amer J Cardiol* 32:449-455, 1073.

286. McLaurin, L. P., Rolett, E. L., Grossman, W.: Impaired left ventricular relaxation during pacing-induced ischemia. *Amer J Cardiol* 32:751-757, 1973.

287. Leaf, A.: On the mechanism of fluid exchange of tissues *in vitro. Biochem J* 62:241-248, 1956.

288. Kowada, M. A., Ames, A., III, Majno, G., et al.: Cerebral ischemia. I. An improved experimental method for study; cardiovascular effects and demonstration of an early vascular lesion in the rabbit. *J Neurosurg* 28:150-157, 1968.

289. Ames, A., Wright, R. L., Kowada, M., et al.: Cerebral ischemia. II. The no-reflow phenomenon. *Amer J Path* 52:437-453, 1968.

290. Chiang, J., Kowada, M., Ames, A., III, et al.: Cerebral ischemia. III. Vascular changes. *Amer J Pathol* 52:455-476, 1968.

291. Flores, J., DiBona, D. R., Beck, C. H., et al.: The role of cell swelling in ischemic renal damage and the protective effect of hypertonic solute. *J Clin Invest* 51:118-126, 1972.

292. Willerson, J. T., Powell, W. J., Guiney, T. E., et al.: Improvement in myocardial function and coronary blood flow in ischemic myocardium after mannitol. *J Clin Invest* 51:2989-2998, 1972.

293. Hutton, I., Watson, J. T., Templeton, G. H., et al.: Influence of hypertonic mannitol on regional myocardial blood flow during acute myocardial ischemia. *Circulation* 48:IV-179, 1973.

294. Powell, W. J., Jr., Flores, J., DiBona, D. R., et al.: The role of cell swelling in myocardial ischemia and the protective effect of hypertonic mannitol. *J Clin Invest:* in press, 1974.

295. Willerson, J. T., Curry, G. C., Atkins, J. M., et al.: The influence of hypertonic mannitol on hemodynamics and coronary blood flow in patients. *Circulation* 48:IV-7, 1973.

296. Koch-Weser, J.: Influence of osmolarity of perfusate on contractility of mammalian myocardium. *Amer J Physiol* 204:957-962, 1963.

297. Wildenthal, K., Mierzwiak, D. S., Mitchell, J. H.: Acute effects of increased serum osmolarity on left ventricular performance. *Amer J Physiol* 216:898-904, 1969.

298. Atkins, J. M., Wildenthal, K., Horwitz, L. D.: Cardiovascular responses to hypertonic mannitol in anaesthetized and conscious dogs. *Amer J Physiol* 225:132-137, 1973.

299. Smithen, C., Christodoulou, J., Keller, N., et al.: Hemodynamic, metabolic and ultrastructural consequences of hyperosmolal mannitol following myocardial anoxia. *Circulation* 48:IV-10, 1973.

300. Willerson, J. T., Crie, J. S., Adcock, R. C., et al.: The influence of calcium on the inotropic effect on cardiac muscle of hyperosmolar agents. *Circ Res* 21:460, 1973.

301. Gould, L., Reddy, C. V., Gomprecht, R. F.: Effect of glucose-insulin-potassium infusion on the human conduction system. *Amer J Cardiol* **33**: 498-506, 1974.

302. Willerson, J. T., Weisfeldt, M. L., Sanders, C. A., et al.: Influence of hyperosmolar agents on hypoxic papillary muscle function. *Cardiovasc Res* **8**:8-17, 1974.

303. Weissler, A. M., Altschuld, R. A., Gibb, L. E., et al.: Effect of insulin on the performance and metabolism of the anoxic isolated perfused rat heart. *Circ Res* **32**:108-116, 1973.

304. Lolley, D. M., Hewitt, R. L., Drapanas, T.: Retroperfusion of the heart with a solution of glucose, insulin, and potassium during anoxic arrest. *J Thoracic Cardiovasc Surg* **67**:364-370, 1974.

305. Ettinger, P. O., Regan, T. J., Oldewurtel, H. A., et al.: Ventricular conduction delay and asystole during systemic hyperkalemia. *Amer J Cardiol* **33**: 876-886, 1974.

306. Gmeiner, R., Kanpp, E., Dienstl, F.: Effect of insulin on the performance of the hypoxic rat heart. *J Mol Cell Cardiol* **6**:201-206, 1974.

307. Rannels, D. E., Kao, R., Morgan, H. E.: Effect of insulin on lysosomal enzyme activity in perfused rat heart. *Circulation* **47-48** (suppl IV): 25, 1974.

308. Ahmed, S. S., Haider, B., Gamboa, B., et al.: Effect of glucose potassium insulin solution on left ventricular function during acute ischemia. *Fed Proc* **33**:396, 1974.

309. Brachfeld, N.: Ischemic myocardial metabolism and cell necrosis. *Bull N Y Acad Med* **50**:261-293, 1974.

310. Matsumoto, S., Tawara, I., Taneichi, Y.: Angina pectoris induced by intravenous administration of 50% glucose. *Jap Heart J* **15**:218-222, 1974.

311. Dixon, S., Jr., Hyde, S., III, Leonard, R. P., et al.: Failure of glucose-insulin-potassium infusion to modify the consequences of acute coronary artery ligation. *J Thoracic Cardiovasc Surg* **49**:762-766, 1965.

312. Lesch, M., Teichholz, L. E., Soeldner, J. S., et al.: Ineffectiveness of glucose, potassium, and insulin infusion during pacing stress in chornic ischemic heart disease. *Circulation* **49**:1028-1037, 1974.

313. Most, A. S., Gorlin, R., Soeldner, J. S.: Glucose extraction by the human myocardium during pacing stress. *Circulation* **45**:92-96, 1972.

314. Chiong, M. A., West, R., Parker, J. O.: Myocardial balance of inorganic phosphate and enzymes in man. Effects of tachycardia and ischemia. *Circulation* **49**:283-290, 1974.

315. Elliott, W. C., Cohen, L. S., Klein, M. D., et al.: Effects of rapid fructose infusion in man. *J Appl Physiol* **23**:865-868, 1967.

316. Gupta, P. R., Sinka, M. K., Dash, R. J., et al.: Insulin, free fatty acids, and glucose response to intravenous glucagon following myocardial infarction. *Circulation* **49**:357-360, 1974.

317. Kjekshus, J. K.: Effect of inhibition of lipolysis on heart failure following acute coronary occlusion in the dog. *Cardiovasc Res* **8**:73-80, 1974.

318. Meerbaum, S., Lang, T-W, Corday, E., et al.: Progressive alterations of cardiac hemodynamic and regional metabolic function after acute coronary occlusion. *Amer J Cardiol* **33**:60-68, 1974.

319. Corday, E., Lang, T-W, Meerbaum, S., et al.: Closed chest model of intracoronary occlusion for study of regional cardiac function. *Amer J Cardiol* **33**:49-59, 1974.

320. Lang, T-W, Corday, E., Gold, H., et al.: Consequences of reperfusion after coronary occlusion. Effects on hemodynamic and regional myocardial metabolic function. *Amer J Cardiol* **33**:69-81, 1974.

321. Braunwald, E., Maroko, P. R.: The reduction of infarct size—An idea whose time (for testing) has come. *Circulation* **50**:206-209, 1974.

322. Maroko, P. R., Davidson, D. M., Libby, P., et al.: Effect of hyaluronidase on myocardial ischemic injury in patients with acute myocardial infarction. *Clin Res* **21**:436, 1973.

323. Braunwald, E., Maroko, P. R., Libby, P.: Reduction of infarct size following coronary occlusion. *Circ Res* **34-35**(suppl III):192-201, 1974.

324. Maroko, P. R., Carpenter, C. B.: Reduction in infarct size following acute coronary occlusion by the administration of cobra venom factor. *Clin Res* **21**:950, 1973.

325. Nikolalva, L. F., Cherpachenko, N. M., Vesselova, S. A., et al.: Mechanisms of drug action on recovery processes of cardiac muscle in myocardial infarction. *Circ Res* **34-35**(suppl III):202-214, 1974.

326. Thomas, J. X., Jones, C. E., Parker, J. C.: Studies of myocardial adenine nucleotides and metabolites following coronary occlusion. *Fed Proc* **33**:363, 1974.

327. Berne, R. M., Rubio, R.: Adenine nucleotide metabolism in the heart. *Circ Res* **34-35**(suppl III):109-118, 1974.

328. Zelis, R., Lee, G., Mason, D. T.: Influence of experimental edema on metabolically determined blood flow. *Circ Res* **34**:482-490, 1974.

329. Bajusz, E.: Interrelationships between reparative processes in myocardium and the development of congestive heart failure. *Rev Can Biol* **27**:45-60, 1968.

330. Lochner, A., Vanderwalt, J. J., Bajusz, E., et al.: Effects of potassium-glucose-insulin treatment on the histology protein synthesis, and mechanical activity of the myopathic hamster heart, in *Cardiomyopathies. Recent Advances in Studies on Cardiac Structure and Metabolism*, edited by Bajusz, E., Rona, G., University Park Press, Baltimore, 1973, Vol. 2, pp 543-555.

331. Hinton, P., Allison, S. P.: Crystalloid administration in shock and surgical trauma. *Lancet* **2**:594-595, 1969.

332. Hinton, P., Allison, S. P., Littlejohn, S., et al.: Insulin and glucose to reduce catabolic response to injury in burned patients. *Lancet* **1**:767-769, 1971.

333. Allison, S. P., Morley, C. J., Burns-Cox, C. J.: Insulin, glucose and potassium in the treatment of congestive heart failure. *Brit Med J* **3**:675-678, 1973.

# APPENDIX

THERMODYNAMICS AND BIOPHYSICAL CHEMISTRY

X    intensive variable
Y    extensive variable
f(x)  function of x
°C   degree Centigrade
°K   degree Kelvin
$dx$   exact differential of x
$đx$   inexact differential of x
E    internal energy of a system
Q    heat
W    work
H    enthalpy
S    entropy
$\mathcal{E}, \mathcal{E}_m$  electrical potential
P    pressure
V    volume
F    charge
F    the Faraday
A    Helmholtz free energy
G    Gibbs free energy
$\mathcal{F}$    total free energy
$G°$   standard free energy
R    the gas constant (1.987 cal/mol/°)
$G_f°$   standard free energy of formation
$G_f^{°\prime}$   standard free energy change at pH = 7.0
$E^{\ddagger}, E^*$  activation energy of a system
NAD⁺   nicotinamide adenine dinucleotide (formerly DPN)
NADP⁺⁺  nicotinamide   adenine   dinucleotide   phosphate
       (formerly TPN)
FAD    flavin adenine dinucleotide
FMN    flavin mononucleotide

## I. THERMODYNAMICS

The principles of thermodynamics are concerned with the study of energy exchanges and constitute the science of heat and temperature. As such, its laws describe the conversion of heat into mechanical, electrical, and other forms of energy.

Thermodynamics is a self-contained logical structure dealing with macroscopic quantities. It is also a phenomenological theory, and is valuable in that relationships between laws of nature may be derived without any knowledge of the laws themselves. One weakness of thermodynamics is the lack of concern for microscopic events and mechanisms. However, this is simultaneously its strength, for molecular theories must conform to the theories of thermodynamics. Since organisms and intracellular reactions obey the laws of thermodynamics, it is appropriate to discuss these in an appendix. The subject of this monograph is, after all, in a broad sense the energy-balance of the heart, its variation in ischemic heart disease, and the potential of ameliorating a poor energy balance metabolically. The reader interested in a more complete discussion is referred to one or more of the standard treatises on the subject.[1-21]

## A. Definitions

A *system* under thermodynamic consideration constitutes the collection of matter under study. The matter in the region not under study comprises the *environment*. For a given thermodynamic system there exist a number of independent thermodynamic *variables* which completely describe the properties of the system. A system is said to be *isolated* if no heat, work or matter can be exchanged with its surroundings. Closed systems can exchange energy with the environment, but not matter. An *open* system can exchange both matter and energy freely with the environments. A process in which no heat is exchanged with the environment is termed *adiabatic;* one in which no work is done, *isochoric;* one in which the temperature is held constant, *isothermal,* and one in which the pressure is held constant, *isobaric.*

Thermodynamic variables fall into two classes: *intensive* and *extensive.* Intensive variables are those whose values reflect a quality of a system under consideration, and do not require any specification of the quantity of the sample. *Extensive variables* are those which are additive and represent a value of a property of a system summed over all its constituents. Energy in a system, or the ability to do work in a general sense, may be expressed as the product of intensity and capacity variables in the form

$$d\mathrm{E}_j = \mathrm{X}_j d\mathrm{Y}_j$$

where $\mathrm{E}_j$ is the energy transferred, $\mathrm{X}_j$ is the intensive variable or force and $\mathrm{Y}_j$ is the extensive or displacement variable (Table I).[22]

### B. The zero[th] law and temperature

Two bodies are said to be of different *temperature* if they change their properties when in contact with each other, even

**Table I** Intensive and extensive variables in a number of systems.

| system | intensive (Xj) | extensive (Yj) | symbol |
|---|---|---|---|
| unavailable energy in irreversible process | temperature | entropy | TdƟ* |
| transfer of material | chemical potential | number of moles | μdn |
| mechanical-gaseous | pressure | volume | PdV |
| mechanical-surfaces | surface tension | area | ɣ dA |
| mechanical - elastic | tension | length | Τdl |
| electrical | electrical potential | charge volume transferred | Ψdq |
| magnetic | field strength | magnetic intensity transferred | $\vec{H}d\vec{I}$ |
| gravitational | gravitational potential | mass | ∅dm |

**\*** Ɵ is used here instead of the conventional "S".

though no interchange of matter, or chemical, mechanical or electrical (or other forms of energy, as specified in Table I, excluding the first horizontal category) interaction is prevented. It is also possible to define temperature in terms of pressure and volume, *i.e.*, $T = f(P,V)$ and rearrange to consider pressure and temperature the independent variables, rather than pressure and volume. When no further changes occur, *thermal equilibrium* is then said to exist. The existence of temperature is a postulate, sometimes called the zero[th] law of thermodynamics, which may be stated:

> For any body there exists a variable, called the temperature, such that two bodies having the same temperature are in thermal equilibrium when brought into contact.

Temperature scales are then defined as follows: $100°$ centigrade by the phase transformation of water at its boiling point at 1 atm pressure, and $0°$ centigrade as its freezing point when saturated with air at 1 atm pressure. The introduction of the absolute or Kelvin temperature ($°K$) is useful because for an ideal gas, Kelvin temperature is directly proportional to the volume when pressure is constant. The Kelvin degree is defined by the assignment of a value of $273.1600°K$ to the temperature at which point the three phases of water—ice, liquid, and vapor—are in equilibrium.

The formal statement of the zero[th] law is also:

$$\frac{T}{T_0} = \lim_{P \to 0} \frac{(PV)_T}{(PV)_{T_0}}$$

where $T_0$ is the reference temperature, usually $273.16°K$, as mentioned.

## C. The first law

A number of variables are necessary to fully characterize a system under consideration. For instance, the number of moles $n$, the temperature T, and the pressure P specify the *state* of a homogeneous gas of a single molecular species. The variables specifying such a state of a system all have unique values for each given state. A statement of the relationships between such variables is an *equation of state.* Several parameters of interest in thermodynamics are exclusively functions of these variables of state. If a system is taken from one thermodynamic state to another, the difference in the state variables will be independent of the process by which the transition was effected and depend solely upon the initial and final states. The infinitesimal increment of change in a variable which depends on the path taken between initial and final states is an inexact differential, denoted by $d$. For an exact differential, the integral over a closed path, that is, over a cyclical change of state, is zero:

$$\int d\mathrm{f}(x,y)=0,$$

whereas

$$\int d\mathrm{f}(x,y)\neq 0.$$

If the differential of a thermodynamic function is exact, then the function is called a *state function.*

For a closed system

$$d\mathrm{E} \equiv d\mathrm{Q} - d\mathrm{W}$$

which states that the change in internal energy of the system, $d\mathrm{E}$ is defined as the heat, $d\mathrm{Q}$, absorbed by the system, less the work, $d\mathrm{W}$, performed by the system on the environment.

The first law of thermodynamics states that

$$\int d\mathrm{E}=0$$

*i.e.,* the internal energy of a system is a state function. A verbal statement of the first law is that in an isolated system the sum of all forms of energy remains constant, or in any transformation taking place in a closed system the increase in internal energy is equal to the work done on the system added to the heat absorbed by it. The first law places no restriction upon the interconversion of various forms of energy.

An important thermodynamic variable, enthalpy, H, may now be defined

$$H \equiv E + PV.$$

Differentiating and substituting $dE = dQ - dW$, we have

$$dH = dQ - dW + PdV + VdP.$$

In systems of interest to the biochemist the pressure is constant and no external work may be performed other than expansion, or

$$dW = PdV,$$

$$dP = 0$$

and

$$dH_p = dQ_p.$$

Enthalpy is also called the heat content because the change in enthalpy (constant pressure) accompanying a reaction is equal to the heat absorbed, or the heat of reaction. Since enthalpy is a state variable, its change is independent of the path a reaction takes from its initial to its final state. Also of interest to biologists is Hess's Law, a corollary of the above, which states that the heats of reaction for a sequence of reactions are additive.

## D. The second law

For the purpose of illustration, consider an ideal gas with the property that

$$dE = C_v dT,$$

where $C_v$ is the heat capacity at constant volume. Substituting, we have

$$dQ = dE + dW$$

$$= C_v T + P dV$$

$$= C_v dT + \frac{RT}{V} dV.$$

Multiplying by $1/T$ and restricting the equation to reversible processes, we may write

$$\frac{dQ_{rev}}{T} = C_v \frac{dT}{T} + R \frac{dV}{V} = d(C_v \ln T + R \ln V),$$

because the equation of state is valid near equilibrium. The expression ($dQ/T$) is an exact differential even though $dQ$ is not, and defines a new thermodynamic variable *entropy* as follows:

$$dS \equiv \frac{dQ_{rev}}{T}.$$

Although discussed here for ideal gases, this expression is true for all systems. There are several equivalent statements of the second law with relevance for biochemists that will be mentioned.

Lord Kelvin said:

> "it is impossible by means of inanimate material agency
> to derive mechanical effect from any portion of matter
> by cooling it below the temperature of the coldest of
> the surrounding objects."

To further explore and illustrate the second law, let us study heat flow from a reservoir at temperature $T_1$ to a reservoir at temperature $T_2$, where $T_1 > T_2$. The changes in entropies are given by

$$dS_1 = -\frac{dQ}{T_1}$$

and

$$dS_2 = +\frac{dQ}{T_2}.$$

The entropy change for the isolated system taken together is positive:

$$dS = dS_1 + dS_2 = dQ\left(\frac{1}{T_2} - \frac{1}{T_1}\right) > 0$$

Kelvin's statement says that heat cannot be simply converted into work unless accompanied by other changes, which may be regarded as energy "payment" for the conversion. Lewis restated the second law:

> "every spontaneous process is capable of doing work; to reverse such a process requires the performance of work."

These statements do *not* mean that heat cannot be converted into useful work. They *do* state that this conversion of heat cannot be made spontaneous, *i.e.*, without an energy expenditure just for the conversion privilege. The Clausius statement of the second law is therefore not surprising:

> "it is impossible to construct a device, that, operating in a cycle, will produce no effect other than the transfer of heat from a cooler to a hotter body."

Implicit in this discussion is the definition of *reversibility* as a process which occurs without a change in entropy. Spontaneous or irreversible reactions necessarily involve an increase in entropy. All actually occurring processes are irreversible. In the *equilibrium state* entropy is a maximum and may serve as one criterion of equilibrium. Remaining close to equilibrium is not a sufficient condition of reversibility, but it is a necessary condition.

For a closed system in contact with a heat source, the second law may be stated as

$$TdS \geq dQ$$

where T is the temperature of the heat source and equality is true by definition for reversible processes, whereas the inequality sign is applicable for irreversible processes. Thus the entropy of a closed system can never decrease during an adiabatic change in state:

$$dS_{(\text{adiabatic})} \geq 0$$

For reversible transformations, the first and second laws may be combined:

$$dE = TdS - dW.$$

The third law, also known as the Nernst heat theorem, states that at the absolute zero of temperature the entropy of an ordered crystal is zero, which would correspond to a state of complete order.

In formal notation, for a reversible temperature change in a substance at constant pressure:

$$d(S)_p = \frac{d(Q)_p}{T} = \frac{C_p dT}{T}$$

where $C_p$ is the isobaric heat capacity. On integration we have

$$S_T = \int_0^T C_p \frac{dT}{T} + S_0.$$

But between temperatures 0 and T, for each phase transition that occurs there is an associated entropy of transition:

$$\Delta S_{tr} = \Delta H_{tr}/T$$

and

$$S_T = \int_0^T C_p d\ln T + \sum \frac{\Delta H_{tr}}{T_{tr}} + S_0,$$

where "phase transition" includes transitions between crystalline forms.

The third law states that the entropy of a pure crystalline substance at $0°K$ is zero:

$$S_0 = \lim_{T \to 0} S_T = 0,$$

and

$$\lim_{T \to 0} (\Delta G - \Delta H) = 0.$$

The third law is usually given less attention than the first two laws, since it is not as important for the understanding of biochemical reactions, and numerous exceptions exist because most substances do not assume a "pure crystalline" form.

## E. Summary and biological implications of the laws

The first law is a statement of the conservation of energy; the second law places a limitation on the conversion of heat into work. The foundations of thermodynamics are three facts of common experience:

(i) bodies are at equilibrium only when they have the same temperature;

(ii) perpetual motion is impossible, and

(iii) reversal of natural processes in their entirety is impossible. In formal terms:

$$dE = dQ + dW;$$
$$dS = dQ/T \text{ for reversible changes;}$$
$$dS \geq 0 \text{ for changes in isolated systems,}$$
$$\text{and } dE = TdS - dW.$$

The principle that entropy can only increase or remain constant applies only to a closed system which is adiabatically isolated. Whenever a system can exchange either heat or matter with the environment an entropy decrease of the system is permitted under the second law. Entire living organisms are open systems [36] and create negative entropy at the expense of ingestion and metabolism of foodstuffs. In this connection entropy is regarded as an index of disorder.[23]

The importance of thermodynamics in biology has been underscored by the appearance of a number of monographs on the subject.[24-27] Since many biological reactions do not occur at equilibrium, several objections to the use of classical thermodynamics [28] in biology have stressed modern addenda dealing exclusively with nonequilibrium thermodynamics.[29-34]

## F. Generalized energy function

Gibbs introduced the useful concept of chemical work, which allows an expression of $dE$ for chemical systems. If $-dn_i$ moles of the $i^{th}$ chemical species are lost from a system, either by chemical reactions or by transport to the environment, an energy change of $-\mu_i dn_i$ occurs where $\mu$ is the intensive variable of chemical work and is sometimes called the *chemical potential*. In a system with electrical potential, $\mathcal{E}_m$, not uncommon in biology, we may write the state function:

$$dW = PdV - Fdl - \mathcal{E}_m dF - \sum_{i=1}^{R} \mu_i dn_i + \ldots$$

where perhaps a muscle shortens through a distance $l$ with force $F$, and F is the charge moving through the electrical potential $\mathcal{E}_m$. The right portion of the equation describes ways in which energy may enter or leave the system. This equation is open ended and a number of different energy terms may be added. It is evident that

$$dE = TdS - PdV + Fdl + \mathcal{E}_m dF + \sum_{i=1}^{k} \mu_i dn_i + \ldots$$

The chemical potential may be defined as the change in energy of a system resulting from the addition of $dn_i$ moles of the $i^{th}$ component to a system while other intensive variables are maintained constant, $j$ denoting all components of the system other than $i$:

$$\mu_i = \left(\frac{\partial E}{\partial n_i}\right)_{S, V, l, F, n_j \quad j \neq 1.}$$

## G. Free energy

Since many biological processes occur under nonadiabatic conditions, and because entropy is difficult to assess experimentally, two new thermodynamic functions have been defined and serve as a practical index of spontaneity. The Helmholtz free energy A, is given by

$$A \equiv E - TS,$$

and the Gibbs free energy, G, is given by

$$G \equiv E + PV - TS = A + PV.$$

Differentiating, we have

$$dA = dE - TdS - SdT.$$

Combining relations for an isochoric isothermal process, we have

$$dA = dQ - TdS \geq 0,$$

as a criterion of spontaneity. Differentiating further,

$$dG = dE + PdV - TdS + VdP - SdT.$$

For an isobaric, isothermal process in which expansion work is the only form of work that occurs:

$$dG = dQ - TdS \leq 0.$$

$dA$ and $dG$ are both thermodynamic functions of state and hence are exact differentials. The expression using Gibbs free energy is more frequently used in biochemical reactions, since isochoric isothermal conditions are less frequently met than isothermal, isobaric conditions. Nonisothermal systems are beyond the scope of this review [17] but may be analyzed thermodynamically as well.[37]

For straightforward homogeneous phase chemical systems at constant pressure and temperature, using the fact that for reversible transformations $dQ = TdS$, then

$$dG = \sum_{i=1}^{k} \mu_i dn_i.$$

At equilibrium,

$$dG = \Sigma \mu_i dn_i = 0.$$

During a chemical reaction in which reactants are converted into products, the change in G from initial to final state at constant temperature and pressure is:

$$\Delta G = \int_{initial}^{final} dG = 0$$

provided there is a reversible pathway from reactants to products such that each state is an equilibrium state. This holds since $dG = 0$ everywhere along the path. Since G is a state variable, $\Delta G$ has the same value for all paths. Therefore chemical reactions taking place reversibly at constant temperature and pressure occur at constant G.

## H. Total free energy

For the analysis of physiological and biochemical processes, the equation $dG = dQ - TdS \leq 0$ is not applicable, and it becomes necessary to define a new thermodynamic variable, the total free energy, denoted $\mathcal{F}$:

$$\mathcal{F} = A - \sum_i Y_i \left( \frac{\partial E}{\partial Y_i} \right),$$

where $Y_i$ represents all the extensive variables in the system $E = f(Y_i)$. Rewriting,

$$dW = -\sum_i \left( \frac{\partial E}{\partial Y_i} \right) dY_i.$$

The intensive variable associated with a given extensive variable is $X_i$ and we may write:

$$X_i = -\left( \frac{\partial E}{\partial Y_i} \right).$$

Differentiating,

$$d\mathscr{F} = \left[ dE - \sum_i \left( \frac{\partial E}{\partial Y_i} \right) dY_i \right] - TdS - \left[ SdT + \sum_i Y_i \left( \frac{\partial E}{\partial Y_i} \right) \right]$$

Thus for any isothermal process in which all forces in a system remain constant,

$$d\mathscr{F} = dQ - TdS \leq 0.$$

From the expression for $d\mathscr{F}$ above, since $d\mathscr{F}$ is an exact differential and a homogeneous function of the first degree, we have

$$\partial\mathscr{F} = 1,$$

$$\frac{\partial\mathscr{F}}{\partial Y_i} = -\frac{\partial E}{\partial Y_i} = X_i,$$

$$\frac{\partial\mathscr{F}}{\partial T} = -S,$$

$$\frac{\partial\mathscr{F}}{\partial S} = -T, \quad \text{and}$$

$$\frac{\partial\mathscr{F}}{\partial X_i} = Y_i.$$

It may also be shown that

$$\left(\frac{\partial X_i}{\partial T}\right) = \frac{\partial^2 \mathcal{F}}{\partial T \partial Y_i}, \quad \text{and}$$

$$-\left(\frac{\partial S}{\partial Y_i}\right) = \frac{\partial^2 \mathcal{F}}{\partial Y_i \partial T}.$$

Then

$$\left(\frac{\partial X_i}{\partial T}\right) = -\left(\frac{\partial S}{\partial Y_i}\right).$$

Other similar relationships, called the Maxwell reciprocity relations, may be shown to be true, for instance

$$\left(\frac{\partial T}{\partial Y_i}\right) = -\left(\frac{\partial X_i}{\partial S}\right).$$

In terms of these partial derivatives of $\mathcal{F}$, a generalized condition of equilibrium may be stated. The complex equation for $d\mathcal{F}$ (page 354) is true for all paths leading to a given equilibrium state, at constant $\{X_i\}$ and T. If $\{X_i\}$ includes all forces that tend to change the $\{Y_i\}$, then at equilibrium $\mathcal{F}$ will be a minimum with respect to the changes in the set $\{Y_i\}$. At internal equilibrium in an isolated system

$$X_i = \frac{\partial \mathcal{F}}{\partial Y_i} = 0 \quad \text{and}$$

$$\frac{\partial X_i}{\partial Y_i} = \frac{\partial^2 \mathcal{F}}{\partial X_i \partial Y_i} \geq 0.$$

## II. CHEMICAL EQUILIBRIA

Consider a generalized reaction:

$$aA + bB \underset{2}{\overset{1}{\rightleftharpoons}} cC + dD$$

where a, b, c, d are the number of molecules participating in the reaction. The free-energy change $\Delta G$ is given by:

$$\Delta G = \Delta G^\circ + RT \ln \frac{[C]^c[D]^d}{[A]^a[B]^b}$$

in which the terms in brackets are the molar concentrations of A, B, C, D and $a$, $b$, $c$, $d$ are the exponents of the concentrations, R is the gas constant (1.987 cal/mole/°), T is the absolute temperature and $G^\circ$ is the standard free energy change.

The free energy of a substance is usually referenced to the standard free energy of formation, $\Delta Gf^\circ$, defined as the change in free energy accompanying the formation of the substance in its standard state from its elements in their standard states or the total free energy yielded on complete decomposition (Table II). The standard state is the most stable form of substance at one atmosphere pressure and 0°C. The standard free energy change, $G^\circ$, for any reaction is the difference between standard free energies of formation of the products less the free energies of formation of the reactants:

$$\Delta G^\circ = \Sigma \Delta Gf^\circ_{(products)} - \Sigma \Delta Gf^\circ_{(reactants)}, \quad \text{or}$$

$$\Delta G^\circ = cG_C^\circ + dG_D^\circ - aG_A^\circ - bG_B^\circ.$$

When this reaction is at equilibrium, the condition of minimum free energy is met and no further net change is possible. We then have

$$\Delta G^\circ + RT \ln \frac{[C]^c[D]^d}{[A]^a[B]^b} = 0.$$

For the reaction under consideration, the velocity of forward reaction is proportional to the concentrations of the reactants raised to the exponents of the number of molecules, or

$$v_1 = k_1[A]^a[B]^b, \qquad \text{and similarly}$$

$$v_2 = k_2[C]^c[D]^d,$$

where $k_1$ and $k_2$ are individual velocity constants. At equilibrium, $v_1 = v_2$, hence

**Table II** Free energies of formation in kcals/mole at 25° and at atmospheric pressure in aqueous solution at one molal activity unless otherwise stated. Reproduced with permission.[82]

| COMPOUND | $\Delta G^0$ | COMPOUND | $\Delta G^0$ |
|---|---|---|---|
| Acetaldehyde | −33.38 | Glyoxylate⁻ | −112.00 |
| Acetic Acid | −95.48 | Hydrogen (ion) | 0.00 |
| anion⁻ | −88.99 | Hydrogen chloride | −31.35 |
| Acetoacetate⁻ | −118.00 | Hydrogen peroxide | −32.67 |
| Acetone | −38.52 | Hydrogen sulfide | −6.54 |
| *cis* Aconitate³⁻ | −220.51 | anion⁻ | +3.00 |
| DL-Alanine | −89.11 | Hydroxide ion | −37.60 |
| L-Alanine | −88.75 | β-Hydroxybutyric acid | −127.00 |
| L-Alanylglycine | −114.57 | anion⁻ | −121.00 |
| Ammonia (gas) | −3.98 | Isocitrate³⁻ | −277.65 |
| Ammonia (NH₃) | −6.37 | Isopropanol | −44.44 |
| (NH₄) | −19.00 | α-Ketoglutarate⁻ | −190.62 |
| L-Asparagine | −125.86 | Lactate | −123.76 |
| L-Aspartic acid | −172.31 | α-Lactose | −362.15 |
| anion⁻ | −166.99 | β-Lactose | −375.76 |
| anion²⁻ | −154.99 | DL-Leucine | −81.76 |
| *n*-Butanol | −41.07 | L-Leucine | −81.68 |
| Butyric acid | −90.86 | DL-Leucylglycine | −110.90 |
| anion⁻ | −84.28 | Lithium ion⁺ | −70.22 |
| Calcium ion²⁺ | −132.18 | L-Malate²⁻ | −201.98 |
| Carbon dioxide (gas) | −94.26 | β-Maltose | −357.80 |
| Carbon dioxide | −92.31 | Mannitol | −225.29 |
| Carbonic acid | −149.00 | Methanol | −41.88 |
| anion⁻ | −140.31 | Nitrate⁻ | −26.41 |
| anion²⁻ | −126.22 | Nitrite⁻ | −8.25 |
| Carbon monoxide (gas) | −32.81 | Oxalacetate²⁻ | −190.53 |
| Chloride ion⁻ | −40.02 | Oxalate²⁻ | −161.30 |
| Citrate³⁻ | −279.24 | Palmitic acid (solid) | −82.9 |
| Creatine | −63.17 | L-Phenylalanine (solid) | −50.6 |
| Creatinine | −6.91 | Potassium ion⁺ | −67.47 |
| L-Cysteine | −81.21 | Potassium chloride | −97.59 |
| L-Cystine | −159.00 | *n*-Propanol | −42.02 |
| Ethanol | −43.39 | Pyruvate⁻ | −113.44 |
| Formaldehyde | −31.20 | Sodium ion⁺ | −62.59 |
| Fructose | −218.78 | Sodium chloride | −93.94 |
| Formic acid | −85.10 | Sorbitol | −225.31 |
| anion⁻ | −80.00 | Succinic acid | −178.39 |
| Fumaric acid | −154.67 | anion²⁻ | −164.97 |
| anion²⁻ | −144.41 | Sucrose | −370.90 |
| α-D-Galactose | −220.73 | Sulfate²⁻ | −177.34 |
| α-D-Glucose | −219.22 | L-Threonine | −123.00 |
| L-Glutamic acid | −171.76 | L-Tryptophane (solid) | −28.5 |
| anion²⁻ | −165.87 | L-Tyrosine (solid) | −92.2 |
| Glycerol | −116.76 | Urea | −48.72 |
| Glycine | −89.26 | Water (gas) | −54.64 |
| Glycogen (per glucose unit) | −158.30 | Water (liquid) | −56.69 |
| Glycolate⁻ | −126.90 | | |

$$k_1[A]^a[B]^b = k_2[C]^c[D]^d, \qquad \text{or}$$

$$K_{eq} = \frac{k_1}{k_2} = \frac{[C]^c[D]^d}{[A]^a[B]^b} \qquad \text{where } K_{eq} \text{ is the}$$

equilibrium constant.

Returning to our equation at equilibrium and substituting, we have

$$\Delta G° = -RT \ln K_{eq} \qquad \text{or}$$

$$\Delta G° = -2.303 \, RT \log_{10} K_{eq} \qquad \text{and at } 37°C,$$

$$\Delta G° = -1420 \log_{10} K_{eq}.$$

This relation enables us to calculate the free energy change of a reaction from its equilibrium constant at a given temperature. If the $K_{eq}$ for a reaction is 1.0, then $\Delta G° = 0$ and no free energy change occurs when 1 mole of reactants completely react to form product at a 1.0 molar concentration. For $K_{eq} < 1.0$, $\Delta G° > 0$, and for $K_{eq} > 1.0$, $\Delta G° < 0$. Chemical reactions with a negative free energy change are called *exergonic* and proceed spontaneously. Reactions with positive standard free energies are termed *endergonic* since the reaction proceeds only if external free energy is made available. The relationship between $\Delta G°$ and $K_{eq}$ is illustrated in Table III and the standard free energies of some reactions appears in Table IV.

## III. ENERGY TRANSFER IN METABOLIC PROCESSES

### A. General principles

Before considering the free energies of particularly illustrative reactions, it is appropriate to observe several features about metabolic processes:

1. The systems under consideration usually can exchange matter with their surroundings, *i.e.*, are open

**Table III** Relationship between the equilibrium constant and the standard free-energy change at 25°.

| $K'_{eq}$ | $\Delta G°$, cal |
|---|---|
| 0.001 | +4089 |
| 0.01 | +2726 |
| 0.1 | +1363 |
| 1.0 | 0 |
| 10.0 | −1363 |
| 100.0 | −2726 |
| 1,000.0 | −4089 |

**Table IV** Standard free-energy changes of some chemical reactions (pH = 7.0; T = 25°).

| Reaction | $\Delta G°'$, kcal |
|---|---|
| **Hydrolysis:** | |
| Acid anhydrides: | |
| Acetic anhydride + $H_2O$ $\longrightarrow$ 2 acetate | −21.8 |
| Pyrophosphate + $H_2O$ $\longrightarrow$ 2 phosphate | − 8.0 |
| Esters: | |
| Ethyl acetate + $H_2O$ $\longrightarrow$ ethanol + acetate | − 4.7 |
| Glucose 6-phosphate + $H_2O$ $\longrightarrow$ glucose + phosphate | − 3.3 |
| Amides: | |
| Glutamine + $H_2O$ $\longrightarrow$ glutamate + $NH_4^+$ | − 3.4 |
| Glycylglycine + $H_2O$ $\longrightarrow$ 2 glycine | − 2.2 |
| Glycosides: | |
| Sucrose + $H_2O$ $\longrightarrow$ glucose + fructose | − 7.0 |
| Maltose + $H_2O$ $\longrightarrow$ 2 glucose | − 4.0 |
| **Rearrangement:** | |
| Glucose 1-phosphate $\longrightarrow$ glucose 6-phosphate | − 1.7 |
| Fructose 6-phosphate $\longrightarrow$ glucose 6-phosphate | − 0.4 |
| **Elimination:** | |
| Malate $\longrightarrow$ fumarate + $H_2O$ | + 0.75 |
| **Oxidation:** | |
| Glucose + $6O_2$ $\longrightarrow$ $6CO_2$ + $6H_2O$ | −686 |
| Palmitic acid + $23O_2$ $\longrightarrow$ $16CO_2$ + $16H_2O$ | −2338 |

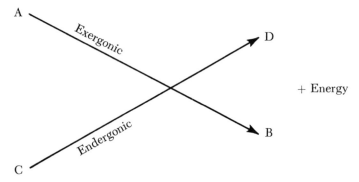

**Figure 1A**  Coupling of an exergonic to an endergonic reaction.[35]

2. The individual reactions are catalyzed enzymatically.
3. Chemical reaction systems are frequently not spatially homogenous and therefore spatial flows of matter and the geometrical constraints of the system are important.
4. Coupling between reactions and between exergonic reactions and endergonic processes, *e.g.*, charge transport, frequently occurs (Figs. 1 and 2).

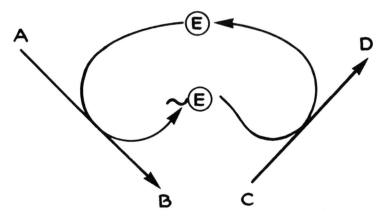

**Figure 1B**  Transference of free energy from an exergonic to an endergonic pathway through formation of a high-energy intermediate compound.[35]

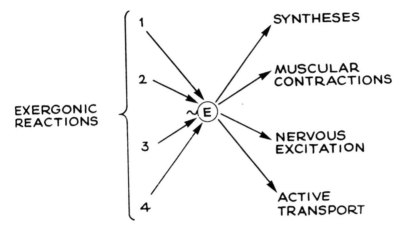

**Figure 2** Transduction of energy through a common high-energy compound to energy-requiring (endergonic) biologic processes.[35]

5. The steady state, rather than equilibrium, is the usual experimental situation encountered.

6. Metabolic conversions in which there is a large change in free energy associated with the overall process tend to occur stepwise with the free energy of each reaction step relatively small, and therefore

7. The number of consecutive reaction steps involved in most metabolic sequences is large.

8. Whenever water is a reactant or product, its thermodynamic activity is set at 1.0, even though the concentration of water is nearly 55.5 molar in the systems considered.

9. pH 7.0 is designated the reference state in biochemical reactions, rather than a pH of 0.0, as is used in physical chemistry. The standard free energy change at pH 7.0 is denoted $\Delta G^{\circ\prime}$.

10. The $\Delta G^{\circ\prime}$ values usually used in biochemistry are based upon the ratio of ionized to unionized substance at pH 7.0. Since the extent of ionization of one or more components of the system may vary with pH, $\Delta G^{\circ\prime}$ may also vary substantially with pH.

## B. Energy-rich compounds

In 1932 Harden and Young [38] reported that the fermentation of glucose by yeast juice abated rapidly in the absence of inorganic phosphate. After addition of phosphate, an abrupt rise in the rate of fermentation occurred coincident with inorganic phosphate disappearance and increase in organic phosphate. About the same time, Lundsgaard [39-41] noted that a muscle poisoned with iodoacetate could contract 40-50 times even though glucose metabolism was inhibited. During these residual contractions phosphorylcreatine and adenosine triphosphate were hydrolyzed as inorganic phosphate was liberated. Muscle exhaustion occurred when all the creatine phosphate had disappeared. Later work by Embden, Meyerhof, Parnes, Cori and others [42, 43] showed that the organic phosphates present in the fermentation of glucose were glucose-6-phosphate, fructose-6-phosphate and fructose-1, 6-diphosphate and were also intermediates in the metabolism of glycogen and glucose in muscle. Fiske and Subbarow [44] and Eggleton and Eggleton [45] demonstrated the breakdown of creatine phosphate during muscle contraction and its resynthesis during recovery from exercise. Meyerhoff and Suranyi [46] reported that the enzymatic breakdown of creatine phosphate was exergonic and that this energy liberated was stored in the N-P bond of the molecule. Meyerhof and Lohmann [47] discovered that arginine phosphate in invertebrate muscle was the counterpart of creatine phosphate in vertebrate muscle, since the N-P bond of arginine phosphate also released much energy when broken. Lohmann [48] isolated adenosine triphosphate (ATP) from muscle, a compound from which phosphate groups may be consecutively removed, yielding adenosine diphosphate (ADP) and adenosine monophosphate (AMP) (Fig. 3). Lohmann [49] further studied the decomposition of ATP and found that it preceded that of creatine phosphate:

$$ATP + H_2O \rightarrow ADP + P_i$$

$$\Delta G' = -8 \text{ kcal/mole.}$$

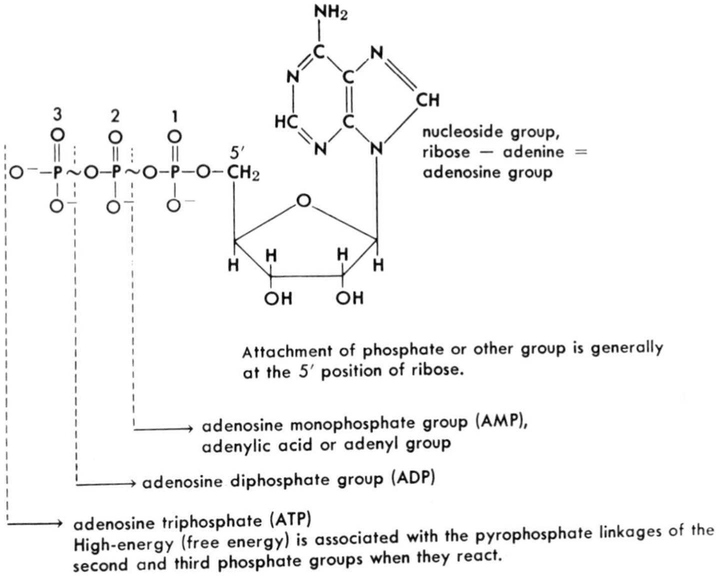

**Figure 3** Structure of ATP with component groups illustrated.

He also observed that the breakdown of creatine phosphate was not due to hydrolysis but to reaction with ADP:

$$\text{creatine phosphate} + \text{ADP} \rightleftharpoons \text{ATP} + \text{creatine}$$

$$\Delta G' = -3 \text{ kcal/mole.}$$

This reaction (also known as the Lohmann reaction) is reversible and serves to replenish the supply of ATP after ATP is used for muscle contraction. Thus creatine phosphate serves as an energy reservoir to restore the N-P bonds of ATP after their hydrolysis.

The use of molecules such as ATP as a driving force for a number of endergonic reactions has led to a classification of some compounds as high energy or energy-rich and others as low-energy substances. The terminal phosphate bond of ATP is "high energy," as denoted $\sim$P, since it releases much energy when broken, whereas ordinary phosphate esters are considered "low energy." Jencks [50] defined a high energy compound as one whose "reaction with a substance commonly present in the environment is accompanied by a large negative free energy change at physiological pH." As a guide, compounds with a $\Delta G^{\circ\prime}$ of hydrolysis at pH 7.0 less than 7 Kcal/mole and compounds exhibiting an oxidation-reduction potential at pH 7.0 less than the oxygen electrode potential by 0.5 V may be considered "energy-rich."

One must mention that the expression "high-energy bond" has a quite different meaning in biochemistry than in physical chemistry. In physical chemistry, a high energy bond is one which requires a large amount of thermochemical energy for dissociation, and therefore is an index of stability. As per the definition given above, a high energy bond in biochemistry refers to the large free energy decreases associated with reactions of that bond, such as hydrolysis or group transfer. Therefore a high energy substance is not one with a high thermochemical dissociation energy, but one whose reactions are associated with large free energy decreases, *i.e.*, they tend to go to completion.

Energy-rich compounds fall into several groups. The prominent phosphate derivatives are of four categories: phosphoric acid anhydrides, phosphoric-carboxylic anhydrides, phosphoguanidines, and enol phosphates (Figs. 3 and 4). In addition, thiol esters, amino acid esters, and dihydropyridines are among the energy rich substances.

## C. Phosphoric acid anhydrides

The best example of this group is ATP itself, well known for the variety of phosphorylating reactions in which it is a participant (Fig. 5).[51] Table 5 indicates that the hydrolysis of one mole of ATP to AMP and inorganic phosphate liberates over 7 kcal of free energy. Other phosphoric acid anhydrides exhibit similar standard free energies of hydrolysis at pH 7.0. Phosphate anhydrides tend to have high energies of activation and are therefore relatively resistant to nonenzymatic hydrolysis. In order to illustrate the reasons for this energy-rich

**Table V**  Standard free energy of hydrolysis of some phosphorylated compounds.

| | $\Delta G^{\circ\prime}$, kcal | Phosphate group transfer potential† |
|---|---|---|
| Phosphoenolpyruvate | −14.80 | 14.8 |
| 1,3-Diphosphoglycerate | −11.80 | 11.8 |
| Phosphocreatine | −10.30 | 10.3 |
| Acetyl phosphate | −10.10 | 10.1 |
| Phosphoarginihe | − 7.70 | 7.7 |
| ATP | − 7.30 | 7.3 |
| Glucose 1-phosphate | − 5.00 | 5.0 |
| Fructose 6-phosphate | − 3.80 | 3.8 |
| Glucose 6-phosphate | − 3.30 | 3.3 |
| Glycerol 1-phosphate | − 2.20 | 2.2 |

† Defined as $-\Delta G^{\circ\prime} \times 10^{-3}$

situation, consider the compound acetic anhydride, with a large free energy of hydrolysis at pH 7.0. First, the electrophilic carbonyl carbon atom is stabilized by electron donation and destabilized by election withdrawal. Since the acetyl moiety tends to withdraw electrons, it destabilizes acetic anhydride with respect to hydrolysis.

A free energy decrease may occur because of a diminution in electrostatic repulsion between groups in a compound. The hydrolysis of pyrophosphate at pH 7.0 and 25°C illustrates this principle:

$$\underset{\text{Pyrophosphate}}{HO-\overset{\overset{O}{\|}}{\underset{\underset{O^-}{|}}{P}}-O\sim\overset{\overset{O}{\|}}{\underset{\underset{O^-}{|}}{P}}-O^-} + 2H_2O \rightarrow \underset{\text{Phosphate}}{2HO-\overset{\overset{O}{\|}}{\underset{\underset{O^-}{|}}{P}}-O^-} + H_3O^+$$

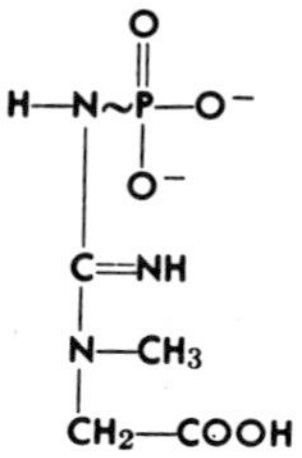

creatine phosphate

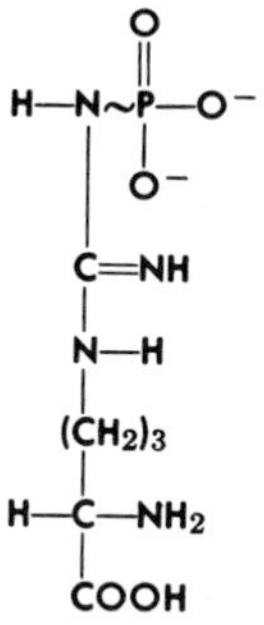

arginine phosphate

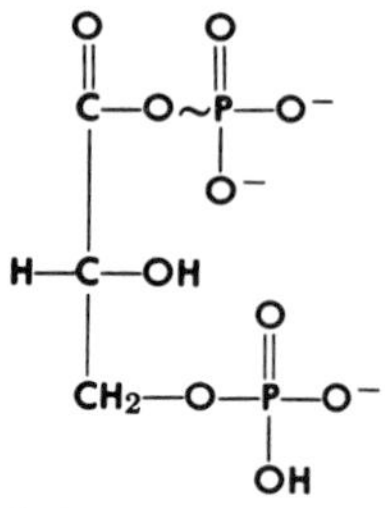

1,3-diphosphoglyceric acid

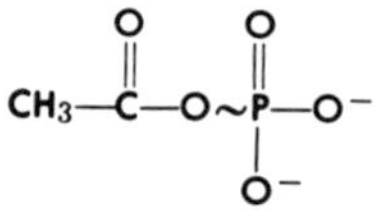

acetyl phosphate

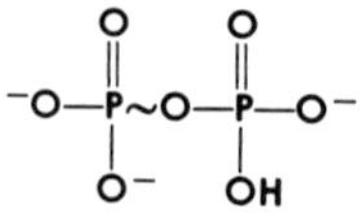

inorganic pyrophosphate

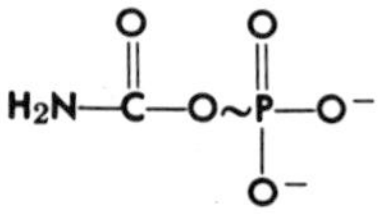

carbamyl phosphate
carbamylating agent

**Fig. 4A** Structures of high energy compounds of biological interest.

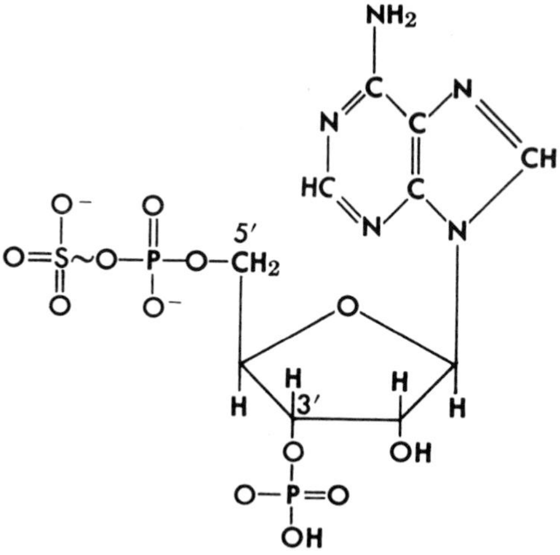

3'-phosphoadenosine-5'-phosphosulfate
"active sulfate"
sulfating agent

Figure 4B.

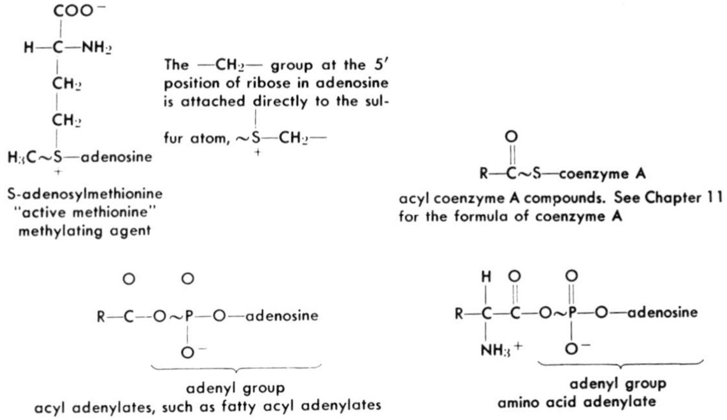

$$
\begin{array}{c}
COO^- \\
| \\
H—C—NH_2 \\
| \\
CH_2 \\
| \\
CH_2 \\
| \\
H_3C\sim S—adenosine \\
+
\end{array}
$$

S-adenosylmethionine
"active methionine"
methylating agent

The —CH$_2$— group at the 5'
position of ribose in adenosine
is attached directly to the sulfur atom, $\sim S—CH_2—$
+

$$
\begin{array}{c}
O \\
\| \\
R—C\sim S—coenzyme\ A
\end{array}
$$

acyl coenzyme A compounds. See Chapter 11
for the formula of coenzyme A

$$
\begin{array}{c}
O \quad\quad O \\
\| \quad\quad \| \\
R—C—O\sim P—O—adenosine \\
| \\
O^-
\end{array}
$$

adenyl group
acyl adenylates, such as fatty acyl adenylates

$$
\begin{array}{c}
H \quad O \quad\quad O \\
| \quad\ \| \quad\quad \| \\
R—C—C—O\sim P—O—adenosine \\
| \quad\quad\quad | \\
NH_3^+ \quad\quad O^-
\end{array}
$$

adenyl group
amino acid adenylate

**Figure 4C.**

The electrostatic repulsion between negative oxygen and phosphate atoms in pyrophosphate is relieved when the compound is hydrolyzed. A similar reaction occurs when ATP is hydrolyzed:

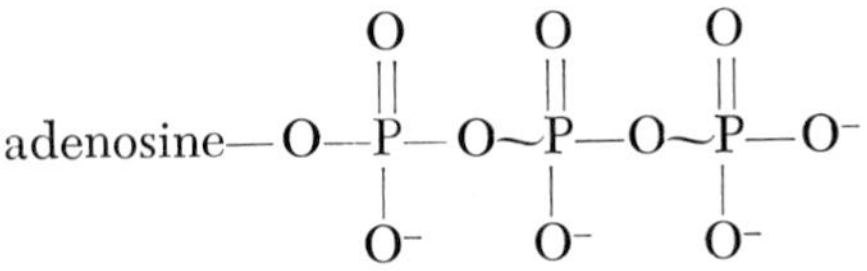

$$
\begin{array}{c}
O \quad\quad O \quad\quad O \\
\| \quad\quad \| \quad\quad \| \\
adenosine—O—P—O\sim P—O\sim P—O^- \\
| \quad\quad | \quad\quad | \\
O^- \quad\ O^- \quad\ O^-
\end{array}
$$

$$ADP + P_i$$
$(\Delta G' = -7\ \text{Kcal/mole})$

$$AMP + PP_i$$
$(\Delta G' = -8.6\ \text{kcal/mole})$

Hydrolysis of the terminal phosphoryl group of ADP at pH 7.4 at 25°C yields a $\Delta G'$ of 6.9 kcal/mole, while hydrolysis of AMP to adenosine and $P_i$ is associated with much less free energy decrease:

$$ADP + H_2O \rightarrow AMP + P_i \quad\quad \Delta G' = -6.9\ \text{kcal/mole}$$

$$AMP + H_2O \rightarrow adenosine + P_i \quad\quad \Delta G' = -3\text{-}4\ \text{kcal/mole}$$

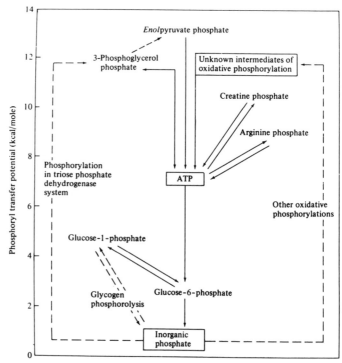

**Figure 5A**    A diagram showing some reactions leading to the formation and utilization of ATP in terms of $\Delta G°$ of the energy-rich compounds involved. Reprinted by permission.[51]

The rapid hydrolysis of ordinary acid anhydrides, such as acetic anhydride, and the relative stability of ATP to hydrolysis has already been mentioned. Lipmann[52] noted that the complete hydrolysis time for acetic anhydride is a few seconds, while that for acetyl phosphate is several hours, and that for pyrophosphate is infinite.

The more stable state of a compound is that form associated with maximum resonance. If hydrolysis converts a substance to a form with greater resonance, the reaction will tend to go to completion, with a decrease in free energy.[53] Considering again the case of acetic anhydride with a resonance energy of 29 kcal/mole, the reaction completes with a resonance energy

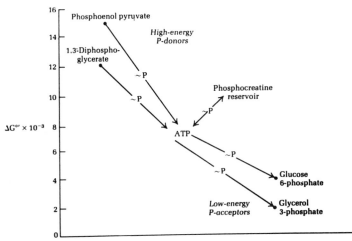

**Figure 5B** Flow of phosphate groups from high-energy phosphate donors to low-energy acceptors via ATP-ADP system.

of two acetate anions at 36 kcal/mole. This loss of resonance energy upon formation of the anhydride results from the fact that the *pi* electrons of the oxygen atom linking the carbonyl carbons cannot satisfy the electronic demand of both carbonyl carbons simultaneously:

$$
\underset{CH_3}{} \overset{\overset{O}{\parallel}}{C} - O - \overset{\overset{O}{\parallel}}{C} - CH_3,
$$

a situation called competing or opposing resonance. Although this mechanism is operative for ATP, the difference in resonance energies between reactants and products is less striking.

Another potential driving force for the hydrolysis of ATP and other polyphosphates is the differential solvation of the reactants and products. If the products are solvated better than the reactants, the reaction will proceed. The relative importance of this mechanism for ATP remains unknown.

The carboxylic-phosphoric anhydrides (exemplified by acetyl phosphate and amino acyl adenylates, Fig. 4) are also energy-rich compounds. The destabilizing influence of the electron-withdrawing phosphate group on the carbonyl moiety, and the decreased resonance energy of the reactants in relation to the products also account for the liberation of much free energy on hydrolysis of these substances.

Phosphoenol pyruvate, an enol phosphate, releases $-14.8$ kcal/mole upon hydrolysis:

$$\begin{array}{ccc} \text{COO}^- & \text{O} & \\ | & \| & \\ \text{C} - \text{O} \sim \text{P} - \text{O}^- + \text{H}_2\text{O} \rightarrow & & \\ \| & | & \\ \text{CH}_2 & \text{O}^- & \end{array} \quad \begin{array}{ccc} \text{O} & \text{COO}^- & \text{COO}^- \\ \| & | & | \\ \text{HO} - \text{P} - \text{O}^- + \text{C} - \text{OH} \rightarrow \text{C} = \text{O} \\ | & \| & | \\ \text{O}^- & \text{CH}_2 & \text{CH}_3 \end{array}$$

phosphopyruvate          enol-     keto-
                        pyruvate  pyruvate

The energy-rich state of phosphoenolpyruvate is due to two factors. The enol of pyruvic acid is less stable than the keto form by approximately 10-12 kcal mole. Thus a free energy decrease is associated with an isomerization of the product of the reaction. The hybridization of the O—P bond in phosphoenol pyruvate is $sp_2$. Such bonds are less stable than $sp_3$ bonds and as a result, enol phosphates are less stable than ordinary phosphate esters.

The phosphoguanides, such as creatine phosphate and arginine phosphate (Fig. 4) are also important biological high energy compounds. The standard free energy of hydrolysis of these substances at physiological pH is approximately $-7$ to $-10$ kcal/mole. Their energy-rich nature is due to the inhibition of the normal resonance of the guanidinium ion. The guanidinium ion, or alkyl guanidinium ion, is a nearly symmetrical species with roughly equal contributions to its stability from each of its valence-bond forms. The large resonance energy associated with this symmetrical species accounts for the very high basicity of the guanidines. The conversion of guanidines to guanidine phosphates destroys the symmetry of this molecule. The resonance form with the positive charge adjacent to the positively charged phosphorus atom is particularly unfavorable:

$$
\begin{array}{ccc}
\overset{\displaystyle H}{\underset{\displaystyle |}{}}\ \overset{\displaystyle N^+H_2}{\underset{\displaystyle \|}{}} & \overset{\displaystyle H}{\underset{\displaystyle |}{}}\ \overset{\displaystyle NH_2}{\underset{\displaystyle |}{}} & \overset{\displaystyle H}{\underset{\displaystyle |}{}}\ \overset{\displaystyle NH_2}{\underset{\displaystyle |}{}} \\
R—N—C & \leftrightarrow R—N^+=C & \leftrightarrow R—N—C \\
\ \ \ |\ & \ \ \ \ \ | & \ \ \ \ \| \\
NH_2 & NH_2 & N^+H_2
\end{array}
$$

$$
\begin{array}{l}
\overset{\displaystyle H}{\underset{\displaystyle |}{}}\ \ \overset{\displaystyle N^+H_2}{\underset{\displaystyle \|}{}}\ \ \ \ \ \overset{\displaystyle O^-}{\underset{\displaystyle |}{}} \\
R—N—C—NH—P^+—O^- \leftrightarrow R—N^+=C—NH—P^+—O^- \\
\ \ \ \ \ \ \ \ \ \ \ \ \ \ |\ \ \ \ \ \ \ \ \ \ \ \ \ \ \ \ \updownarrow \ \ \ \ \ \ \ \ \ | \\
\ \ \ \ \ \ \ \ \ \ \ \ \ \ O^- \ \ \ \ \ \ \ \ \ \ \ \ \ \ \ \ \ \ \ \ \ \ \ \ \ \ \ \ O^-
\end{array}
$$

$$
\begin{array}{l}
\ \ \ \ \ \ \ \ \ \ \ \ \ \ \ \ \ \overset{\displaystyle H}{\underset{\displaystyle |}{}}\ \ \overset{\displaystyle NH_2}{\underset{\displaystyle |}{}}\ \ \ \ \overset{\displaystyle O^-}{\underset{\displaystyle |}{}} \\
\ \ \ \ \ \ \ \ \ \ \ \ \ \ \ \ R—N—C=N^+H—P^+—O^- \\
\ \ \ \ \ \ \ \ \ \ \ \ \ \ \ \ \ \ \ \ \ \ \ \ \ \ \ \ \ \ \ \ \ \ \ | \\
\ \ \ \ \ \ \ \ \ \ \ \ \ \ \ \ \ \ \ \ \ \ \ \ \ \ \ \ \ \ \ \ \ \ O^-
\end{array}
$$

Thiol esters, especially those involving coenzyme A, are important energy-rich compounds, particularly in acyl-group transfer reactions. The diminished resonance interaction between the *pi* electrons of the sulfur atom and the carbonyl group, compared with such interaction in ordinary oxygen esters or in carboxylate anions, provides a driving force for the hydrolysis compared with oxygen esters. Some studies suggest that the sulfur atom not only does not act as an effective electron donor to the carbonyl group, but may actually act as an electron acceptor.[54]

$$
\begin{array}{cc}
\overset{\displaystyle O}{\underset{\displaystyle \|}{}} & \overset{\displaystyle O^-}{\underset{\displaystyle |}{}} \\
R_1—C—O—R_2 & \leftrightarrow R_1—C=O^+—R_2
\end{array}
$$

$$
\begin{array}{ccc}
\overset{\displaystyle O}{\underset{\displaystyle \|}{}} & \overset{\displaystyle O^-}{\underset{\displaystyle |}{}} & \overset{\displaystyle O^+}{\underset{\displaystyle |}{}} \\
R_1—C—S—R_2 & \leftrightarrow R_1—C=S^+R & \leftrightarrow R_1—C=S^-—R
\end{array}
$$

Therefore the inhibition of resonance in the thiol esters provides an explanation for the energy rich nature of these compounds. The increased free energy released on the hydrolysis of acetoacetyl thiol esters as compared with ordinary thiol ester results from destabilization of the thiol esters by the strongly electron withdrawing acetyl substituent in the acyl portion of the molecule.

The amino acid esters are another category of energy-rich compounds, and are important in the biosynthesis of proteins. These compounds release a large amount of free energy on hydrolysis, probably due to destabilization of the ester by the electron-withdrawing ammonium group.

Reduced pyridine nucleotides are the final group of energy-rich substances to be considered here. The transfer of an electron pair from the pyridine nucleotide coenzymes (nicotinamide adenine dinucleotide and nicotinamide adenine dinucleotide phosphate) to oxygen yields energy, since the standard redox potential for the pyridine nucleotides is approximately $-0.32$V. The corresponding free energy change is of the order of 40 kcal/mole, which may be used to synthesize three molecules of ATP.

## D. Thermodynamic analysis of high energy compounds

Oesper [55] noted that an additional free energy change occurred whenever an acid reactant (or an acid hydrolysis product) produced an acid and anion. In general terms:

$$X\!-\!PO_3H^- \overset{k_1}{\rightleftharpoons} X\!-\!PO_3^{-2} + H_2O \overset{k_h}{\rightleftharpoons} HX + HPO_4^{-2}$$
$$\qquad\qquad\quad \updownarrow k_2 \qquad\qquad +$$
$$\qquad\qquad\quad H^+ \qquad\qquad H^+$$
$$\qquad\qquad\quad + \qquad\qquad \updownarrow k_3$$
$$\qquad\qquad\quad X^- \qquad\qquad H_2PO_4^-$$

Hill and Morales [56] reported that the free energy change for the actual equilibrium mixture of the various forms of reactants and products, $\Delta G'$, is given by

$$\Delta G' = \Delta G'_h + \Delta G'_2 + \Delta G'_3 - \Delta G'_1.$$

These investigators found that the free energy contribution from the ionization of the carboxyl group could be written

$$\Delta G_2 = -RT \ln (1 + k_2/[H^+]).$$

For $[H^+] \gg k_2$, $\Delta G_2 = O$. For $[H^+] \ll k_2$,

$$\Delta G_2 = RT \ln\left(\frac{[H^+]}{k_2}\right).$$

Therefore the actual free energy contribution of the hydrolysis reaction is a function of the equilibrium constant of the hydrolysis reaction and the pH of the reaction mixture. Under physiological conditions, the free energy of hydrolysis must be corrected for the concentrations of reactants and products:

$$\Delta G = \Delta G' + RT \ln \frac{[ADP][P_i]}{[ATP]}.$$

For energy-rich compounds with an N—P bond, the greater stability of the O—P bond as compared with the N—P bond (approximately 28 kcal/mole) is nearly exactly offset by the greater stability of the O—H bond in the product (approximately 26.5 kcal/mole). In addition to the free energy contributions of resonance stabilization and ionization, Hill and Morales [56] proposed a contribution from electrostatic repulsion of negative charges on neighboring phosphorus atoms of polyphosphates. Such a contribution would be on the order of magnitude of $-3$ to $-4$ kcal/mole for ADP or phosphoenolpyruvate and $-5$ to $-6$ kcal/mole for ATP.

A different treatment was given by George and Rutman.[57] ATP hydrolysis may be written

$$ATP + H_2O \rightarrow ADP + P_i + \Psi H^+$$

where $\Psi$ may be positive or negative. Since the cleavage of a pyrophosphate linkage releases two ionizing groups, the number of $[H^+]$ produced or consumed will depend on the p$k$'s of the new ionizing groups and upon the pH of the hydrolytic reactions. The observed free energy change is then:

$$\Delta G_{observed} = [\Delta H - T\Delta S] + \Psi RT \ln [H^+].$$

These relationships are depicted in Figure 6, where it will be

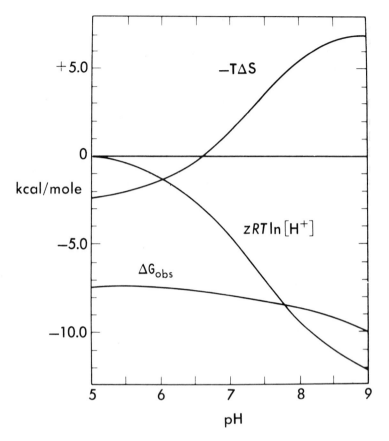

**Figure 6**  The variation of $\Delta F_{observed}$, $\phi RTln[H^+]$, and $-T\Delta S$ for the hydrolysis of ATP yielding ADP over the pH range 5-9.

noted that at pH 7.5, most of the $\Delta G_{observed}$ for ATP hydrolysis is contributed by $\psi RT \ln [H^+]$, while at pH 7.0, the hydrogen ion term contributes about 50% of the total $\Delta G_{observed}$. The unfavorable entropy changes at such pH's is offset by favorable values of $\Delta H$.

### E. Adenosine triphosphate

The value of $\Delta G^{\circ\prime}$ for the hydrolysis of ATP might be calculated from knowledge of the equilibrium constant with use of the relationship

$$\Delta G^{\circ\prime} = -2.303 \, RT \log K'_{eq}.$$

Experimentally, direct measurement of $K'_{eq}$ for this reaction is not easy because of the difficulty in precisely defining equilibrium in a reaction going to completion with a large $\Delta G^{\circ\prime}$. However, since we noted that overall $\Delta G^{\circ\prime}$ for a series of reactions is the sum of individual $\Delta G^{\circ\prime}$ for each, a value of $\Delta G^{\circ\prime}$ for ATP hydrolysis may be indirectly determined.

Consider the reaction

$$ATP + glucose \xrightarrow{\text{hexokinase}} ADP + glucose\text{-}6\text{-}phosphate \quad \text{with}$$

measured values $K'_{eq} = 661$ and $G_1{}^{\circ\prime} = -4.0$ kcal/mole, and

$$H_2O + glucose\text{-}6\text{-}phosphate \xrightarrow{\text{phosphatase}} glucose + P_i$$

with measured values $K'_{eq} = 171$ and $G_2{}^{\circ\prime} = -3.3$ kcal/mole. Then for the reaction

$$ATP + HOH \xrightarrow{\text{Mg}^{++}} ADP + P_i \qquad \text{we have}$$

$$\Delta G^{\circ\prime}{}_{ATP} = \Delta G_1{}^{\circ\prime} + G_2{}^{\circ\prime} = -4.0 + (-3.3) = -7.3 \text{ kcal/mole}$$

at pH 7.0 and $T = 37^\circ$. The free energies of hydrolysis of the two remaining phosphate bonds are

$$ADP + HOH \rightleftharpoons AMP + P_i$$
$$\Delta G^{\circ\prime} = -7.3 \text{ kcal/mole}$$

and

$$AMP + HOH \rightleftharpoons adenosine + P_i$$
$$\Delta G^{\circ\prime} = -3.4 \text{ kcal/mole}$$

The variation in $\Delta G^{\circ\prime}_{ATP}$ with pH has already been mentioned (Figs. 6 and 7). However, since $Mg^{++}$ complexes with each phosphate:

$$Mg^{++} + ATP^{-4} \rightleftharpoons Mg\ ATP^{-2}$$

$$Mg^{++} + ADP^{-3} \rightleftharpoons MgADP^{-}$$

$$Mg^{++} + HPO_4^{-2} \rightleftharpoons MgHPO_4$$

it is apparent that $G^{\circ\prime}_{ATP}$ varies with $[Mg^{++}]$ and even furthers its pH-dependency, since the affinities of each phosphate for $Mg^{++}$ increases with pH. Last, the concentrations of these reactants within intracellular compartments is significantly different than the "standard" conditions at which $\Delta G^{\circ\prime}$ is defined (1.0M). When appropriate corrections are made for pH,

**Effect of pH on free energy of hydrolysis of ATP (25°C).**

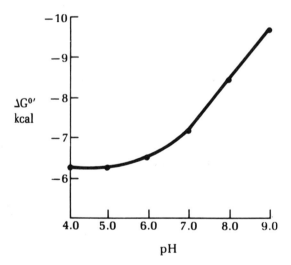

**Figure 7**   Effect of pH on free energy of hydrolysis of ATP (25°C).

[$Mg^{+2}$], and the actual concentrations of ATP, ADP and $P_i$, the $\Delta G_{ATP}$ is nearly $-12.5$ kcal/mole. This value for actual $\Delta G_{ATP}$ need not be spatially homogeneous within the cell for the reasons discussed.

A great many reactions involve the cleavage of the terminal phosphate of a high energy compound:

$$A—R—P{\sim}P{\sim}P \rightarrow A—R—P{\sim}P + P_i,$$

the so-called orthophosphate cleavage. However, in some reactions the two terminal phosphate groups may be removed as a single unit:

$$A—R—P{\sim}P{\sim}P \rightarrow A—R \cdot P + P{\sim}P,$$

the so-called pyrophosphate cleavage. These reactions are but a special case of a class of "group transfer" reactions.[51]

High energy phosphates corresponding to ATP and ADP in which the phosphate groups are linked to nucleosides such as inosine, uridine, cytidine, and guanosine also exist naturally and are called "inosine triphosphate" (ITP), "uridine diphosphate" (UDP), etc. These 5'-di- and 5'-triphosphates of the various ribonucleosides serve as precursors in RNA synthesis but also channel high-energy phosphate groups into specific reactions (Fig. 8A). All channels interconnect with ATP by means of a number of reactions catalyzed by the enzyme nucleoside diphosphokinase (Fig. 8B).

While the reactions responsible for ATP cleavage have been discussed, there are several mechanisms by which ATP may be regenerated. The activity of the enzyme inorganic pyrophosphatase ensures the return of $PP_i$ to the phosphate pool:

$$PP_i + H_2O \rightarrow 2P_i$$

The orthophosphate ($P_i$) so produced becomes available for the resynthesis of ATP (Fig 9). Another enzyme, adenylate kinase or myokinase, catalyzes the regeneration of ADP from AMP:

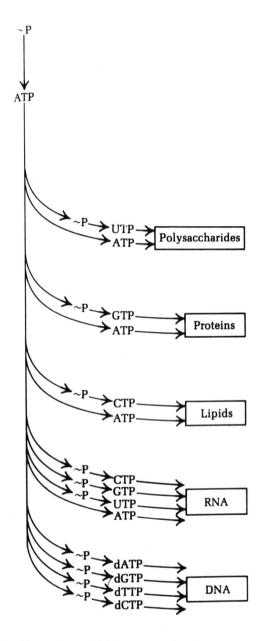

**Figure 8A** Channeling of high-energy phosphate groups into different biosynthetic pathways via the ribonucleoside and deoxyribonucleoside 5′-triphosphates.

## Nucleoside diphosphokinase reactions

$$ATP + UDP \rightleftharpoons ADP + UTP$$

$$ATP + GDP \rightleftharpoons ADP + GTP$$

$$ATP + CDP \rightleftharpoons ADP + CTP$$

$$GTP + UDP \rightleftharpoons GDP + UTP$$

$$ATP + dCDP \rightleftharpoons ADP + dCTP$$

$$GTP + dADP \rightleftharpoons GDP + dATP$$

**Figure 8B** Nucleoside diphosphokinase reactions.

$$ATP + AMP \rightarrow 2ADP.$$

Various other nucleoside (X) monophosphokinases also catalyze the formation of other XDP's from the corresponding XMP's:

$$ATP + XMP \rightleftharpoons ADP + XDP.$$

For completeness it should be mentioned that the notion of a high energy phosphate bond has not been completely accepted and controversy continues.[58] Gillespie, Maw and Vernon [59] and more recently Banks [60] and Banks and Vernon [61] held that cleavage of a bond requires energy and "the 'energetic' interpretation of the function of ATP is totally erroneous and that free energy changes, either actual or standard, are of little relevance." [61] The thermodynamic arguments proposed by these workers were countered by Pauling,[62] Huxley,[63] and Wilkie [64] but no clear conclusion to the dispute emerged.[65, 66]

## IV. REACTION KINETICS

### A. Distribution of energy

In a given population of molecules, distribution of kinetic energy is "random" and is illustrated in Figure 10.[68, 69] In

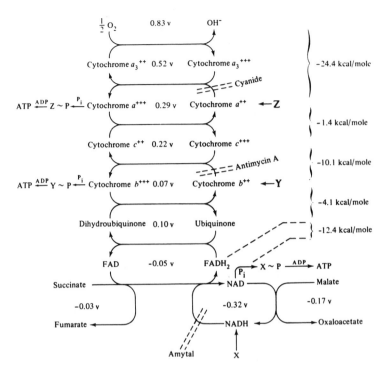

**Figure 9** A schematic representation of a hypothetical organization of the sequential electron transport in mitochondria. The apparent sites of action of various inhibitors are also shown. Approximate values for E' and ΔG' are given for the various reactions. X, Y, and Z are hypothetical intermediates supposedly involved in the coupling of oxidation and phosphorylation.[85]

this plot the fraction of the molecules $\left[ (dn/dv)\left( \dfrac{1}{n_T} \right) \right]$ with mean velocities between $v$ and $v + dv$ (on the ordinate) is shown as a function of $v$ (on the abscissa). Restricting our discussion to two dimensions, we may write

$$\frac{dn}{n_T dv} = \frac{mv}{KT}\exp -\left( \frac{mv^2}{2KT} \right),$$

where $m$ is molecular mass, $\frac{1}{2}mv^2$ is kinetic energy, K is the Boltzmann constant (K = R/N where R is the gas constant

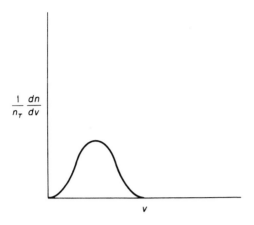

$$\frac{1}{n_T}\frac{dn}{dv}$$

$v$

**Figure 10**    Distribution of velocities of gas molecules or of molecules in an ideal solution. $dn/n_t$ is the fraction of molecules possessing a velocity in the range of $v$ to $v+dv$. The area under the curve has a value of unity.[69]

and N is Avogadro's number) and T is temperature. Defining E, kinetic energy,*

$$E=\frac{mv^2}{2},$$

$$dE=mvdv \qquad\qquad \text{and}$$

$$\frac{dn}{n_T}=\frac{1}{KT}e^{(-E/KT)}dE.$$

In order to determine the fraction of molecules with energy greater than a given value of E we integrate over E to $\infty$:

$$\int_0^n \frac{dn}{n_T}=\frac{1}{KT}\int_E^\infty e, \qquad\qquad \text{or}$$

$$\frac{n}{n_T}=e^{-E/KT} \qquad\qquad \text{which becomes}$$

---

* Notation of E changes for the purpose of this discussion.

$$\ln(n/n_T) = -\frac{E}{KT}.$$

The probability of molecules reacting is a function of their kinetic energy, and for this and other reasons it is common to speak of an activation energy which is required for the reactants to proceed to completion. For a given chemical reaction, a compound may be in a so-called metastable state (Fig. 11, panel a, position 1). An energy of activation, $E^{\dagger}$ must be imparted to the reactant to move it to position 2 (Fig. 11, panel a), following which the reaction proceeds with an increase in entropy and/or decrease in free energy to the equilibrium state. For simple systems with a given amount of energy, some molecules will have sufficient energy to exceed $E^{\dagger}$ (Fig. 11, panel b). The addition of external energy to a system will shift the distribution curve to the right (Fig 11, panel c). In practice the reaction rate constant, $K_T$, proportional to $n/n_T$, is more closely described by another equation because of other variables affecting reaction rate:

$$K_T = e^{-E/KT}a(KT/h)$$

where a is a constant and h is Planck's constant.

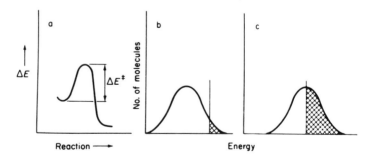

**Figure 11**    $\Delta E^{\dagger}$ corresponds to the activation energy.[69]

## B. Chemical kinetics

### 1. Order of reactions

Chemical reactions may be classified according to the number of reactant molecules whose concentrations influence the velocity of a reaction. In the hypothetical reaction:

$$n_1A + n_2B + n_3C + \ldots \rightarrow m_1X + m_2Y + m_3Z + \ldots$$

there is a velocity of disappearance or formation of each species, *e.g.*, the velocity of disappearance of A is $-d[A]/dt$ and of B, $-d[B]/dt$, etc. If the concentration of A is plotted against time, the slope is the rate constant for component A at a given time (Fig 12).

The order of a reaction is the number of molecules participating in the reaction whose concentrations influence its velocity. In a zero order reaction the velocity is independent of the concentrations of any and all reactants and the reaction velocity is given by

$$\frac{d[A]}{dt} = -k$$

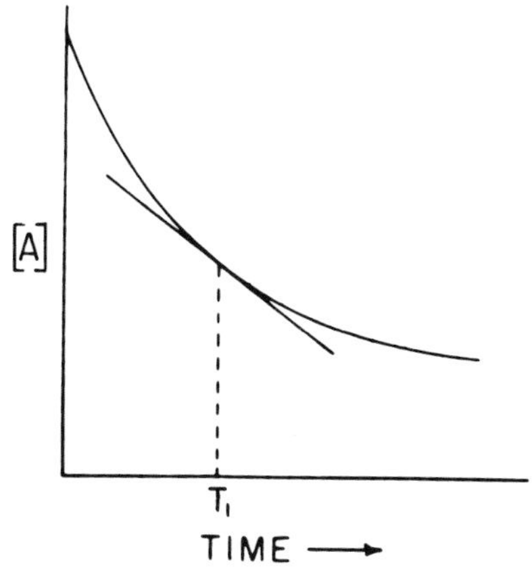

**Figure 12** Hypothetical plot of the concentration [A] against time. The velocity of the reaction after a given time, t, is equal to the slope of the curve.

Integrating, we have

$$[A] = -kT + [A]_0.$$

Plotting A *versus* t describes a linear function whose slope is $-k$ with dimensions $L^{-3}t^{-1}$ (Fig. 13). The time required for one half of the components to react, the $t_{1/2}$, is $= [A]_0/2k$ in zero order reactions. Zero order kinetics are characteristic of surface reactions at substrate concentrations in excess of that required to saturate the surface.

Reactions with a velocity proportional to the concentration of only one component are first-order reactions, and their velocity is described by

$$\frac{d[A]}{dt} = -k[A],$$

for the simplest reaction: $A \rightarrow P$.
Upon integration

$$\ln[A] = \ln [A]_0 - kt, \quad \text{or}$$

$$[A] = [A]_0 e^{-kT}$$

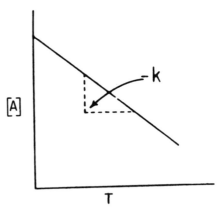

**Figure 13**  Plot of a zero order reaction. The slope of the line is equal to $-k$.

where [A] is the concentration of the rate-controlling reactant at time t and $[A]_0$ is the concentration at $t=0$. $k$ has the dimensions of $t^{-1}$ in first order reactions, and is equal to the reciprocal of the time required for $1/e^{th}$ part of the reactant to react, from the following expression:

$$\frac{[A]}{[A]_0} = \frac{1}{e^{kt}}.$$

Converting to logarithms to the base 10:

$$\log [A] = -\frac{kt}{2.303} + \log_{10}[A]_0.$$

If $\log [A]$ *versus* time is plotted, a straight line will be described (Fig. 14). Plotting [A] *versus* time gives the curve illustrated in Figure 15. The $t_{1/2}$ of first order reactions is given by

$$t_{1/2} = \frac{0.693}{k}$$

from which it is noted that $t_{1/2}$ is independent of the initial concentration of the reactant, $[A]_0$. As an example of a first

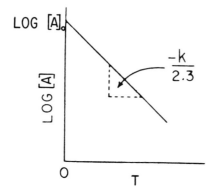

**Figure 14** Hypothetical plot of a first order reaction. The slope of the line is $-k/2.303$.

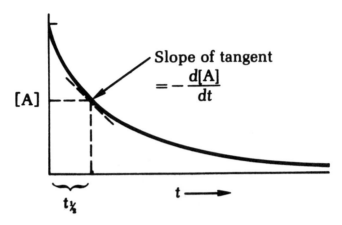

**Figure 15**   Plot of the course of a first-order reaction. The half-time ($t_{1/2}$) is the time required for one-half of the initial reactant to be consumed.

order reaction, we need only cite the diffusion of a substance across a uniplanar surface as per Fick's laws.

The rate of second order reactions depends upon the concentrations of two reactant molecules which may be identical or different. For the reaction:

$$A + B \rightarrow P$$

we have

$$\frac{d[A]}{dt} = \frac{d[B]}{dt} = -\frac{d[P]}{dt} = k[A][B].$$

Letting X be the moles of [A] that have reacted at time t, then the values of [A] and [B] at time t will be $([A]_0 - x)$ and $([B]_0 - rx)$ where $r$ is a factor related to the stoichiometry of the reaction. Substituting,

$$\frac{d[A]}{dt} = -k([A]_0 - x)([B]_0 - rx).$$

Integrating, and evaluating the constant of integration by sub-stituting the initial conditions, $x = 0$ at $t = 0$:

$$kt = \frac{1}{[B]_0 - r[A]_0}\left[\ln\left(\frac{[A]_0}{[A]_0 - x}\right) - \ln\left(\frac{[B]_0}{[B]_0 - rx}\right)\right]$$

$$t = \frac{2.303}{k(r[A]_0 - [B]_0)}\log\frac{[B]_0([A]_0 - x)}{[A]_0([B]_0 - rx)}$$

A plot of $\log [B]_0([A]_0 - x)/[A]_0([B]_0 - rx)$ *versus* t yields a straight line whose slope is $-k([A]_0 - [B]_0)/2.303$. For the special case where

$$2A \rightarrow P, \text{ we have}$$

$$\frac{-d[A]}{dt} = k[A]^2 \qquad \text{which gives}$$

$$\frac{1}{[A]} = kt + \frac{1}{[A]_0}.$$

A plot of $1/[A]$ *versus* time gives a straight line (Fig. 16) with slope $k$. The $t_{1/2}$ for this reaction is

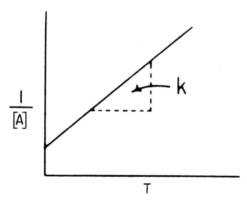

**Figure 16** Second order reaction plot for the condition that the initial concentrations of A and B are equal or that two molecules of A are reacting together. Slope of the line is equal to $k$, the reaction constant.

$$t_{1/2} = \frac{1}{k[\text{A}]_0}.$$

In second order reactions, $k$ has the dimensions of $L^3t^{-1}$. For reactions of the type

$$a\text{A} + b\text{B} + c\text{C} + \ldots \rightarrow \text{P}$$

The reaction velocity is

$$\frac{d[\text{A}]}{dt} = -k[\text{A}]^a[\text{B}]^b[\text{C}]^c \ldots$$

## 2. Reversible reactions

Considering the reversible reactions

$$\text{A} + \text{B} \underset{k_2}{\overset{k_1}{\rightleftharpoons}} \text{C} + \text{D},$$

the rate of reaction, $v$, is given by

$$v = -\frac{d[\text{A}]}{dt} = \frac{d[\text{C}]}{dt} = k_1[\text{A}][\text{B}] - k_2[\text{C}][\text{D}].$$

At equilibrium, as previously mentioned, the reactions occur with equal velocities and there is no net change in any reactant, *i.e.*, $d[\text{A}]/dt = 0$ and therefore as derived:

$$K_{eq} = \frac{k_1}{k_2} = \frac{[\text{C}][\text{D}]}{[\text{A}][\text{B}]}.$$

Integrating and evaluating the constant of integration at the initial equilibrium conditions when $[\text{A}]_0 = [\text{B}]_0$ and $[\text{C}]_{eq} = [\text{D}]_{eq}$:

$$k_1 t = \frac{[\text{C}]_{eq}}{[\text{A}]_0{}^2 - [\text{C}]_{eq}{}^2} \ln\left(\frac{[\text{A}]_0{}^2[\text{C}]_{eq} - [\text{C}]_{eq}[\text{C}]}{[\text{A}]_0{}^2[\text{C}]_{eq} - [\text{A}]_0{}^2[\text{C}]}\right).$$

For the special case in which

$$A + B \underset{k_2}{\overset{k_1}{\rightleftharpoons}} I \xrightarrow{k_3} P,$$

then three equations describe the system as follows:

$$\frac{d[A]}{dt} = \frac{d[B]}{dt} = k_2[I] - k_1[A][B],$$

$$\frac{d[I]}{dt} = k_1[A][B] - (k_2 + k_3)[I],$$

$$\frac{d[P]}{dt} = k_3[I].$$

At time t:

$$[A]_0 - [A] = [B]_0 - [B].$$

One solution for these equations appears in Figure 17. For the situation $k_2 \gg k_3$,

$$\frac{d[P]}{dt} = -\frac{d[A]}{dt} = k_3 K_{eq}[A][B],$$

$$K_{eq} = \frac{k_1}{k_2}.$$

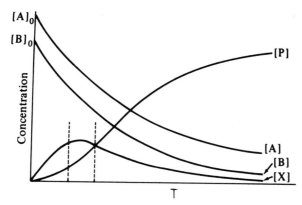

**Figure 17** Progress curve for the reaction sequence mentioned in the text. Reproduced with permission.[84]

For the situation $k_3 \gg k_2 \approx k_1$, P forms quickly and relatively little [I] goes back to A and B, *i.e.*, the formation of [I] is rate-limiting:

$$\frac{d[I]}{dt} = k_1[A][B].$$

## 3. Simultaneous reactions

For the instance in which a reactant may form two products:

$$
\begin{array}{ccc}
 & A & \\
k_1 \swarrow & & \searrow k_2 \\
B & & C
\end{array}
$$

The rate of decomposition is given by:

$$-\frac{d[A]}{dt} = (k_1 + k_2)[A].$$

Upon integration:
$$\ln\frac{[A]_0}{[A]} = (k_1 + k_2)t$$

and rearranging,
$$[A] = [A]_0 e^{-(k_1+k_2)t}.$$

The rate of formation of B is

$$\frac{d[B]}{dt} = k_1[A] = k_1[A]_0 e^{-(k_1+k_2)t}.$$

Integrating, we have

$$[B] = -\frac{k_1[A]_0}{k_1+k_2} e^{-(k_1+k_2)t} + \lambda$$

where $\lambda$ can be evaluated at $t = 0$:

$$\lambda = \frac{k_1[A]_0}{k_1+k_2},$$

and therefore

$$[B] = \frac{k_1[A]_0}{k_1 + k_2} [1 - e^{-(k_1+k_2)t}].$$

Similarly,

$$[C] = \frac{k_2[A]_0}{k_1 + k_2} [1 - e^{-(k_1+k_2)t}],$$

and

$$\frac{[B]}{[C]} = \frac{k_1}{k_2}.$$

### 4. *Consecutive reactions*

Reaction sequences are particularly important in intermediary metabolism. Consider a relatively simple sequence of two consecutive reactions in which the rate constants are of similar magnitude:

$$A \xrightarrow{k_1} B \xrightarrow{k_2} P. \qquad \text{Then}$$

$$\left.\begin{array}{l} \dfrac{d[A]}{dt} = -k_1[A] \\[2em] \dfrac{d[B]}{dt} = k_1[A] - k_2[B] \\[2em] \dfrac{d[P]}{dt} = k_2[B]. \end{array}\right\}$$

Integrating the first expression,

$$[A] = [A]_0 e^{-k_1 t}$$

and substituting in the second:

$$\frac{d[B]}{dt} = k_1[A]_0 e^{-k_1 t - k_2[B]}$$

Then integrating:

$$[B] = \left(\frac{k_1[A]_0}{k_2 - k_1}\right) e^{-k_1 t} - e^{-k_2 t},$$

which is plotted in Figure 18. For all values of t,

$$[A] + [B] + [P] = [A]_0$$

and combining

equations,

$$[P] = [A]_0 - [A]_0 e^{-k_1 t} - \frac{k_1[A]_0}{k_2 - k_1}$$

and rearranging,

$$[C] = \frac{[A]_0}{k_2 - k_1} [k_2(1 - e^{-k_1 t}) - k_1(1 - e^{-k_2 t})].$$

## C. Activated complex and transition state

Continuing with concepts introduced in the section on distribution of energy, we wish to formalize our thoughts as follows.

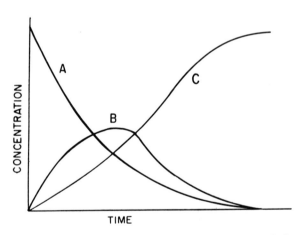

**Figure 18** Hypothetical plots of the concentrations of the reactants in consecutive reactions.

The energy of a reacting system can be described by potential energy surfaces (Fig 19). For a reaction to occur there must be a "saddle point" in the contour of such a descriptive surface which leads to a lower energy state. To pass over the saddle point the molecules must exist in an *activated state* with an energy content greater than that of the reactants in their "normal" state. The average of the increment in energy required to produce the activated state is called the activation energy. Only a fraction of molecules comprising a system with an internal energy greater than a threshold value enter into a reaction via the activated state. The Arrhenius expression for a reaction rate constant, $k_T$, proportional to the number of molecules attaining the activated state, is:

$$k_T = Ze^{-E^*/RT} \text{ or } \frac{d \ln k_T}{dt} = -\frac{E^*}{RT^2}$$

where $E^*$ is the energy of activation, and Z is the frequency factor such that $0 < Z < 1$. The velocity of a reaction is equal to the number of molecules reacting per second in unit volume

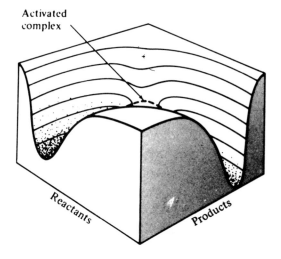

**Figure 19A** Three-dimensional contour model for the energy relations of the reaction sequence mentioned in the text.

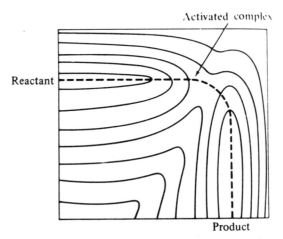

**Figure 19B**  Contour map of Figure 19A showing the reaction path (dotted line) from the reactants, via the activated complex, to the products.

(Z) multiplied by the chance that the colliding particles have sufficient energy to react, $(e^{-E^*/RT})$. The plot of this equation appears in Figure 20. The plot of $\ln k_T$ versus $1/T$ theoretically describes a linear relation, but in practice this is not always

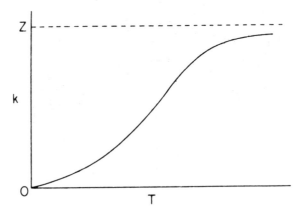

**Figure 20**  Variation of the specific rate constant of a reaction with temperature according to the Arrhenius equation.

true. Not all activated collisions result in reaction because the entire molecular surface is not reactive and therefore the colliding molecules must be properly oriented. We may then write

$$k_T = PZe^{-E^*/RT}$$

where P is the steric factor, $0 \leq P \leq \infty$.

For the hypothetic sequence

$$AB + C \rightleftharpoons ABC^* \rightleftharpoons AC + B,$$
$$_1 \qquad _2 \qquad _3$$

where ABC* is the active complex, we may picture the energy events along a two dimensional cross section of the contour, potential energy as the ordinate (Fig 21). The activated complex ABC* at energy position 2 obeys previously derived relations:

$$\Delta G^* = \Delta H^* - T\Delta S^* = -RT \ln K^*$$

where K* is the equilibrium constant and $\Delta G^*$, $S\Delta^*$, $\Delta H^*$ are the usual thermodynamic variables associated with the formation of ABC*. If M* represents the number of activated complexes per unit volume along distance $\delta$ and $v$ is the mean velocity of ABC* across $\delta$, then the frequency of crossing the energy barrier is $v/\delta$. Only half ABC* moves in either direction:

$$\text{reaction rate} = k[AB][C] = \tfrac{1}{2}M^* \frac{v}{\delta} c,$$

where c is a transmission coefficient and represents the probability of the activated system at position 2 progressing to products (AC + B) at energy level 3. The function c is complex but is commonly close to one for reactions in a homogeneous medium involving simple bond rearrangements, *e.g.*, hydrolysis and group transfers. From statistical mechanics we can say:

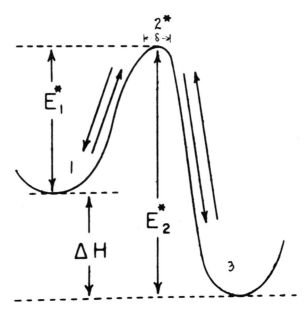

**Figure 21**   Energy pass of a reaction. A diagrammatic representation of the cross-section of pass, $2^*$, leading from one energy valley, 1, which represents the normal state of the reactants, into a second valley, 3, which is the energy level of the products of the reaction. $E_1^*$ represents the energy of activation of the forward reaction and $E_2^*$ that of the opposing reaction. The molecules pass from the normal state, 1, to the activated state, $2^*$, and back again to the normal state, 1. Between the normal reactants and the activated complex an equilibrium is established, which is continually being disturbed by the activated complex proceeding on to 3. The number of such molecules passing over the energy barrier is related to the concentration of activated complex, and the mean velocity of crossing the barrier is related to the energy of the activated molecules.

$$M^* = [ABC](2\pi m^* kT)^{1/2}(\delta/h),$$

where $k$ is Boltzmann's constant ($1.38 \times 10^{-16}$ erg/degree/molecule), h is Planck's constant ($6.62 \times 10^{-27}$ erg-sec), and $m^*$ is the mass of the activated complex.[67] The velocity $v$ is given by

$$v = \left(\frac{2kT}{\pi m^*}\right)^{\frac{1}{2}}.$$

Since ABC* is in equilibrium with the reactants AB + C,

$$K^* = \frac{[ABC]}{[AB][C]},$$

The reaction rate $= k_T[AB][C]$

and combining we have

$$k_T = c\left(\frac{kT}{h}\right)K^*$$

where $kT/h$ is a frequency and T is the absolute temperature. Assuming $c = 1$,

$$\Delta G^* = -RT \ln \frac{k_T h}{kT} = \Delta H^* - T\Delta S^*$$

or

$$k_T = \left(\frac{kT}{h}\right)e^{-\Delta G^*/RT} = \frac{kT}{h}e^{\Delta S^*/R}e^{-\Delta H^*/RT}$$

And assuming $\Delta S^*$ is independent of T,

$$\frac{d \ln k_T}{dT} = \frac{\Delta H^*}{RT^2} = \frac{1}{T} = \frac{\Delta H^* + RT}{RT^2},$$

which leads us to

$$E^* = \Delta H^* + RT$$

or the energy of activation, $E^*$, is equal to the sum of $\Delta H^* + RT$. At lower temperatures and substantial values of $E^*$, $\Delta H^* \approx E^*$ and we may rewrite

$$PZ \approx \frac{kT}{h} e^{\Delta S^*/R}.$$

The smaller the decrease in entropy required to form the activated complex, the faster the reaction will proceed. If $\Delta S^*$ is not large, the reaction will advance slowly, even if $\Delta H^\circ$ is large. Conversely, even if $\Delta H^\circ$ is small, the reaction may proceed rapidly if $\Delta S^\circ$ is considerable. We may further subdivide the components of the above approximation as follows:

$$Z \approx \frac{kt}{h} \qquad \text{and}$$

$$P \approx e^{\Delta S^*/R}$$

where P, the steric factor of collision, is related to the entropy of activation.

## V. ENZYMES AND ENZYME KINETICS

### A. Introduction

Enzymes, as do all catalysts, decrease the free energy of activation and thereby accelerate chemical reactions (Fig 22). By lowering the energy required for activation, a greater proportion of molecules have internal energies in excess of the threshold value. While enzymes clearly increase the velocities of reactions (by factors of $10^1$ to $10^{12}$ times), the $\Delta G$ and therefore the overall tendency of the reaction to occur remains unchanged.

Enzymes are proteins generally ranging from 10,000-500,000 amu in molecular weight. They are usually named according to the reaction they catalyze, sometimes by adding the suffix -ase to one of the names of the substrates. An enzyme which is part protein conjugated to a non-amino acid group is termed a holoenzyme, the protein moiety is termed the apoenzyme and the remainder is called a prosthetic group. When the dissociation constant of a prosthetic group is large, and the prosthetic group only associates with the enzyme when acting on

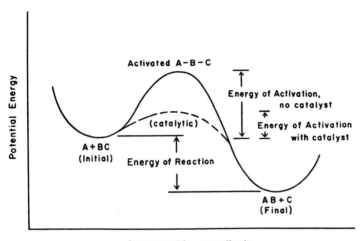

**Figure 22** Potential energy diagram for a reaction occurring in one case in the absence and in another case in the presence of a catalyst. Before reacting, the molecules must accumulate sufficient kinetic energy (energy of activation) to pass over the energy barrier represented by the rising curve, even though the reaction occurs with a loss in free energy (approximately indicated by the heat of reaction). In the presence of a catalyst the energy of activation is considerably less than in its absence.[76]

the substrate, the prosthetic group is called a cofactor or coenzyme. Two prosthetic groups known for dehydrogenases deserving of mention are coenzyme I, or nicotinamide adenine dinucleotide ($NAD^+$), formerly known as diphosphopyridine nucleotide ($DPN^+$) (Fig 23), and coenzyme II, or nicotinamide adenine dinucleotide phosphate ($NADP^+$), formerly known as triphosphopyridine nucleotide ($TPN^+$). Another prosthetic group is flavin adenine dinucleotide (Fig 24). The various types of enzymes appear in Table VI.

## B. Active site and specificity

While an enzyme acts like an inorganic catalyst, it is much more specific. Enzymes are thought to form an association

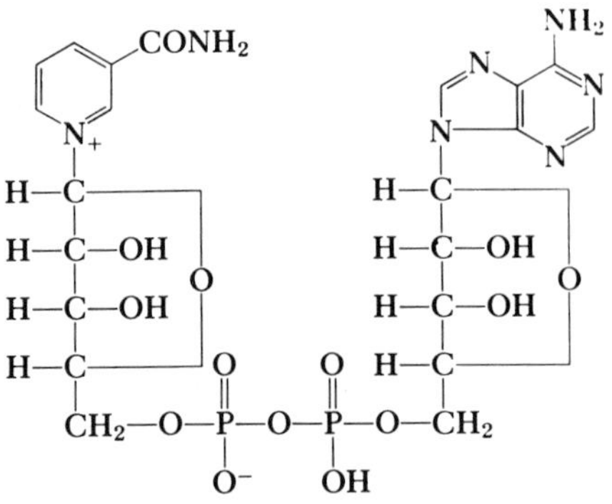

**Figure 23**  Nicotinamide adenine dinucleotide (NAD), the coenzyme or prosthetic group of some of the dehydrogenases. Nicotinamide adenine dinucleotide phosphate (NADP) is similar in structure except that it has an extra phosphoric acid residue attached to the pentose of adenosine (right side of the molecule). The reduced form of NAD may be designated $NADH_2$ or $NADH + H^+$ when it is desirable to show the release of an $H^+$ ion in the reduction. If the latter designation is employed, then the oxidized form of NAD should be given as $NAD^+$. The same conventions are to be used with NADP.

with their substrates, leading to a decrease in energy of activation. Adsorption of reactant molecules to an enzyme may be the stress equivalent of several hundred atmospheres pressure. The precision with which this occurs led to the so-called "lock and key" analogy for enzyme and substrate (Fig 25). According to this hypothesis, the correct shape of substrate (key) can only combine with the enzyme with the complementary shaped hole (lock) (Fig 26). Interaction with substrate involves the three-dimensional structure of the enzyme molecule as well as the catalyst groups. This view is supported by the observation that enzymes lose their activity when their tertiary structure is destroyed and is also consistent with the notion that specific enzymes must have at least three points of attachment to their substrates in order to explain their unsymmetrical action on symmetrical substrates. This concept also explains how enzymes distinguish between stereoisomers of

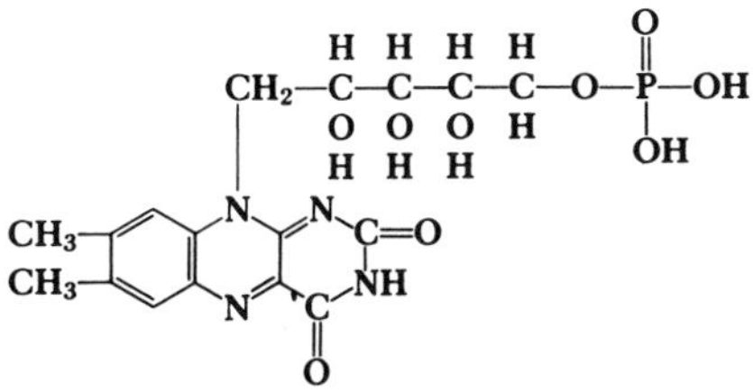

Riboflavin phosphate
(flavin mononucleotide)

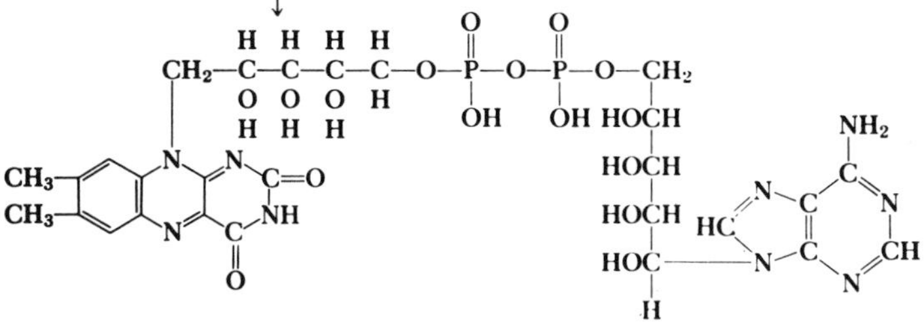

Flavin adenine dinucleotide (FAD)

DPNH + FMN ⟶ DPN + FMNH₂
or                    or
FAD                 FADH₂

**Figure 24** Riboflavin prosthetic groups of "yellow" enzymes. Both yellow enzymes participate primarily in transport of hydrogen ions and electrons from prosthetic groups of one of the dehydrogenases (*e.g.*, nicotinadmide adenine dinucleotide) to the cytochromes. Each prosthetic group has specific functions, *e.g.*, FMN is the prosthetic group of lactic dehydrogenase and FAD is the prosthetic group of aldehyde oxidase,D-amino oxidase and fatty acyl-CoA dehydrogenases.

substrates as well, and helps visualize how inhibitors could compete with substrate for association with enzymes.

Only a small portion of the enzyme complexes with the substrate and interacts with cofactors (if they are involved in a given reaction). Such a critical area of the enzyme molecule is called an active site, and its small size implies that only a given number of groups on the enzyme molecule are involved in catalysis (Fig 27). As such, low molecular weight analogues of the substrate may be bonded to a single active site on an

**Table VI**　International classification of enzymes (class names, code numbers, and types of reactions catalyzed).

| | |
|---|---|
| 1.　Oxido-reductases | 3.2　Glycosidic bonds |
| 　　(Oxidation-reduction reactions) | 3.4　Peptide bonds |
| | 3.5　Other C—N bonds |
| 　　1.1　Acting on —CH—OH | 3.6　Acid anhydrides |
| | 4.　Lyases |
| 　　1.2　Acting on —C=O | 　　(Addition to double bonds) |
| 　　1.3　Acting on —CH=CH— | |
| | 　　4.1　—C=C— |
| 　　1.4　Acting on —CH—NH₂ | |
| | 　　4.2　—C=O |
| 　　1.5　Acting on —CH—NH— | |
| 　　1.6　Acting on NADH; NADPH | 　　4.3　—C=N— |
| 2.　Transferases | 5.　Isomerases |
| 　　(Transfer of functional groups) | 　　(Isomerization reactions) |
| 　　2.1　One-carbon groups | 　　5.1　Racemases |
| 　　2.2　Aldehydic or ketonic groups | 6.　Ligases |
| 　　2.3　Acyl groups | 　　(Formation of bonds |
| 　　2.4　Glycosyl groups | 　　with ATP cleavage) |
| 　　2.7　Phosphate groups | 　　6.1　C—O |
| 　　2.8　S-containing groups | 　　6.2　C—S |
| 3.　Hydrolases | 　　6.3　C—N |
| 　　(Hydrolysis reactions) | 　　6.4　C—C |
| 　　3.1　Esters | |

* From Lehninger, 1970: Biochemistry. Worth Publishers, New York, p. 148.

enzyme and destroy its activity. In addition, when an enzyme is combined with substrate, x-ray crystallography electron density maps show increased electron density at a small site, presumably the active one.[71] The role of the remainder of the enzyme molecule (other than the active site) is less defined. However, in many instances the amino acids involved in the attachment of the substrate are not located near each other, and a given conformation of the polypeptide chain is necessary to orient these attachment sites properly for a reaction to occur. The portion of the molecule surrounding the active site may also protect against unproductive enzyme-substrate combinations and thereby aid in conferring specificity. Independ-

(a)

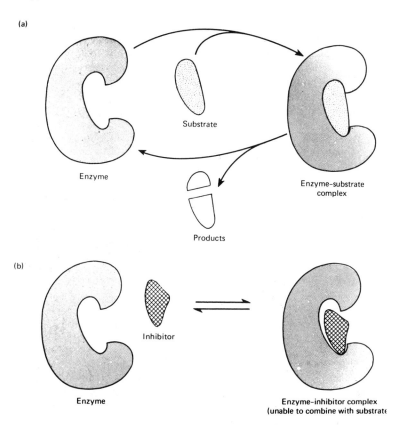

(b)

**Figure 25** Lock-and-key model for the binding of substrates and inhibitors by enzymes. (a) Formation of an enzyme-substrate complex. This may either dissociate or result in the conversion of the substrate into products. (b) A competitive inhibitor can also combine with the enzyme and prevent it from reacting with the substrate. Reproduced with permission.[69]

ent of the relative roles of active site and the remainder of the enzyme molecule, it is likely that the enzyme orients the substrate(s) and coenzyme in a manner most conducive for reaction. One may regard this as an increase in the order of the system, associated with a greater probability of reaction (Fig 27B).

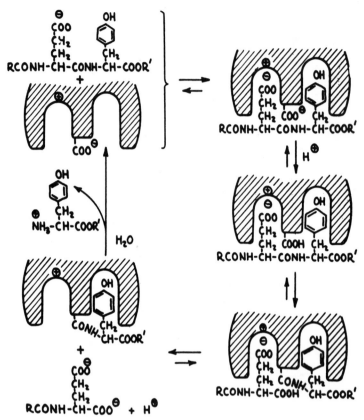

**Figure 26** A proposed hypothetical mechanism of action of pepsin; N-acyl-L-glutamyl-L-tyrosine ester represented as substrate. (From Boyer *et al.*, 1960: *The Enzymes.* Vol. 4. Academic Press, New York.) The sequence of amino acids, their 3-dimensional arrangement and the nature of the active spots have now been determined for trypsin, chymotrypsin and elastase (D.M. Chatton, unpublished).

Recently, in order to account for small structural changes that occur when enzymes complex with their substrates, Koshland [72-74] proposed an induced-fit mechanism for enzyme-substrate interaction, in which the substrate effects a definite change in the enzyme molecule (Fig 28). This hypothesis has

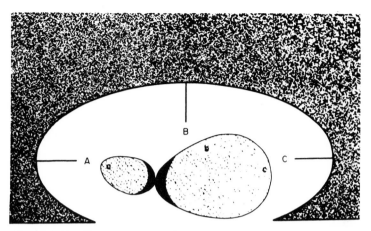

**Figure 27A** Representation of an enzyme reaction. A, B, and C represent reactive groups of the enzyme. The egg-shaped molecules represent substrate molecules. The shaded areas in the molecules represent the reactive groups of the substrates. a, b, and c are groups in the substrate which can interact with A, B, and C. Reproduced with permission.[70]

been buttressed by the crystallographic studies of Phillips [75] of lysozyme combined with polysaccharide substrate. In this system, the region available for binding the substrate can accommodate six amino sugar units of the polysaccharide sur-

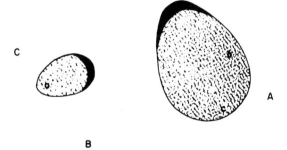

**Figure 27B** The reaction of Figure 27A without the enzyme molecule. The reactive groups A, B, and C are no longer attached. The probability of all reactive groups becoming appropriately oriented is much diminished. Reproduced with permission.[70]

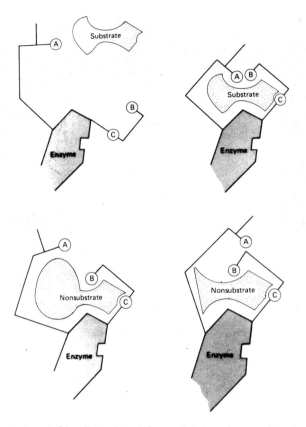

**Figure 28**  Koshland's induced-fit model for the combination of enzyme and substrate. The upper two sketches show that in the presence of an appropriately shaped substrate the catalytically important groups A and B are brought together; this alignment allows the reaction to occur. In the lower two sketches the nonsubstrate molecules are capable of attaching to binding group C, but they do not have the correct shape to give the proper alignment of A and B and so they act as competitive inhibitors. Reproduced with permission.[69]

face. Binding of the enzyme and substrate distorts the enzyme slightly in such a way that cleavage of the polysaccharide is favored. The actions of the side chains of glutamic acid 35 and aspartic acid 52 are responsible for the reaction, which are separated by 16 amino acids in the primary structure of the enzyme, but are close to one another in its three-dimensional structure (Fig 29).

## Inhibitors

Since enzymes and their substrates combine during catalysis, it is appropriate to consider activators and inhibitors of enzyme action in a qualitative manner at this point. Figure 25b

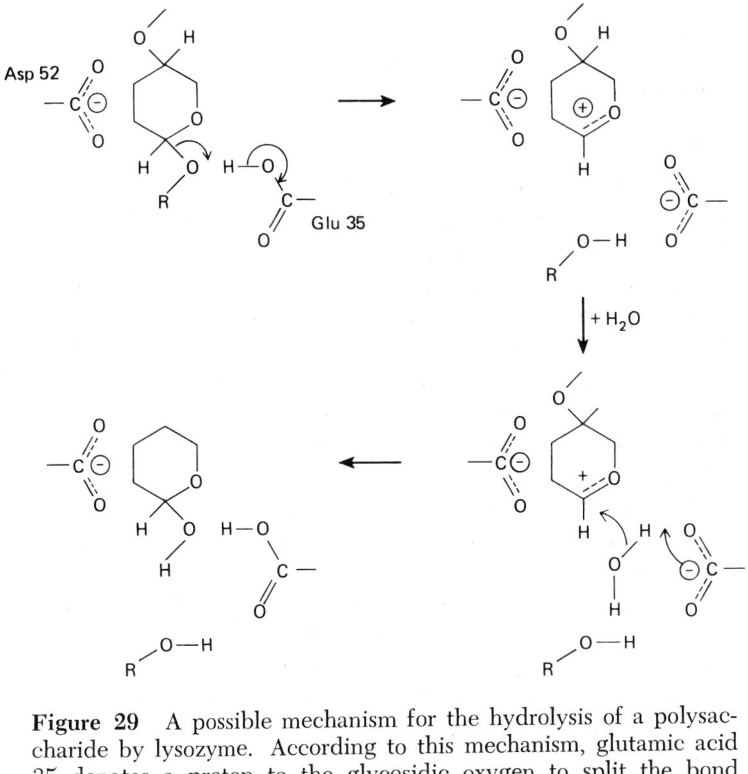

**Figure 29** A possible mechanism for the hydrolysis of a polysaccharide by lysozyme. According to this mechanism, glutamic acid 35 donates a proton to the glycosidic oxygen to split the bond between the two sugars. This leaves the terminal hydroxyl of the glutamic acid ionized and means that the sugar residue at the top will be in the form of a positively charged carbonium ion. The latter is thought to be stabilized by the negatively charged aspartic acid 52. The participation of water completes the reaction with the addition of a hydroxyl ion to the sugar residue and a proton to the ionized glutamic acid 35. Reproduced with permission.[69]

depicts the mechanism by which a competitive inhibitor may prevent substrate-enzyme interaction according to the "lock and key" hypothesis. Figure 28 shows how an inhibitor similar to a substrate may gain "entry" to the active site area of the enzyme molecule according to the induced-fit hypothesis. However, if the inhibitor is not identical with the substrate, the inhibitor cannot induce the correct orientation of catalytic groups to complete a reaction.

A noncompetitive inhibitor cannot occupy the same position on the enzyme as does a competitive inhibitor, since it is dissimilar enough in structure to prevent access to the active site. The induced-fit theory may be used to explain the action of noncompetitive inhibitors (Fig 30). The inhibitor combines with the enzyme at an area other than the active site, and changes the position of a part of the enzyme which contains one of the catalytic groups ( B ), thus preventing the substrate from inducing it into correct alignment for reaction. In other words, noncompetitive inhibitors appear to act by altering the conformation of enzymes. The induced-fit hypothesis may also help explain the influence of activators on enzyme catalyzed reactions. By forming an association with the catalytically active groups in the "correct" position for reaction, the complex is stabilized (Fig 30c-d). A summary of these various alterations of enzyme activity appears in Figure 31.

The influence of various substances which modify enzyme activity provides a means for metabolic control. Substantial changes in reaction kinetics may result, since a small change in enzyme activity may result in a major change in the rate of the catalyzed reaction. This effect is illustrated in Figure 32. A small shift in the curve reaction velocity *versus* substrate concentration creates an amplified change in the reaction rate if the substrate concentration is fixed at S.

In summary, the actual mechanisms responsible for enzyme action remain unknown. However, the general principles involved are similar to those governing other organic reaction mechanisms.[77] An enzyme may fix the substrates in correct position for reaction, as discussed. Some component of the active site may function as a nucleophilic (electron-donating)

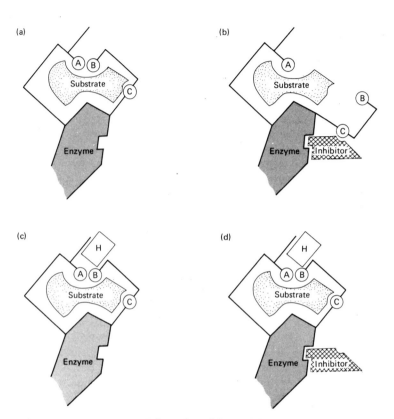

**Figure 30** Extension of the induced-fit model for enzyme-substrate combination to explain the effects of an inhibitor and activator (H). (a) A and B are catalytically important groups which must be in the correct alignment for enzyme activity. (b) When the inhibitor binds group C, the enzyme cannot achieve an active conformation. The inhibitor would be noncompetitive if its presence did not alter the binding of substrate, but it would be competitive if the chain containing B and C were significantly involved in substrate binding. (c) The activator stabilizes the active conformation. (d) The activator could overcome the effects of the inhibitor. Reproduced with permission.[69]

**Figure 31**   Enzyme inhibition and activation. Reproduced with permission.[76]

*Enzyme Inhibition and Activation*

⌣ = enzyme surface
S  = substrate
I   = inhibitor
A  = activator.   This might consist of a salt in hydrolyses or of an electron acceptor
(second substrate) in oxidations.
● = active spot on enzyme
x  = auxiliary active spot

*Note:* Interaction (electron transport) between ● and x might occur through a protein.

Competitive inhibition:

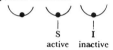

S       I
active   inactive

Noncompetitive (independent) inhibition—no interference of I with the attachment of S:

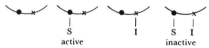

S        I       S   I
active            inactive

Independent activation:

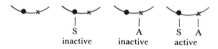

S        A       S   A
inactive   inactive   active

Activation through binding:

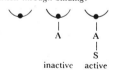

A        A
|
S
inactive   active

Activation through removal (e.g., pepsinogen to pepsin):

S
inactive     active

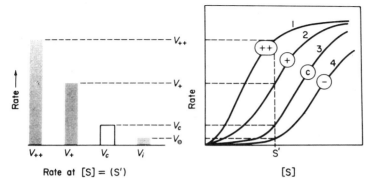

**Figure 32** Generalized substrate response curve for an enzyme which is regulated by positive effectors (+) or negative effectors (−). The control (no effectors) is indicated by the letter c. From D. E. Atkinson, *Science* **150**: 851-857 (1965). Copyright 1965 by the American Association for the Advancement of Science.

or electrophilic (electron-withdrawing) group, as may be the case for the transfer of a phosphate group to creatine (Fig 33). The displacement of a group from the substrate may lead to covalent bond formation with the enzyme and subsequently to transfer to an acceptor. The catalytically active group may function as an acid or base. The substrate may also be altered by a nonpolar group at the active site, which, because of a low dielectric constant at a hydrophobic site, might change the ionization of the substrate. Finally, the possibility that the enzyme-substrate interaction might induce a conformational change in the enzyme, substrate, and/or enzyme-substrate complex has been considered.

## C. Kinetics of enzyme-catalyzed reactions

### 1. *The Michaelis-Menton equation*

In the previous action selected qualitative aspects of enzyme function were discussed. We now seek to describe these inter- actions in quantitative terms. The reader who desires a more exhaustive treatment than that given here is referred to the

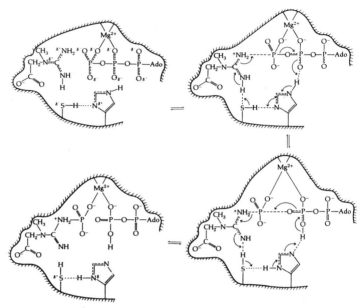

**Figure 33**  Schematic representation of a model for the transfer of a phosphate group from ATP to creatine, catalyzed by creatine kinase. Ado represents adenosine. The first diagram (top left) shows all groups at the instant of binding by the two substrates. The last diagram (bottom left) represents the completion of the reaction before detachment. The complexed $Mg^{2+}$ holds the phosphate component in place. The electrophilic attack of the histidine residue of the enzyme on the phosphate, together with the nucleophilic attack by the sulfhydryl group of the enzyme on the creatine, breaks the terminal phosphate bond of the ATP and simultaneously transfers the phosphate to the creatine. Detachment of the two molecules from the enzyme's active site completes the reaction. Reproduced with permission.[78]

discussions in Netter,[79] Mahler and Cordes [80] and Dixon and Webb [81] where additional references may be obtained as well.

Consider the reaction

$$E + S \underset{k_2}{\overset{k_1}{\rightleftharpoons}} ES \underset{k_4}{\overset{k_3}{\rightleftharpoons}} P + E$$

in which E is enzyme, S is substrate,, ES the enzyme-substrate complex or intermediate, and P the product, (Fig 34). The velocities of reaction are:

$$\frac{d[S]}{dt} k_2[ES] - k_1[S][E]$$

$$\frac{d[ES]}{dt} = k_1[E][S] - (k_2 + k_3)[ES]$$

$$\frac{d[E]}{dt} = (k_2 + k_3)[ES] - k_1[S][E]$$

$$\frac{d[P]}{dt} = k_3[ES].$$

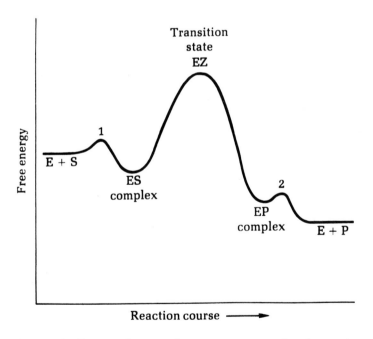

**Figure 34** Energy diagram for an enzyme-catalyzed reaction. Small energy barriers exist at points 1 and 2.

It is obvious that the total amount of enzyme is constant if none is synthesized nor inactivated, and

$$[E]_o = [E] + [ES].$$

There are no easy and explicit solutions to these equations. It is trivial to observe that the instantaneous values of $[E]$, $[ES]$, and $[P]$ will be a function of $[S]$, $[E]$, $k_1$, $k_2$, and $k_3$. Two situations may be considered. In the first instance, $[S]$ and $[E]$ are comparable, $k_3 \lessdot k_1/k_2$, and hence the concentrations of all components change significantly with time and exhibit transient state kinetics (Fig 35A). The actual solution of the equations in this instance may be provided with computer assistance (Fig 36).

In the second situation, when $[S] \gg [E]$ and/or $k_3 \ll k_1/k_2$, then after the initial period of reaction and until equilibrium is attained, the slopes of the progress curves for $[ES]$ and $[E]$ are nearly zero. In addition, the larger the ratio $[S]_o/[E]_o$, the shorter the period necessary to reach a steady concentration of ES (Fig 35B). This steady state situation leads to the well known Michaelis-Menton equation as follows.

Assuming the steady state approximation $d[ES]/dt = 0$ and $d[E]/dt = 0$ hold, then

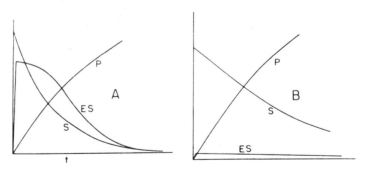

**Figure 35** A. Transient state kinetics. B. Steady state kinetics. Reproduced with permission.[82]

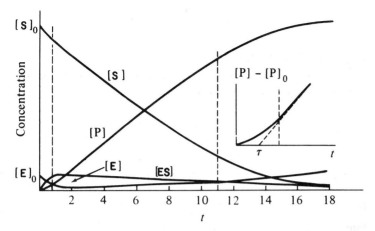

**Figure 36** Progress curve for a reaction sequence with computer assistance. (Program from Cleland, W. W. *Nature* **198**: 463 (1963); *Advan. Enzymol.*, **29**: 1 (1967)).

$$k_1[\text{E}][\text{S}] = (k_2 + k_3)[\text{ES}], \qquad \text{which gives}$$

upon substitution:

$$[\text{ES}] = \frac{k_1[\text{S}][\text{E}]_0}{k_1[\text{S}] + k_2 + k_3}, \qquad \text{and the rate}$$

of disappearance of S in the steady state is given by

$$v = -\frac{d[\text{S}]}{dt} = \frac{d[\text{P}]}{dt} = k_3[\text{ES}]$$

$$= \frac{k_1 k_3[\text{S}][\text{E}]_0}{k_1[\text{S}] + k_2 + k_3},$$

$$= \frac{k_3[\text{S}][\text{E}]_0}{(k_2 + k_3)/k_1 + [\text{S}]}$$

Then $\qquad [\text{E}]_0 = \left(\dfrac{k_{\text{m}}}{[\text{S}]} + 1\right)[\text{ES}].$

setting $k_{\text{m}} = (k_2 + k_3)/k_1$ and defining $V_{\text{m}} = k_3[\text{E}]_0$:

$$v = \frac{V_m [S]}{k_m + [S]},$$

which is the Michaelis-Menton equation.

$k_m$ is not a true dissociation constant as defined because [ES] is varying continually during the reaction:

$$k_m = \frac{k_2 + k_3}{k_1} = \frac{[E][S]}{[ES]}.$$

The dissociation constant of the complex, $k_c$, is actually given by $k_2 / k_1$, and therefore

$$k_m = k_c + \frac{k_3}{k_1}.$$

If $k_3 / k_1 \ll k_c$ then $k_m \rightarrow k_c$. The constant $V_m$ is directly proportional to the amount of enzyme present, and $k_m$ is a property of the enzyme under consideration.

## 2. Forms of the Michaelis-Menton equation

When plotting velocity versus substrate concentration, one notes that the value of [S] when $v = V_m / 2$ is really $k_m$. As seen in Figure 37, $v$ approaches $V_m$ asymptotically as [S] increases. When [S] is low, this term may be neglected in the denominator of the Michaelis-Menton equation, and $v = (V_m / k_m)[S]$ approximates the beginning of the curve in Figure 37a. When [S] is large, deletion of $k_m$ from the equation leaves $v = V_m$, *i.e.*, the reaction velocity is independent of the substrate concentration because the enzyme is entirely complexed to the substrate. The distinctive feature exhibited by reactions behaving in this manner is *saturation*.

There are a number of ways the equation may be rearranged to yield linear plots. Taking the reciprocal of both sides,

$$\frac{1}{v} = \frac{1}{V_m [S] / (k_m + [S])} = \frac{k_m + [S]}{V_m [S]},$$

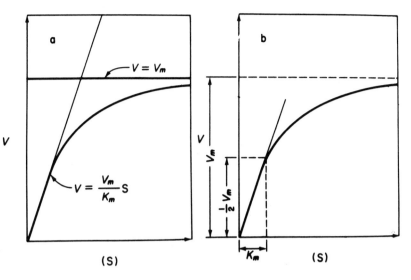

**Figure 37** Relationship between the various kinetic parameters in an enzyme catalyzed reaction. (a) Rate of the reaction (V) as a function of substrate concentration (S). Initial slope and asymptote. (b) Rate of the reaction (V) as a function of substrate concentration (S).

which upon rearranging becomes

$$\frac{1}{v} = \frac{k_m}{V_m[S]} + \frac{[S]}{V_m[S]}, \text{ or}$$

$$\frac{1}{v} = \left(\frac{k_m}{V_m}\right)\left(\frac{1}{[S]}\right) + \frac{1}{V_m},$$

also known as the Lineweaver-Burk equation. The intercept of this plot is $1/V_m$ on the ordinate, $-1/k_m$ on the abscissa, and its slope is $k_m/V_m$ (Fig 38). $V_m$ may be derived with greater ease using Lineweaver-Burk plots.

Multiplying both sides of the equation by $vV_m$,

$$v = -k_m\left(\frac{v}{[S]}\right) + V_m.$$

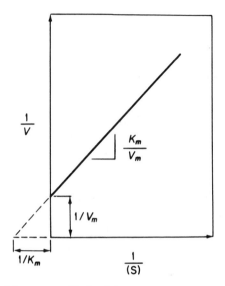

**Figure 38**    Lineweaver-Burk plot.

Plotting $v$ *versus* $\left(\dfrac{v}{[S]}\right)$ gives Figure 39, the Eadie-Hofstee

plot. Finally, the Michaelis-Menton equation may be written

$$\frac{[S]}{v} = \frac{[S]}{V_m} + \frac{k_m}{V_m},$$    which is

plotted in Figure 40. Or it can be written

$$\frac{k_m d[S]}{[S]} + d[S] = -V_m dt \quad \text{which becomes}$$

$$[S] + k_m \ln [S] = -V_m t + \mathcal{M}_0$$

upon integration. Evaluating the constant $\mathcal{M}_0$, at $t = 0$ ($\mathcal{M}_0 = [S]_0 + k_m \ln [S]_0$) substituting and converting to the base 10:

$$[S]_0 - [S] + 2.3 k_m \log \frac{[S]_0}{[S]} = V_m t$$

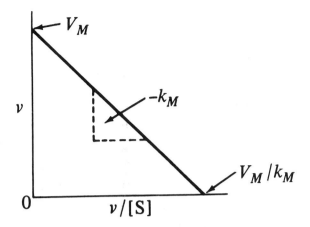

**Figure 39** Eadie-Hofstee plot.

From this equation, it is seen that an enzyme-catalyzed reaction in the steady state is a "mixed" zero order and first order reaction. For small $[S]_0$,

$$\log\frac{[S]_0}{[S]}=\left(\frac{V_m}{2.3k_m}\right)t$$

describes a first order reaction, and for large $[S]_0$:

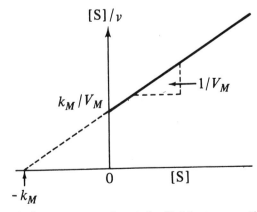

**Figure 40** Another plot of the Michaelis-Menton equation.

$$[S]_0 - [S] = V_m t$$

describes a zero order reaction.

The velocities of reactions may be expressed in moles/sec/mole-enzyme or the "turnover number," the maximum number of substrate molecules transformed per unit time by a single enzyme molecule ($V_m / [E]$).

### 3. *Two substrate reactions*

Most enzymic reactions really occur between two substrate molecules. Sometimes one substrate will be present in great excess as compared with the other. The sequence of binding between substrate(s) and enzyme may be random or be sequential.[84, 85] Consider the reactions:

for which

$$E + A \rightleftharpoons EA \qquad\qquad k_A = \frac{[E][A]}{[EA]}$$

$$E + B \rightleftharpoons EB \qquad " \qquad k_B = \frac{[E][B]}{[EB]}$$

$$EA + B \rightleftharpoons EAB \qquad " \qquad k'_B = \frac{[EA][B]}{[EAB]}$$

$$EB + A \rightleftharpoons EAB \qquad " \qquad k'_A + \frac{[EB][A]}{[EAB]}$$

$$EAB \rightarrow E + Products$$

$$[E]_0 = [E] + [EA] + [EB] + [EAB].$$

where the overall velocity of the reaction is given by

$$v = k[EAB], \quad \text{and}$$

$$V_m = k[E]_0.$$

Eliminating [E], [EA], and [EB] from these equations,

$$V_m = \left| \left( \frac{k_A k'_B}{[B]} + k'_A \right) \frac{1}{[A]} + \frac{k'_B}{[B]} + 1 \right| v$$

or

$$\frac{1}{v} = \left( \frac{k_A k'_B}{B} + k'_A \right) \frac{1}{V_m[A]} + \left( \frac{k'_B}{[B]} + 1 \right) \frac{1}{V_m}$$

If $[B] \gg k'_B$, these two equations are approximated by the Michaelis-Menton equation. If $[B]$ is held constant, the plot $1/v$ *versus* $1/[A]$ for different values of $[B]$ describes a family of straight lines (Fig 41). This assumes the two substrates combine independently with their active sites, $k_A \approx k'_A$ and $k_B \approx k'_B$ and

$$\frac{v}{V_M} = \frac{\left( \frac{[A]}{k_A} \right) \left( \frac{[B]}{k_B} \right)}{\left( 1 + \frac{[A]}{k_A} \right) \left( 1 + \frac{[B]}{k_B} \right)}$$

which is the product of two Michaelis-Menton equations.

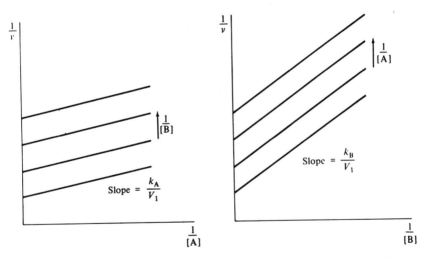

**Figure 41**  Plots of bisubstrate enzyme reactions.  Reproduced with permission.[86]

### D. Inhibitors

Excluding enzyme inhibition by destruction, there are two major types of enzyme inhibition—competitive and noncompetitive, as previously mentioned. If a substance inhibits an enzyme by combining with the same active site as does the substrate, it is said to "compete" with the substrate and the inhibition may be overcome with excess substrate. Competitive inhibition is described by

$$E + I \underset{k_2}{\overset{k_1}{\rightleftharpoons}} EI$$

where the enzyme-inhibitor complex [EI] cannot go on to form product, as does the ES complex. An inhibitor constant may be defined by

$$k_I = \frac{k_2}{k_1} = \frac{[E][I]}{[EI]}$$

The Lineweaver-Burke plot, $\dfrac{1}{v}$ *versus* $\dfrac{1}{[S]}$ at varying concentrations of I, demonstrates straight lines of differing slope intersecting at a common intercept on the ordinate (Fig 42A). $V_m$ is not changed by the presence of an inhibitor, but the apparent $k_m$ will be greater than the actual $k_m$. The slope of the uninhibited reaction is $k_m/V_m$, whereas the slope of the inhibited reaction is $(k_m/V_m)\left(1 + \dfrac{[I]}{k_I}\right)$.

Noncompetitive inhibition is not reversed by increasing the substrate concentration, since the inhibitor binds at a locus on the enzyme other than the active site:

$$E + I \rightleftharpoons EI.$$

The inhibitor may also combine with ES:

$$ES + I \rightleftharpoons ESI$$

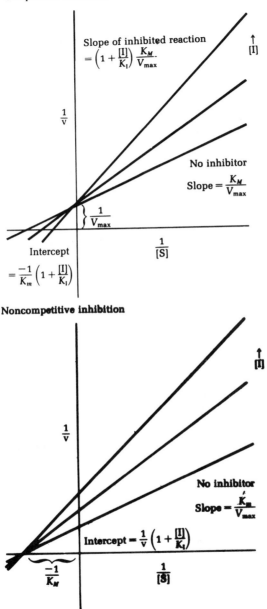

Competitive inhibition

Slope of inhibited reaction
$$= \left(1 + \frac{[I]}{K_I}\right) \frac{K_M}{V_{max}}.$$

$\frac{1}{v}$

$\uparrow$
$[I]$

No inhibitor

Slope $= \frac{K_M}{V_{max}}$

$\left\{ \frac{1}{V_{max}} \right.$

Intercept

$= \frac{-1}{K_m}\left(1 + \frac{[I]}{K_I}\right)$

$\frac{1}{[S]}$

**Noncompetitive inhibition**

$\frac{1}{v}$

$\uparrow$
$[I]$

No inhibitor

Slope $= \frac{K'_m}{V_{max}}$

Intercept $= \frac{1}{v}\left(1 + \frac{[I]}{K_I}\right)$

$\underbrace{\quad}$

$\frac{-1}{K_M}$

$\frac{1}{[S]}$

**Figure 42**  a. b Lineweaver-Burk plots of competitive and non-competitive inhibition.

where the forms EI and ESI are inactive. The Lineweaver-Burke plots in this instance (Fig 42B), do not intersect the $1/v$ axis at a common point, but the intercept is greater on the $1/v$ axis for the inhibited than the noninhibited enzyme. $V_m$ is diminished by the inhibitor and cannot be restored by increasing the substrate concentration. Another plot illustrating the kinetics of competitive and noncompetitive inhibition—in this instance $v$ *versus* $[S]$—appears in Figure 43.

## VI. OXIDATION-REDUCTION POTENTIALS

The loss of electrons from a molecule is termed *oxidation* and raises the oxidation state of the species. Similarly, *reduction* refers to the gain of electrons by a molecule, resulting in a lowered oxidation state. An *oxidizing agent* effects the oxidation of another species, during which reaction the oxidizing agent is itself reduced:

$$\text{oxidant}^z + ne^{-1} \rightleftharpoons \text{reductant}^{z-n}$$

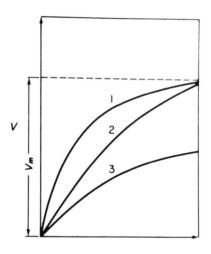

(S)

**Figure 43** Rate of a reaction (V) as a function of substrate concentration (S). Control, curve 1. Competitive inhibition, curve 2. Noncompetitive inhibition, curve 3.

where $z$ is the oxidation state, or valence, and $n$ is the number of electrons transferred per mole. In reactions in which one reactant is an electron donor and another is an electron acceptor, the ability to exchange electrons may be imbodied in an oxidation-reduction (redox) potential. If two molecular species—1 and 2—can exist in at least two oxidation states, *i.e.*, in an "oxidized" and "reduced" form, the two reactions may be coupled:

$$\frac{\begin{array}{r} red_1 \rightleftharpoons ox_1{}^{n+} + ne^- \\ ox_2{}^{n+} + ne^- \rightleftharpoons red_2 \end{array}}{red_1 + ox_2 \rightleftharpoons ox_1 + red_2}$$

If connected as illustrated in Figure 44 via a KCl bridge, an electromotive force may be recorded on the galvanometer. The system is composed of two "half-cells," each of which consists of an element or substance in two oxidation states; the most common situation is an element immersed in a solution of its own ion. The hydrogen half-cell is the standard against which all other half-cells are compared with respect to the ability to release (or gain) electrons (Table 7). The normal hydrogen half cell is defined as having zero electrode potential at unit

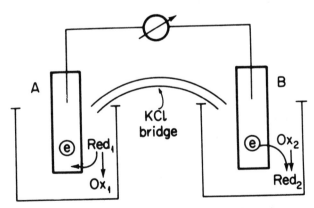

**Figure 44** An electrochemical cell, composed of two molecular species (1 and 2), each with two oxidation states. By convention, electrons travel from the left half-cell (A) to the right half-cell (B).

**Table VII**  Normal electrode potentials at 25°C.  Reproduced with permission.[87]

| ELECTRODE | ELECTRODE REACTION | NORMAL[†] ELECTRODE POTENTIAL (VOLTS) AGAINST HYDROGEN ELECTRODE |
|---|---|---|
| Li⁺, Li | Li $= Li^+ + e$ | −2.9595 |
| Na⁺, Na | Na $= Na^+ + e$ | −2.7146 |
| Zn⁺⁺, Zn | Zn $= Zn^{++} + 2e$ | −0.7618 |
| Fe⁺⁺, Fe | Fe $= Fe^{++} + 2e$ | −0.441 |
| Pb⁺⁺, Pb | Pb $= Pb^{++} + 2e$ | −0.122 |
| H⁺, H₂ (1 atm.) | ½H₂ $= H^+ + e$ | 0.0000[‡] |
| Cu⁺⁺, Cu | Cu $= Cu^{++} + 2e$ | +0.3441 |
| Ag⁺, Ag | Ag $= Ag^+ + e$ | +0.7978 |
| Au⁺⁺⁺, Au | Au $= Au^{+++} + 3e$ | +1.36 |

* Data from West, 1956. The electrode potential is the reduction potential and measures the free energy of reduction; its sign is arbitrary and follows the scheme of Clark, 1952. When the opposite sign is used for the electrode potentials the values represent the oxidation potentials or their readiness to be oxidized and measure the free energy of oxidation (e.g., Lewis and Randall, 1961). This convention is now followed by biologists the world over and by European physical chemists.

† All salts 1 N in activity (standard state).

‡ At pH 0.0 (1 N H⁺).

activity of hydrogen ion at 760 mm Hg pressure.  When the hydrogen half cell donates electrons, the potential is positive. Since all the redox potentials are compared with the same reference, one may consider the difference between redox potentials of two half cells.  For example, consider two half cells with electrode potentials of $\mathcal{E}_1$ and $\mathcal{E}_2$ for the reactions

$$AH_2 + B \rightleftharpoons BH_2 + A$$
$$AH_2 \rightleftharpoons A + 2H^+ + 2e^- \qquad (\mathcal{E}_1)$$

$$B + 2H^+ + 2e^- \rightleftharpoons BH_2 \qquad (\mathcal{E}_2)$$

The actual voltage recorded will be $(\mathcal{E}_1 - \mathcal{E}_2)$ or the electromotive force is the algebraic sum of the component electrodes of the cell.

## A. Thermodynamics of redox reactions

We previously discussed the equation

$$dW = PdV - F^*dl - \mathcal{E}dF - \sum_{i=1}^{k} \mu_i dn_i + \ldots$$

where $\mu_i$ is the chemical potential of the $i^{th}$ species present in $-dn_i$ moles, $-\mathcal{E}dF$ is the electrical work performed by charge

* F denotes force—note change in notation for this equation only.

$-dF$ moving through a potential $\mathcal{E}$. An extensive variable $\theta_i$ may be defined as the extent of advancement of the $i^{th}$ reaction," such that in a closed system

$$\sum_i m_{ij}\frac{d\theta_i}{dt}=\frac{dn_j}{dt}$$

where $n_j$ is the number of moles of the $j^{th}$ species present and $m_{ij}$ is the stoichiometric coefficient of the $j^{th}$ species in the $i^{th}$ reaction, $m_{ij}>0$ for products and $m_{ij}<0$ for reactants. The total free energy $\mathcal{F}$ is given by

$$\mathcal{F}=E-TS-\Sigma X_iY_i-\Sigma\mu_jn_j$$

where E, T, S, $X_i$ and $Y_i$ have their previous meanings, the mole numbers $n_j$ specify the number of moles of each species present in the system, $\{Y_i\}$ the set of extensive variables does not include $\{n_j\}$, and $\mu_j$ is the chemical potential of the $j^{th}$ species.

The rate of change of $\mathcal{F}$ due to all chemical reactions is

$$\left(\frac{d\mathcal{F}}{dt}\right)_{chemical}=\sum_j\left(\frac{\partial\mathcal{F}}{\partial n_j}\right)\frac{dn_j}{dt}$$

$$=\sum_j\sum_i m_{ij}\left(\frac{d\theta}{dt}\right)\frac{\partial\mathcal{F}}{\partial n_j}$$

The coefficient of $(d\theta_i/dt)$ gives $(\partial\mathcal{F}/\partial\theta_i)$:

$$\frac{\partial\mathcal{F}}{\partial\theta_i}=\sum_j m_{ij}\frac{\partial\mathcal{F}}{\partial n_{ij}}$$

From these the following relation may be derived:

$$dW_{rev}=-(dG)_{T,P}=-z\mathcal{E}Fd\theta \qquad \text{where}$$

F is the Faraday (96,494 coulombs), $\mathcal{E}$ is the voltage across the cell, $z$ reflects the number of electrons, and $dW$ is the useful, reversible electric work performed by the cell. In connection with another half cell at equilibrium

$$\Delta G = -z\mathcal{E}F,$$

where by convention $\mathcal{E} > 0$ for a spontaneously discharging cell and therefore the free energy change is negative as well.

The dependence of the cell potential on temperature is derived considering the relation $(\partial \mathcal{G}/\partial T) = -S$ and

$$\left(\frac{\partial \mathcal{E}}{\partial T}\right)_P = \frac{\Delta S}{zF}$$

From this and the equation $G = A + PV = E + PV - TS$ an expression for enthalpy as a function of temperature may be derived:

$$\Delta H = zF\left[T\left(\frac{\partial \mathcal{E}}{\partial T}\right)_P - \mathcal{E}\right] = zFT^2\left(\frac{\partial[\mathcal{E}/T]}{\partial T}\right)_P,$$

and

$$\Delta G - \Delta H = T\left(\frac{\partial(\Delta G)}{\partial T}\right)_P,$$

from which we have

$$\mathcal{E} = -(\Delta H/zF) + T\left(\frac{d\mathcal{E}}{dT}\right).$$

The chemical and electrical energies are equal when $T\left(\dfrac{d\mathcal{E}}{dT}\right) = 0$, either at absolute 0 or when $\dfrac{d\mathcal{E}}{dT} = 0$.

## B. Chemical cells

Expressions for the voltages of electrodes and cells derive from the relation

$$\Delta G = \mu_2 - \mu_1 = -RT \ln\left(\frac{a_1}{a_2}\right)$$

where $\mu_1$ and $\mu_2$ are the chemical potentials and $a_1$ and $a_2$ are the activities of the substances involved in the half-cells. Since

$$\Delta G = -z\mathcal{E}F \qquad , \quad \text{we have}$$

$$\mathcal{E} = \frac{RT}{zF} \ln\left(\frac{a_1}{a_2}\right).$$

As mentioned, we may also express this equation as the algebraic sum of two electrode potentials, each of the form

$$\mathcal{E}° + \left(\frac{RT}{zF}\right) \ln a,$$

where $\mathcal{E}°$ is the standard electrode potential when the activities of involved substances are unity.

For the reaction

$$aA + bB \rightleftharpoons cC + dD$$

The free energy change may be written

$$\Delta G = \Delta G° + RT \ln\frac{(a_C)^c(a_D)^d}{(a_A)^a(a_B)^b}.$$

In a soluble oxidation-reduction system the free energy change may be expressed

$$\Delta G = \Delta G° + RT \ln \frac{a_{\text{oxidant}}}{a_{\text{reductant}}},$$

or if the reaction creates a reversible potential:

$$\mathcal{E} = \mathcal{E}° + RT \ln \frac{a_{\text{oxidant}}}{a_{\text{reductant}}},$$

where $\mathcal{E}°$ is the standard redox potential and $\mathcal{E}° = \mathcal{E}$ when $\frac{\text{ox}}{\text{red}} = 1$. At 30° this equation reduces to

$$\mathcal{E} = \mathcal{E}^\circ + \frac{0.06}{z} \log \frac{[\text{oxidant}]}{[\text{reductant}]}.$$

Table 8 indicates $\mathcal{E}^\circ$ values for some systems of biological interest. Each "system" consists of the oxidized and reduced forms of a substance, *e.g.*, pyruvate-lactate. Just as the Henderson-Hasselbach equation expresses the relationship between the dissociation constant of an acid, the pH, and the concentration of a proton donor and acceptor species, the above equations quantitatively depict the relation between the standard redox potential of a given system, the observed potential, and the activity or concentration ratio of the electron donor (reductant or reducing agent) and electron acceptor (oxidant or oxidizing agent). Just as the Henderson-Hesselbach equation describes a titration curve, the plot of the redox potential as a function of percent oxidation yields an S-shaped titration curve (Fig 45). At 100% reductant, the observed potential is maximally negative. As the reaction proceeds, a greater percentage of the reductant appears in its oxidized form. At the midpoint of the titration, the ratio [oxidant]/[reductant]=1, at which point $\mathcal{E} = \mathcal{E}^{\circ\prime}$. Continuing the analogy, this midpoint "corresponds" to the midpoint of the acid-base titration curve, at which the pK' of an acid equals the pH. The titration curves for a single and double electron transfer are composed in Figure 46, and some actual titration curves of biological significance are illustrated in Figure 47. It will be noted that in the electrochemical series appearing in Tables VII and VIII that if an electrode potential is greater (*i.e.*, more positive) for a chosen system B than for system A, system B will oxidize system A. Since the redox potential reflects free energy changes of a reaction, it also follows that a system of lower redox potential (A) can never spontaneously oxidize a system of greater redox potential (B). Knowledge of the values of $\mathcal{E}^{\circ\prime}$ for various biological systems allows the prediction of electron flow, just as the phosphate-group transfer potential allows prediction of group transfer, and also permits calculation of the free energy involved and equilibrium values of interest.

**Table VIII** Normal oxidation-reduction potentials of some biologically important systems at pH 7.0. Reproduced with permission.[87]

| System | $E_0'$ | T IN °C. |
|---|---|---|
| Ketoglutarate $\rightleftharpoons$ succinate $+ CO_2 + 2H^+ + 2e$ | $-0.68$ | —‡ |
| Ferredoxin reducing substance | $-0.60$ | —** |
| Isocitrate $\rightleftharpoons$ $\alpha$-ketoglutarate $+ CO_2$ | $-0.48$ | — |
| Ferredoxin | $-0.432$ | —§ |
| Formate $\rightleftharpoons$ $CO_2 + H_2$ | $-0.420$ | 38 |
| $H_2 \rightleftharpoons 2H^+ + 2e$ | $-0.414$ | 25 |
| $NADH + H^+ \rightleftharpoons NAD^+ + 2H^+ + 2e$ | $-0.317$ | 30† |
| $NADPH + H^+ \rightleftharpoons NADP^+ + 2H^+ + 2e$ | $-0.316$ | 30† |
| Horseradish oxidase | $-0.27$ | —† |
| $FADH_2 \rightleftharpoons FAD + 2H^+ + 2e$ | $-0.219$ | 30† |
| $FMNH_2 \rightleftharpoons FMM + 2H^+ + 2e$ | $-0.219$ | 30† |
| Lactate $\rightleftharpoons$ pyruvate $+ 2H^+ + 2e$ | $-0.180$ | 35 |
| Malate $\rightleftharpoons$ oxaloacetate $+ 2H^+ + 2e$ | $-0.102$ | 37 |
| Reduced flavin enzyme $\rightleftharpoons$ flavin enzyme $+ 2H^+ + 2e$ | $-0.063$ | 38 |
| Vitamin K | $-0.060$ | —†† |
| Luciferin* $\rightleftharpoons$ oxyluciferin $+ 2H^+ + 2e$ | $-0.050$ | ?* |
| Ferrocytochrome $b$ $\rightleftharpoons$ ferricytochrome $b + e$ | $-0.04$ | 25 |
| Succinate $\rightleftharpoons$ fumarate $+ 2H^+ + 2e$ | $-0.015$ | 30 |
| Plastoquinone | $0.00$ | —** |
| Decarboxylase | $+0.19$ | —† |
| Ferrocytochrome $c$ $\rightleftharpoons$ ferricytochrome $c + e$ | $+0.26$ | 25 |
| Ferrocytochrome $a$ $\rightleftharpoons$ ferricytochrome $a + e$ | $+0.29$ | 25 |
| Ferrocytochrome $a_3$ $\rightleftharpoons$ ferricytochrome $a_3 + e$ | ? | —‡ |
| Plastocyanin | $+0.36$ | —** |
| $P_{700}$ | $+0.40$ | —** |
| Coenzyme Q (in ethanol) | $+0.54$ | — |
| $H_2O \rightleftharpoons \frac{1}{2}O_2 + 2H^+ + 2e$ | $+0.815$ | 25 |

Data from Goddard, 1945. Potentials in all cases are at or near neutrality, except:

* From McElroy and Strehler, 1954: Bact. Rev. *18*.

† From Clark, 1960.

‡ From Goddard and Bonner, 1960: *In Plant Physiology, a Treatise.* Steward, ed. Academic Press, New York. Goddard and Bonner give the NADPH/NADP$^+$ system as $-0.324$, and NADH/NAD$^+$ as $-0.320$.

§ From Tagawa and Arnon, 1962: Nature *195*:537-543. The value cited is for spinach ferredoxin.

** Rabinowitch and Govindjee, 1971: Photosynthesis. Wiley, New York. The relative positions of Cyt f (preceding plastocyanin) and Cyt $b_3$ (preceding plastoquinone) in green plant cells have been determined but the exact values have not.

†† Lehninger, 1965: The Mitochondrion. W. A. Benjamin, New York.

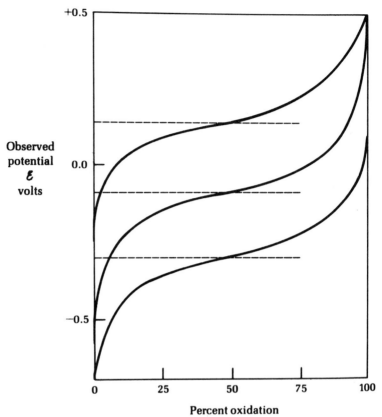

**Figure 45**  Oxidation-reduction titration curves of three reducing agents, showing midpoint potential $\mathscr{E}$ values (at pH = 7.0, T = 25°C).

## C. Redox potential and pH

In many biological systems the reduced form of a substance may exist as an anion which, upon accepting a hydrogen ion, may lose charge and hence change the potential. For two-electron reductions represented by

$$ox + 2e^- \rightarrow red^=,$$

the electrode potential is given by

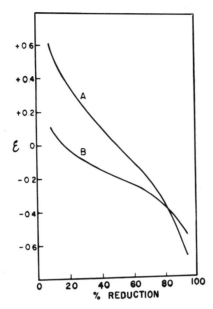

**Figure 46** Red-ox potentials as functions of the percentage of reductant present. A is for a single electron transfer and B is for a two electron transfer.

$$\mathcal{E} = \mathcal{E}° + \frac{RT}{2F} \ln \frac{ox}{red^=}$$

but the reduced form may ionize as follows:

$$\left\{ \begin{array}{l} H_2 \, red \overset{k_1}{\rightleftharpoons} H \, red^- + H^+ \\ H \, red^- \underset{k_2}{\rightleftharpoons} H^+ + red^= \end{array} \right\}.$$

We may write

$$k_1 = \frac{[H^+][H \, red^-]}{[H_2 \, red]},$$

$$k_2 = \frac{[H^+][red^=]}{[H \, red^-]}.$$

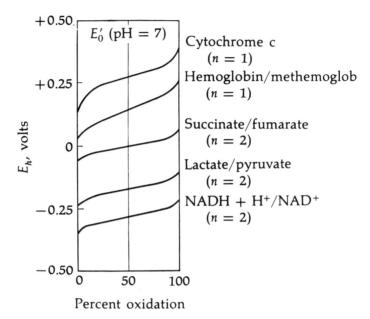

Figure 47  Potentiometric titration curves. $\mathcal{E}_h$=observed potential difference (in volts); $n$=number of electrons transferred per mole oxidized.

But the total reduced form may only take one of three forms, or

$$\text{red}_{\text{total}} = H_2 \, \text{red} + H \, \text{red}^- + \text{red}^= ,$$

and combining all equations we have

$$\mathcal{E} = \mathcal{E}^\circ + \frac{RT}{2F} \ln \frac{[\text{ox}]}{[\text{red}]} + \frac{RT}{2F} \ln \frac{[H^+]^2 + k_1[H^+] + k_1 k_2}{k_1 k_2}$$

when $[\text{ox}]/[\text{red}] = 1$,

$$\mathcal{E} = \mathcal{E}' + \frac{RT}{2F} \ln \{[H^+]^2 + k_1[H^+] + k_1 k_2\}.$$

For $k_1 \ll [H^+]$ and $k_2 \ll [H^+]$    we approximate at

$$\mathcal{E} = \mathcal{E}' + \frac{RT}{F} \ln [H^+] = \mathcal{E}' - 0.06 \text{ pH,}$$

but if $k_2 \ll [H^+] \ll k_1$, at $30°$ we have

$$\mathcal{E} = \mathcal{E}'' + \frac{RT}{2F} \ln [H^+] = \mathcal{E}'' - 0.03 \text{ pH.}$$

## D. Biological oxidations

Three major classes of redox reactions occur biologically and are catalyzed by enzymes in the overall pathway of electrons from substrate to oxygen:

1. The pyridine-linked dehydrogenases, requiring either NAD or NADP as coenzymes;
2. flavin-linked dehydrogenases, containing either FAD or FMN as a prosthetic group; and
3. the cytochromes, containing an iron-porphyrin ring system.

In general, the first process in electron transport involves the activation of specific hydrogen atoms by the dehydrogenases. During the second process hydrogen atoms are transferred from metabolites to carriers, and finally combine with oxygen via a "terminal respiratory chain."

Respiration or biological oxidation occurs by means of small oxidation-reduction steps. The final multienzyme system that transports reducing equivalents to oxygen involves still smaller potential jumps, thus permitting more efficient recovery of free energy (Fig 48). Respiration may be aerobic, during which the ultimate hydrogen acceptor is oxygen; or it may be anaerobic, in which case the ultimate hydrogen acceptor is an organic oxidant. The oxidation chain for aerobic respiration is illustrated in Table IX. Two views exist regarding the physical organization of the system depicted. On the one hand, Chance and Williams,[90] proposed that the components of the chain were restricted in movement but reacted wtih one another by thermal collision. In their view, the unit of respiration was the "oxysome," a macromolecular assembly arranged in such a manner that any one redox component could react

**Table IX** Diagram of the mitochondrial respiratory chain. The metabolite system, $M/MH_2$ indicated with an $E_0 = -0.35$ volts is oxaloacetate/malate. $Q/QH_2$ represents the coenzyme Q system. Cyt.$b^{3+}$ represents ferricytochrome b, and cyt.$b^{2+}$ ferrocytochrome b. Representations for the other cytochromes are similar. The ferricytochromes are the oxidants of the systems, and the ferrocytochromes are the reductants. Two functional cytochromes are shown at each cytochrome step because the oxidation of $Fe^{2+}$ to $Fe^{3+}$ in the cytochromes is a one-equivalent oxidation-reduction; the diagram implies that a net two-equivalent transfer occurs at each oxidation-reduction system, although this has not been definitely established, and it would be required to describe different redox potentials for a system of univalent oxidation-reductions. Nonheme iron (nh Fe) and copper are both shown at the approximate sites at which they undergo oxidation-reduction by the preceding redox carrier, but their position has not at this time been completely established and they are shown in parentheses. The oxidation of succinate to fumarate by succinic dehydrogenase in the chain is catalyzed by the nonheme iron-containing flavoprotein, succinic dehydrogenase, which appears to be linked to the oxidation-reduction of cytochrome b without involving coenzyme Q. It is important to note that a net of three ATP molecules is formed by the oxidation of one NADH, whereas a net of only two ATP molecules is formed by the oxidation of succinate. Not all of the redox potentials of respiratory chain carriers are known with certainty; where uncertainty exists, these values have not been given in the row labeled $E_0$ (volts). The voltage difference between the $M/MH_2$ and $\frac{1}{2}O_2/H_2O$ half-cells is 1.14 volts; this, as shown in the calculation, is equivalent to a free energy change of 52.636 calories, or the free energy of hydrolysis of seven ATP molecules; three ATP molecules are actually formed as a result of the overall process. Reproduced with permission.[89]

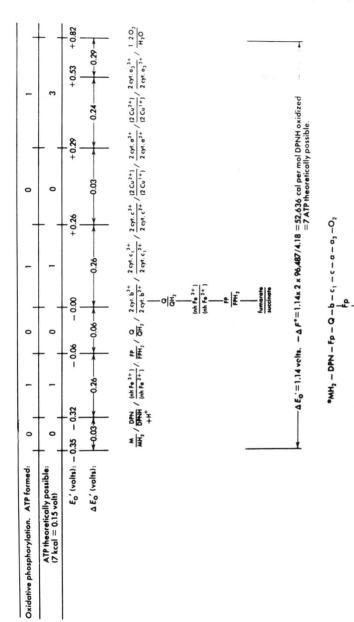

Oxidative phosphorylation. ATP formed:

| | 0 | 1 | 0 | 1 | 0 | 1 |
|---|---|---|---|---|---|---|

ATP theoretically possible:
(7 kcal = 0.15 volt)

| | 0 | 1 | 0 | 1 | 0 | 3 |
|---|---|---|---|---|---|---|

$E_0'$ (volts):   −0.35   −0.32   −0.06   −0.00   +0.26   +0.29   +0.53   +0.82

     −0.03    −0.26    −0.06    0.26    0.03    0.24    0.29

$\Delta E_0'$ (volts):

$$\frac{M}{MH_2} \Big/ \frac{DPN}{DPNH+H^+} \Big/ \frac{(nh\,Fe^{3+})}{(nh\,Fe^{2+})} \Big/ \frac{FP}{FPH_2} \Big/ \frac{Q}{QH_2} \Big/ \frac{2\,cyt.\,b^{3+}}{2\,cyt.\,b^{2+}} \Big/ \frac{2\,cyt.\,c_1^{3+}}{2\,cyt.\,c_1^{2+}} \Big/ \frac{2\,cyt.\,c^{3+}}{2\,cyt.\,c^{2+}} \Big/ \frac{(2\,Cu^{2+})}{(2\,Cu^{1+})} \Big/ \frac{2\,cyt.\,a^{3+}}{2\,cyt.\,a^{2+}} \Big/ \frac{(2\,Cu^{2+})}{(2\,Cu^{1+})} \Big/ \frac{2\,cyt.\,a_3^{3+}}{2\,cyt.\,a_3^{2+}} \Big/ \frac{1\;2\,O_2}{H_2O}$$

$$\frac{Q}{QH_2}$$

$$\frac{(nh\,Fe^{3+})}{(nh\,Fe^{2+})}$$

$$\frac{FP}{FPH_2}$$

$$\frac{fumarate}{succinate}$$

$$\Delta E_0' = 1.14 \text{ volts.} \quad -\Delta F° = 1.14 \times 2 \times 96{,}487/4.18 = 52{,}636 \text{ cal per mol DPNH oxidized} = 7 \text{ ATP theoretically possible.}$$

$$°MH_2 - DPN - Fp - Q - b - c_1 - c - a - a_3 - O_2$$

$$\begin{array}{c} | \\ Fp \\ | \\ S \end{array}$$

Simplified representation

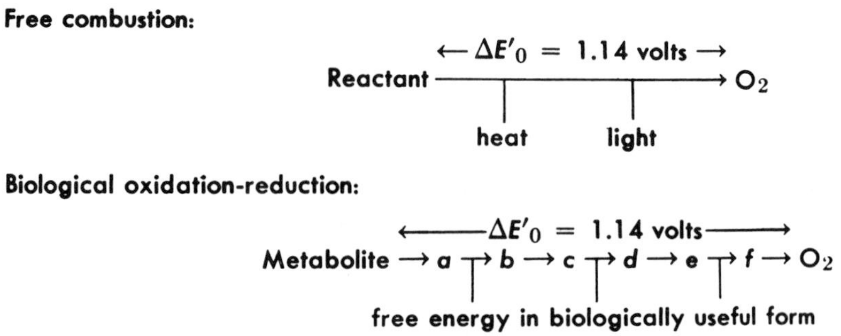

**Free combustion:**

$$\leftarrow \Delta E'_0 = 1.14 \text{ volts} \rightarrow$$

Reactant ——————————→ $O_2$

heat        light

**Biological oxidation-reduction:**

$$\longleftarrow \Delta E'_0 = 1.14 \text{ volts} \longrightarrow$$

Metabolite $\rightarrow a \rightarrow b \rightarrow c \rightarrow d \rightarrow e \rightarrow f \rightarrow O_2$

**free energy in biologically useful form**

**Figure 48** Biological and nonbiological oxidation compared. Note the many intermediary steps in the former involving small potential changes.

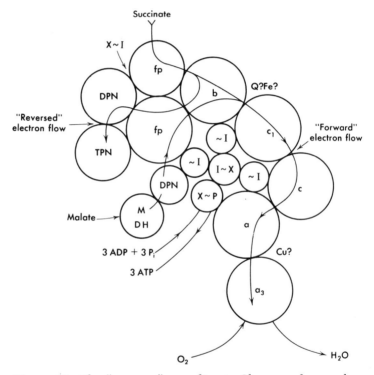

**Figure 49** The "oxysome," according to Chance and co-workers. The diagram gives the flow pattern for reducing equivalents in the respiratory chain indicating the functional relationship of the carriers. This model does not require that "elementary particles" exist as a physical entity. Reproduced with permission.[90]

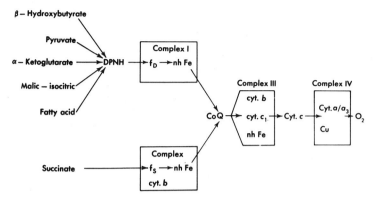

**Figure 50** Diagrammatic representation of the components of the "elementary particle" of respiration, showing functional complexes and their components. The following abbreviations are used: $f_D$, DPNH dehydrogenase; $f_S$, succinic dehydrogenase; nhFe, nonheme iron; Q, coenzyme Q. Reproduced with permission.[91]

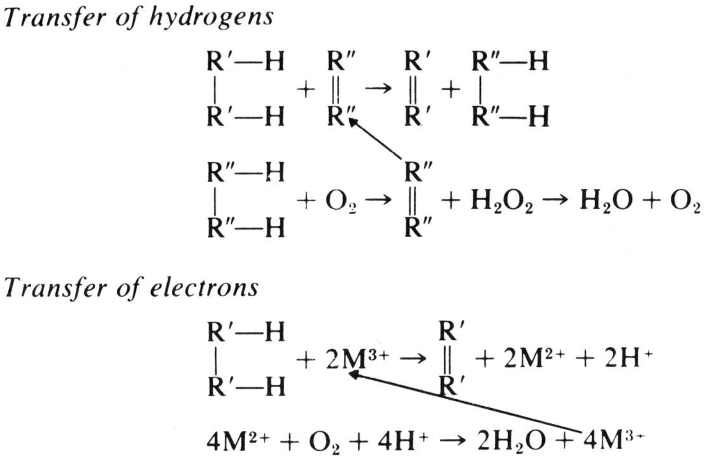

*Transfer of hydrogens*

$$\begin{array}{c} R'{-}H \\ | \\ R'{-}H \end{array} + \begin{array}{c} R'' \\ \| \\ R'' \end{array} \rightarrow \begin{array}{c} R' \\ \| \\ R' \end{array} + \begin{array}{c} R''{-}H \\ | \\ R''{-}H \end{array}$$

$$\begin{array}{c} R''{-}H \\ | \\ R''{-}H \end{array} + O_2 \rightarrow \begin{array}{c} R'' \\ \| \\ R'' \end{array} + H_2O_2 \rightarrow H_2O + O_2$$

*Transfer of electrons*

$$\begin{array}{c} R'{-}H \\ | \\ R'{-}H \end{array} + 2M^{3+} \rightarrow \begin{array}{c} R' \\ \| \\ R' \end{array} + 2M^{2+} + 2H^+$$

$$4M^{2+} + O_2 + 4H^+ \rightarrow 2H_2O + 4M^{3+}$$

**Figure 51** The transfer of hydrogens and/or electrons during oxidation.

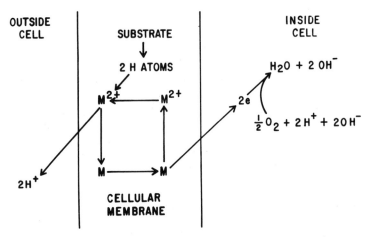

**Figure 52** Hypothetical red-ox ion pump. $M^{2+}$ represents the oxidized red-ox system and M the reduced form; e is the electron.

with several other components (Fig 49). On the other hand, Green [91, 92] suggested that the fundamental unit was the "elementary particle," which contained four organized lipoprotein complexes containing definite parts of the respiratory chain, connected by mobile redox components, primarily coenzyme Q and cytochrome C (Fig 50).

The mechanism of oxidation and reduction need not be an actual transfer of hydrogen ions. Hydrogen atoms may yield electrons to the cytochrome system during a change to hydrogen ions. The iron of the cytochrome system may then be reduced by the electrons and the oxygen activated by the cytochrome oxidase may accept the electrons from the cytochrome system. Alternatively, electrons may be primarily transported (Fig 51). In either case, water is formed from the reactions. An ion pump from redox reactions is also of interest and appears schematically in Figure 52.

### References

1. Rosenbaum, E. J.: *Physical Chemistry,* Appleton-Century-Crofts, New York, 1970.
2. Dickerson, R. E.: *Molecular Thermodynamics,* W. A. Benjamin, Inc., New York, 1969.

3. Guggenheim, E. A.: *Thermodynamics—An Advanced Treatment for Chemists and Physicists,* North-Holland Publishing Co., Amsterdam, 1967.
4. Kirkwood, J. G., Oppenheim, I.: *Chemical Thermodynamics,* McGraw-Hill Book Co., New York, 1961.
5. Caldin, E. F.: *An Introduction to Chemical Thermodynamics,* Oxford University Press, London, 1958.
6. Callen, H. B.: *Thermodynamics,* John Wiley & Sons, New York, 1960.
7. Fong, P.: *Foundations of Thermodynamics,* Oxford University Press, New York, 1963.
8. Wilks, J.: *The Third Law of Thermodynamics,* Oxford University Press, London, 1961.
9. Bent, H. A.: *The Second Law: An Introduction to Classical and Statistical Thermodynamics,* Oxford University Press, New York, 1965.
10. Denbigh, K.: *The Principles of Chemical Equilibrium,* Cambridge University Press, 3rd Edition, 1971.
11. Glasstone, S.: *Textbook of Physical Chemistry,* D. Van Nostrand Company, Princeton, N.J., 2nd Edition, 1959.
12. Castellan, G. W.: *Physical Chemistry,* Addison-Wesley Publishing Company, Reading, Mass. 2nd Edition, 1971.
13. Kestin, J., Dorfman, J. R.: *A Course in Statistical Thermodynamics,* Academic Press, New York, 1971.
14. Hill, T. L.: *An Introduction to Statistical Thermodynamics,* Addison-Wesley Publishing Co., Reading, Mass., 1960.
15. Hill, T. L.: *Thermodynamics of Small Systems,* parts I and II, W. A. Benjamin Inc., New York, 1963.
16. Penner, S. S.: *Thermodynamics for Scientists and Engineers,* Addison-Wesley Publishing Co., Reading, Mass., 1968.
17. Lewis, G. N., Randall, M.: *Thermodynamics,* revised by Pitzer, K. S., Brewer, L., McGraw Hill Book Co., New York, 2nd Edition, 1961.
18. Finkelstein, R. J.: *Thermodynamics and Statistical Physics,* W. H. Freeman Co., San Francisco, 1969.
19. Rock, P. A.: *Chemical Thermodynamics: Principles and Applications,* The Macmillan Company, Toronto, 1969.
20. Denbigh, K. C.: *The Thermodynamics of the Steady State,* Methuen & Co., Ltd., London, 1951.
21. Bray, H. G., White, K.: *Kinetics and Thermodynamics in Biochemistry,* J. & A. Churchill Ltd., London, 1966.
22. Kones, R. J.: Topics in biological transport. I. Particular and ionic diffusion. *J Mol Cell Cardiol* **3**:179-192, 1971.
23. Kones, R. J.: Entropy: qualitative aspects. *Draper Digest* **4**:24-26, 1958 (NYU Dept. of Chemistry).
24. Morowitz, H. J.: *Energy Flow in Biology:* Biological organization as a problem in thermal physics, Academic Press, New York, 1968.
25. Klotz, I. M.: *Energy Changes in Biochemical Reactions,* Academic Press, New York, 1967.
26. Szent-Györgi, A.: *Bioenergetics,* Academic Press, New York, 1957.

27. Hill, T. L.: *Thermodynamics for Chemists and Biologists*, Addison-Wesley Publishing Co., Reading, Mass., 1968.
28. Ciures, A., Margineau, D.: Thermodynamics in biology: an intruder? *J Theoret Biol* **28**:147-150, 1970.
29. Fitts, D. D.: *Nonequilibrium Thermodynamics: a phenomenological theory of irreversible processes in fluid systems*, McGraw Hill Book Co., New York, 1962.
30. Katchalsky, A., Curran, P. F.: *Nonequilibrium Thermodynamics in Biophysics*, Harvard University Press, Cambridge, 1967.
31. DeGroot, S. R., Mazur, P.: *Non-equilibrium Thermodynamics*, North-Holland Publishing Co., Amsterdam, 1963.
32. Gyarmati, I.: *Non-equilibrium Thermodynamics: field theory and variational principles*, Springer-Verlag, Berlin, 1970.
33. DeGroot, S. R.: *Thermodynamics of Irreversible Processes*, North-Holland Publishing Co., Amsterdam, 1966.
34. Prigogine, I.: *Introduction to the Thermodynamics of Irreversible Processes*, Interscience Publishers, New York, 1955.
35. Harper, H. A.: *Review of Physiological Chemistry*, Lange Medical Publications, Los Altos, Calif., 14th Edition, 1973.
36. Ishida, K.: Non-equilibrium thermodynamics of marginal and conditional-open chemical systems. *J Theoret Biol* **40**:301-327, 1973.
37. Wilkie, D. R.: Free energy of non-isothermal systems, *Nature* **245**:457-458, 1973.
38. Robison, R.: *The Significance of Phosphoric Esters in Metabolism*, New York University Press, New York, 1932.
39. Lundsgaard, E.: Untersuchungen über Muskulkontraktionen ohne Milchsäurebildung. *Biochem Z* **217**:162-177, 1930.
40. Lundsgaard, E.: Weitere Untersuchungen über Muskelukontraktionen ohne Milchsäürebildung. *Biochem Z* **227**:51-83, 1930.
41. Lundsgaard, E.: Über die Energetik der anaeroben Muskelkontraktion. *Biochem Z* **233**:322-343, 1931.
42. Barron, E. S. G.: Mechanisms of carbohydrate metabolism. Essay on comparative biochemistry. *Adv Enzym* **3**:149-189, 1943.
43. Cori, C. F., Cori, G. T.: Mechanism of formation of hexosemonophosphate in muscle and isolation of new phosphate ester. *Proc Soc Exp Biol Med* **34**:702-705, 1936.
44. Fiske, C. H., Subbarow, Y.: Phosphocreatine. *J Biol Chem* **81**:629-679, 1929.
45. Eggleton, P., Eggleton, G. P.: Inorganic phosphate and labile form of organic phosphate in gastrocnemius of frog. *Biochem J* **21**:190-195, 1927.
46. Myerhof, O., Suranyi, J.: Über die Warmetönungen der chemischen Reaktionsphasen im Muskel. *Biochem Z* **191**:106-124, 1927.
47. Meyerhof, O., Lohmann, K.: Über die natürlichen guanidinophosphorsäuren (Phosphagene) in der quergestreiften Muskulatur; die physikalischchemischen Eigenschaften der Guanidinophosphorsäuren. *Biochem Z* **196**:49-72, 1928.
48. Lohmann, K.: Darstellung der Adenylprophosphorsäure aus Muskulatur *Biochem Z* **233**:460-469, 1931.

49. Lohmann, K.: Konstitution der Adenylpyrophosphorsäure und Adenosindiphosphorsäure. *Biochem Z* **282**:120-123, 1935.
50. Jencks, W. P.: Coenzyme A transferases, in *The Enzymes*, edited by Paul, D., Boyer, A., et al., Academic Press, New York, 1973, Vol. 9, p. 483-496.
51. Atkinson, M. R., Morton, R. K.: Free energy and the biosynthesis of phosphates, in *Comparative Biochemistry, A Comprehensive Treatise*, edited by Florkin, M., Mason, H. S., Academic Press, New York, 1960, Vol. 2, p. 74.
52. Lipmann F.: The chemistry and thermodynamics of phosphate bonds, in *Phosphorus Metabolism*, edited by McElroy, W. B., Glass, B., Johns Hopkins Press, Baltimore, 1951, vol. 1, p. 521.
53. Kalckar, H. M.: The nature of energetic coupling in biological synthesis. *Chem Rev* **28**:71-178, 1941.
54. Baker, A. W., Harris, G. H.: Physical and chemical effects of substituent groups on multiple bonds. II. Thiolesters. *J Amer Chem Soc* **82**:1923-1928, 1960.
55. Oesper, P.: Sources of the high energy content in energy-rich phosphate. *Arch Biochem* **27**:255-270, 1950.
56. Hill, T. L., Morales, M. F.: On "high energy phosphate bonds" of biochemical interest. *J Amer Chem Soc* **73**:1656-1660, 1951.
57. George, P., Rutmann, R. J.: The high energy phosphate bond concept. *Progr Biophys* **10**:1-52, 1960.
58. McClare, C. W. F.: In defence of the high energy phosphate bond. *J Theoret Biol* **35**:233-246, 1972.
59. Gillespie, R. J., Maw, G. A., Vernon, C. A.: The concept of phosphate bond-energy. *Nature* **171**:1147-1149, 1953.
60. Banks, B. E. C.: Thermodynamics and biology. *Chemy Br* **5**:514-519, 1969.
61. Banks, B. E. C., Vernon, C. A.: Reassessment of the role of ATP in vivo. *J Theoret Biol* **20**:301-326, 1970.
62. Pauling, L.: Structure of high-energy molecules. *Chemy Br* **6**:468-472, 1970.
63. Huxley, A. F.: Energetics of muscle. *Chemy Br* **6**:477-479, 1970.
64. Wilkie, D. R.: Thermodynamics and biology. *Chemy Br* **6**:472-476, 1970.
65. Banks, B. E. C., Vernon, C. A.: A reply to Linus Pauling and A. F. Huxley. *Chemy Br* **6**:541-542, 1970.
66. Ross, R. A., Vernon, C. A.: A reply to Douglas Wilkie. *Chemy Br* **6**:539-540, 1970.
67. Hanna, M. W.: *Quantum mechanics in Chemistry*, W. A. Benjamin, Inc., New York, 1969, 2nd edition, pp. 39–42.
68. Bronk, J. R.: *Chemical Biology: an introduction to biochemistry*, The Macmillan Company, New York, 1973.
69. Tedeschi, H.: *Cell Physiology: molecular dynamics*, Academic Press, New York, 1974, p. 379.
70. Schoellman, G., Shaw, E.: Direct evidence for the presence of histidine in the active center of chymotrypsin. *Biochemistry* **2**:252-255, 1963.
71. Ludwig, M. L., Hartsuck, J. A., Steitz, T. A., et al.: The structure

of carboxypeptidase A. IV. Preliminary results of 2.8 Å resolution and a substrate complex at 6Å resolution. *Proc Natl Acad Sci USA* **57**:511-517, 1967.

72. Koshland, D. E., Neet, K. E.: The catalytic and regulatory properties of enzymes. *Ann Rev Biochem* **37**:359-410, 1968.

73. Koshland, D. E., Jr.: Conformation changes at the active site during enzyme action. *Fed Proc* **23**:719-726, 1964.

74. Koshland, D. E.: Molecular geometry in enzyme action. *J Cell Comp Physiol* **47** (suppl 1): 217-234, 1956.

75. Phillips, D. C.: The three-dimensional structure of an enzyme molecule. *Scientific American* **215**:78-90, 1966.

76. Giese, A. C.: *Cell Physiology*, W. B. Saunders Co., Philadelphia, 1973, 4th edition, p. 390.

77. Breslow, R.: *Organic Reaction Mechanisms*, W. A. Benjamin, Inc., New York, 2nd edition, 1969.

78. White, A., Handler, P., Smith, E. L.: *Principles of Biochemistry*. McGraw-Hill Co., New York, 5th edition, 1973.

79. Netter, H.: *Theoretical Biochemistry*, Wiley-Interscience Division, New York, 1969, pp. 590-690.

80. Mahler, H. R., Cordes, E. H.: *Biological Chemistry*, Harper and Row, New York, 2nd edition, 1971, pp. 267-384.

81. Dixon, M., Webb, E. C.: *The Enzymes*, Academic Press, New York, 3rd edition, 1967, Chapters 2, 4, 8, and 9.

82. Bull, H. B.: *An Introduction to Physical Biochemistry*, F. A. Davis Co., Philadelphia, 1971, p. 401.

83. Bull, H. B.: *An Introduction to Physical Biochemistry*, F. A. Davis Co., Philadelphia, 1971, pp. 405-407.

84. Cleland, W. W.: The kinetics of enzyme-catalyzed reactions with two or more substrates or products. I. Nomenclature and rate equations. II. Inhibition: nomenclature and theory. III. Prediction of initial velocity and inhibition patterns by inspection. *Biochem Biophys Acta* **67**:104-137, 173-187, 188-196, 1963.

85. Dowben, R. M.: *General Physiology: a molecular approach*, Harper and Row, New York, 1969.

86. Netter, H.: *Theoretical Biochemistry*, Wiley-Interscience Division, New York, 1969, pp. 479-510.

87. Giese, A. C.: *Cell Physiology*, W. B. Saunders Co., Philadelphia, 1973, 4th edition, pp. 421, 427.

88. de Donder, T., van Rysselberghe, P.: *Thermodynamic Theory of Affinity*, Stanford University Press, Stanford, Calif., 1936.

89. West, E. S., Todd, W. R., Mason, H. S., et al.: *Textbook of Biochemistry*, The MacMillan Co., New York, 4th edition, 1966, p. 945.

90. Chance, B., Williams, G. R.: The respiratory chain and oxidative phosphorylation. *Adv Enzyme* **17**:65-134, 1956.

91. Green, D. E., Wharton, D. C.: Stoichiometry of the fixed oxidation-reduction components of the electron transfer chain of beef heart mitochondria. *Biochem Z* **338**:335-348, 1963.

92. Green, D. E., Wharton, D. C., Tzagaloff, A., et al.: Oxidases and related redox systems, in *International Symposium on Oxidases and Related Oxidation-Reduction Systems, Proceedings*, edited by King, T. E., John Wiley & Sons, New York, 1965.

# INDEX

(appendix excluded)